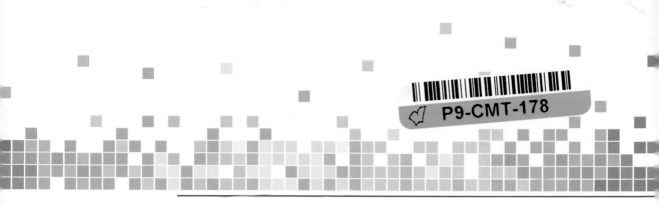

Essentials of Nursing Leadership and Management

SIXTH EDITION

Essentials of
Nursing Leadership
and Management

SIXTH EDITION

Sally A. Weiss, MSN, EdD, RN, CNE, ANEF
Professor of Nursing
Nova Southeastern University Nursing Department
Fort Lauderdale, Florida

Ruth M. Tappen, EdD, RN, FAAN
Christine E. Lynn Eminent Scholar and Professor
Florida Atlantic University College of Nursing
Boca Raton, Florida

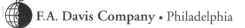 F.A. Davis Company • Philadelphia

F. A. Davis Company
1915 Arch Street
Philadelphia, PA 19103
www.fadavis.com

Printed in the United States of America

Last digit indicates print number: 10 9 8 7 6 5 4 3 2 1

Acquisitions Editor, Nursing: Megan Klim
Developmental Editor: Laurie Sparks
Director of Content Development: Darlene D. Pedersen
Content Project Manager: Echo Gerhart
Electronic Project Editor: Katherine Crowley
Design and Illustration Manager: Carolyn O'Brien

As new scientific information becomes available through basic and clinical research, recommended treatments and drug therapies undergo changes. The author(s) and publisher have done everything possible to make this book accurate, up to date, and in accord with accepted standards at the time of publication. The author(s), editors, and publisher are not responsible for errors or omissions or for consequences from application of the book, and make no warranty, expressed or implied, in regard to the contents of the book. Any practice described in this book should be applied by the reader in accordance with professional standards of care used in regard to the unique circumstances that may apply in each situation. The reader is advised always to check product information (package inserts) for changes and new information regarding dose and contraindications before administering any drug. Caution is especially urged when using new or infrequently ordered drugs.

Library of Congress Control Number: 2014945714

Dedication

To my granddaughter Sydni and my grandson Logan,
who remind me how important it is to nurture our young nurses
and help them learn and grow.
—SALLY A. WEISS

To students, colleagues, family, and friends,
who have taught me so much about leadership.
—RUTH M. TAPPEN

Dedication

Preface

We are delighted to bring our readers this Sixth Edition of *Essentials of Nursing Leadership and Management*. This new edition has been updated to reflect the dynamic health care environment, safety initiatives, and changes in nursing practice. As in our previous editions, the content, examples, and diagrams were designed with the goal of assisting the new graduate to make the transition to professional nursing practice.

The Sixth Edition of *Essentials of Nursing Leadership and Management* focuses on the necessary knowledge and skills needed by the staff nurse as an integral member of the interprofessional health-care team and manager of patient care. Issues related to setting priorities, delegation, quality improvement, legal parameters of nursing practice, and ethical issues are updated for this edition.

This edition focuses on the current quality and safety issues and initiatives impacting the current health-care environment. We continue to bring you comprehensive, practical information on developing a nursing career. Updated information on leading, managing, followership, and workplace issues continue to be included.

Essentials of Nursing Leadership and Management provides a strong foundation for the beginning nurse leader. We would like to thank the people at F. A. Davis for their assistance and our contributors, reviewers, and students for their guidance and support.

    —SALLY A. WEISS
    —RUTH M. TAPPEN

Contributor

PATRICIA BRADLEY, MeD, PhD, RN
Coordinator, Internationally Educated Nurses Program
Faculty, Nursing Department
York University
Toronto, Ontario, Canada

Reviewers

WENDY GREENSPAN, MSN, RN, CCRN, CNE
Assistant Professor
Rockland Community College
Suffern, New York

PAULA HOPPER, MSN, RN, CNE
Professor of Nursing
Jackson Community College
Jackson, Mississippi

CLAIRE MEGGS, MSN, RN
Associate Professor
Lincoln Memorial University
Harrogate, Tennessee

LUISE SPEAKMAN, PhD, RN
Adjunct Faculty, Nursing
Cape Cod Community College
West Barnstable, Massachusetts

JENNIFER SUGG, RN, BSN, MSN, CCRN
Nursing Instructor
Wayne Community College
Goldsboro, North Carolina

Table of Contents

Appendices

Professional Considerations

Leadership and Followership

Nurses study leadership to learn how to work well with other people. We work with an extraordinary variety of people: technicians, aides, unit managers, housekeepers, patients, patients' families, physicians, respiratory therapists, physical therapists, social workers, psychologists, and more. In this chapter, the most prominent leadership theories are introduced. Then, the characteristics and behaviors that can make you, a new nurse, an effective leader and follower are discussed.

Leadership

Are You Ready to Be a Leader?

You may be thinking, "I'm just beginning my career in nursing. How can I be expected to be a leader now?" This is an important question. You will need time to refine your clinical skills and learn how to function in a new environment. But you can begin to assume some leadership functions right away within your new nursing roles. In fact, leadership should be seen as a dimension of nursing practice (Scott & Miles, 2013). Consider the following example:

Billie Thomas was a new staff nurse at Green Valley Nursing Care Center. After orientation, she was assigned to a rehabilitation unit with high admission and discharge rates. Billie noticed that admissions and discharges were assigned rather haphazardly. Anyone who was "free" at the moment was directed to handle them. Sometimes, unlicensed assistant personnel were directed to admit or discharge residents. Billie believed that this was inappropriate because they are not prepared to do assessments and they had no preparation for discharge planning.

Billie had an idea how discharge planning could be improved but was not sure that she should bring it up because she was so new. "Maybe they've already thought of this," she said to a former classmate. They began to talk about what they had learned in their leadership course before graduation. "I just keep hearing our instructor saying, 'There's only one manager, but anyone can be a leader.'"

"If you want to be a leader, you have to act on your idea. Why don't you talk with your nurse manager?" her friend asked.

"Maybe I will," Billie replied.

Billie decided to speak with her nurse manager, an experienced rehabilitation nurse who seemed not only approachable but also open to new ideas. "I have been so busy getting our new electronic health record system on line before the surveyors come that I wasn't paying attention to that," the nurse manager told her. "I'm glad you brought it to my attention."

Billie's nurse manager raised the issue at the next executive meeting, giving credit to Billie for having brought it to her attention. The other nurse managers had the same response. "We were so focused on the new electronic health record system that we overlooked that. We need to take care of this situation as soon as possible. Billie Thomas has leadership potential."

Leadership Defined

Successful nurse leaders are those who engage others to work together effectively in pursuit of a shared goal. Examples of shared goals in nursing would be providing excellent care, reducing infection rates, designing cost-saving procedures, or challenging the ethics of a new policy.

Leadership is a much broader concept than is management. Although managers need to be leaders, management itself is focused specifically on achievement of organizational goals. Leadership, on the other hand:

> *... occurs whenever one person attempts to influence the behavior of an individual or group—up, down, or sideways in the organization—regardless of the reason. It may be for personal goals or for the goals of others, and these goals may or may not be congruent with organizational goals. Leadership is influence (Hersey & Campbell, 2004, p. 12).*

In order to lead, one must develop three important competencies: (1) diagnose: ability to understand the situation you want to influence, (2) adapt: make changes that will close the gap between the current situation and what you are hoping to achieve, and (3) communicate. No matter how much you diagnose or adapt, if you cannot communicate effectively, you will probably not meet your goal (Hersey & Campbell, 2004).

What Makes a Person a Leader?

Leadership Theories

There are many different ideas about how a person becomes a good leader. Despite years of research on this subject, no one idea has emerged as the clear

winner. The reason for this may be that different qualities and behaviors are most important in different situations. In nursing, for example, some situations require quick thinking and fast action. Others require time to figure out the best solution to a complicated problem. Different leadership qualities and behaviors are needed in these two instances. The result is that there is not yet a single best answer to the question, "What makes a person a leader?"

Consider some of the best-known leadership theories and the many qualities and behaviors that have been identified as those of the effective nurse leader (Pavitt, 1999; Tappen, 2001):

Trait Theories

At one time or another, you have probably heard someone say, "She's a born leader." Many believe that some people are natural leaders, while others are not. It is true that leadership may come more easily to some than to others, but everyone can be a leader, given the necessary knowledge and skill.

An important 5-year study of 90 outstanding leaders by Warren Bennis published in 1984 identified four common traits. These traits hold true today:

1. Management of attention. These leaders communicated a sense of goal direction that attracted followers.
2. Management of meaning. These leaders created and communicated meaning and purpose.
3. Management of trust. These leaders demonstrated reliability and consistency.
4. Management of self. These leaders knew themselves well and worked within their strengths and weaknesses (Bennis, 1984).

Behavioral Theories

The behavioral theories focus on what the leader does. One of the most influential behavioral theories is concerned with leadership style (White & Lippitt, 1960) (Table 1-1).

The three styles are:

1. **Autocratic leadership** (also called *directive, controlling,* or *authoritarian*). The autocratic leader gives orders and makes decisions for the group. For example, when a decision needs to be made, an autocratic leader says, "I've decided that this is the way we're going to solve our

table 1-1			
Comparison of Autocratic, Democratic, and Laissez-Faire Leadership Styles			
	Autocratic	**Democratic**	**Laissez-Faire**
Amount of freedom	Little freedom	Moderate freedom	Much freedom
Amount of control	High control	Moderate control	Little control
Decision making	By the leader	Leader and group together	By the group or by no one
Leader activity level	High	High	Minimal
Assumption of responsibility	Leader	Shared	Abdicated
Output of the group	High quantity, good quality	Creative, high quality	Variable, may be poor quality
Efficiency	Very efficient	Less efficient than autocratic style	Inefficient

Source: Adapted from White, R.K., & Lippitt, R. (1960). Autocracy and democracy: An experimental inquiry. New York: Harper & Row.

problem." Although this is an efficient way to run things, it squelches creativity and may reduce team member motivation.

2. **Democratic leadership** (also called *participative*). Democratic leaders share leadership. Important plans and decisions are made with the team (Chrispeels, 2004) Although this appears to be a less efficient way to run things, it is more flexible and usually increases motivation and creativity. In fact, involving team members, giving them "permission to think, speak and act" brings out the best in them and makes them more productive, not less (Wiseman & McKeown, 2010, p. 3). Decisions may take longer to make, but once made everyone supports them (Buchanan, 2011).

3. **Laissez-faire leadership** (also called *permissive* or *nondirective*). The laissez-faire ("let someone do") leader does very little planning or decision making and fails to encourage others to do it. It is really a lack of leadership. For example, when a decision needs to be made, a laissez-faire leader may postpone making the decision or never make the decision at all. In most instances, the laissez-faire leader leaves people feeling confused and frustrated because there is no goal, no guidance, and no direction. Some mature, self-motivated individuals thrive under laissez-faire leadership because they need little direction. Most people, however, flounder under this kind of leadership.

Pavitt summed up the differences among these three styles: a democratic leader tries to move the group toward its goals; an autocratic leader tries to move the group toward the leader's goals; and a

laissez-faire leader makes no attempt to move the group (1999, pp. 330ff).

Task Versus Relationship

Another important distinction is between a task focus and a relationship focus (Blake, Mouton, & Tappel, 1981). Some nurses emphasize the tasks (e.g., administering medication, completing patient records) and fail to recognize that interpersonal relationships (e.g., attitude of physicians toward nursing staff, treatment of housekeeping staff by nurses) affect the morale and productivity of employees. Others focus on the interpersonal aspects and ignore the quality of the job being done as long as people get along with each other. The most effective leader is able to balance the two, attending to both the task and the relationship aspects of working together.

Motivation Theories

The concept of motivation seems simple: we will act to get what we want but avoid whatever we don't want to do. However, motivation is still surrounded in mystery. The study of motivation as a focus of leadership began in the 1920s with the historic Hawthorne studies. Several experiments were conducted to see if increasing light and, later, improving other working conditions would increase the productivity of workers in the Hawthorne, Illinois, electrical plant. This proved to be true, but then something curious happened: when the improvements were taken away, the workers continued to show increased productivity. The researchers concluded that the explanation was found not in the *conditions* of the experiments but in the *attention* given to the workers by the experimenters.

Frederick Herzberg and David McClelland also studied factors that motivated workers in the workplace. Their findings are similar to the elements in Maslow's Hierarchy of Needs. Table 1-2 summarizes these three historical motivation theories that continue to be used by leaders today (Herzberg, 1966; Herzberg, Mausner, & Snyderman, 1959; Maslow, 1970; McClelland, 1961).

Emotional Intelligence

The relationship aspects of leadership are also the focus of the work on emotional intelligence and leadership (Goleman, Boyatzes, & McKee, 2002). From the perspective of emotional intelligence, what distinguishes ordinary leaders from leadership "stars" is that the "stars" are consciously addressing the effect of people's feelings on the team's emotional reality.

How is this done? First, the emotionally intelligent leader recognizes and understands his or her own emotions. When a crisis occurs, he or she is able to manage them, channel them, stay calm and clearheaded, and suspend judgment until all the facts are in (Baggett & Baggett, 2005).

Second, the emotionally intelligent leader welcomes constructive criticism, asks for help when needed, can juggle multiple demands without losing focus, and can turn problems into opportunities.

Third, the emotionally intelligent leader listens attentively to others, recognizes unspoken concerns, acknowledges others' perspectives, and brings people together in an atmosphere of respect, cooperation, collegiality, and helpfulness so they can direct their energies toward achieving the team's goals. "The enthusiastic, caring, and supportive leader generates those same feelings throughout the team," wrote Porter-O'Grady of the emotionally intelligent leader (2003, p. 109).

Situational Theories

People and leadership situations are far more complex than the early theories recognized. Situations can also change rapidly, requiring more complex theories to explain leadership (Bennis, Spreitzer, & Cummings, 2001).

Instead of assuming that one particular approach works in all situations, situational theories recognize the complexity of work situations and encourage the leader to consider many factors when deciding what action to take. Adaptability is the key to the situational approach (McNichol, 2000).

Situational theories emphasize the importance of understanding all the factors that affect a particular group of people in a particular environment. The most well-known is the Situational Leadership Model by Dr. Paul Hersey. The appeal of this model is that it focuses on the task and the follower.

table 1-2	

Leading Motivation Theories

Theory	Summary of Motivation Requirements
Maslow, 1954	Categories of Need: Lower needs (listed first below) must be fulfilled before others are activated. *Physiological* *Safety* *Belongingness* *Esteem* *Self-actualization*
Herzberg, 1959	Two factors that influence motivation. The absence of hygiene factors can create job dissatisfaction, but their presence does not motivate or increase satisfaction. **1.** *Hygiene factors:* Company policy, supervision, interpersonal relations, working conditions, salary **2.** *Motivators:* Achievement, recognition, the work itself, responsibility, advancement
McClelland, 1961	Motivation results from three dominant needs. Usually all three needs are present in each individual but vary in importance depending on the position a person has in the workplace. Needs are also shaped over time by culture and experience. **1.** *Need for achievement:* Performing tasks on a challenging and high level **2.** *Need for affiliation:* Good relationships with others **3.** *Need for power:* Being in charge

Source: Adapted from Hersey, P., & Campbell, R. (2004). *Leadership: A behavioral science approach.* Calif.: Leadership Studies Publishing.

The key is to marry the readiness of the follower with the tasks at hand. "Readiness is defined as the extent to which a follower demonstrates the ability and willingness to accomplish a specific task" (Hersey & Campbell, 2004, p. 114). "The leader needs to spell out the duties and responsibilities of the individual and the group" (Hersey & Campbell, 2004).

Followers' readiness levels can range from unable, unwilling, and insecure to able, willing, and confident. The leader's behavior will focus on appropriately fulfilling the followers' needs, which are identified by their readiness level and the task. Leader behaviors will range from telling, guiding, and directing to delegating, observing, and monitoring.

Where did you fall in this model during your first clinical rotation? Compare this with where you are now. In the beginning, the clinical instructor gave you clear instructions, closely guiding and directing you. Now, she or he is most likely delegating, observing, and monitoring. As you move into your first nursing position, you may return to the needing, guiding, and directing stage. But, you may soon become a leader/instructor for new nursing students, guiding and directing them.

Transformational Leadership

Although the situational theories were an improvement over earlier theories, there was still something missing. Meaning, inspiration, and vision were not given enough attention (Tappen, 2001). These are the distinguishing features of transformational leadership.

The transformational theory of leadership emphasizes that people need a sense of mission that goes beyond good interpersonal relationships or an appropriate reward for a job well done (Bass & Avolio, 1993). This is especially true in nursing. Caring for people, sick or well, is the goal of the profession. Most people chose nursing in order to do something for the good of humankind; this is their vision. One responsibility of nursing leadership is to help nurses see how their work helps them achieve their vision.

Transformational leaders can communicate their vision in a manner that is so meaningful and exciting that it reduces negativity (Leach, 2005) and inspires commitment in the people with whom they work (Trofino, 1995). Dr. Martin Luther King Jr. had a vision for America: "I have a dream that

box 1-1
BHAGs, Anyone?

This is leadership on the very grandest scale. BHAGs are Big, Hairy, Audacious Goals. Coined by Jim Collins, BHAGs are big ideas, visions for the future. Here is an example:

Gigi Mander, originally from the Philippines, dreams of buying hundreds of acres of farmland for peasant families in Asia or Africa. She would install irrigation systems, provide seed and modern farming equipment, and help them market their crops. This is not just a dream, however; she has a business plan for her BHAG and is actively seeking investors.

Imagination, creativity, planning, persistence, audacity, courage: these are all needed to put a BHAG into practice.

Do you have a BHAG? How would you make it real?

Adapted from Buchanan, L. (2012). The world needs big ideas. INC Magazine, 34(9), 57–58.

one day my children will be judged by the content of their character, not the color of their skin" (quoted by Blanchard & Miller, 2007, p. 1). A great leader shares his or her vision with his followers. You can do the same with your colleagues and team. If successful, the goals of the leader and staff will "become fused, creating unity, wholeness, and a collective purpose" (Barker, 1992, p. 42). See Box 1-1 for an example of a leader with visionary goals.

Moral Leadership

A series of highly publicized corporate scandals redirected attention to the values and ethics that underlie the practice of leadership as well as that of patient care (Dantley, 2005). Moral leadership involves deciding how one ought to remain honest, fair, and socially responsible (Bjarnason & LaSala, 2011) under any circumstances. Caring about one's patients and the people who work for you as people as well as employees (Spears & Lawrence, 2004) is part of moral leadership. This can be a great challenge in times of limited financial resources.

Molly Benedict was a team leader on the acute geriatric unit (AGU) when a question of moral leadership arose. Faced with large budget cuts in the middle of the year and feeling a little desperate to figure out how to run the AGU with fewer staff, her nurse manager suggested that reducing the time that unlicensed assistive personnel (UAP) spent ambulating patients would enable UAPs to care for 15 patients, up from the current 10 per UAP.

"George," responded Molly, "you know that inactivity has many harmful effects, from emboli to disorientation, in our very elderly population. Let's try to figure out how to encourage more self-care and even family involvement in care so the UAPs can still have time to walk patients and prevent their becoming nonambulatory."

Molly based her action on important values, particularly those of providing the highest quality care possible. Stewart and colleagues (2012) urge that caring not be sacrificed at the altar of efficiency (p. 227). This example illustrates how great a challenge that can be for today's nurse leaders. The American Nurses Association Code of Ethics (2001) provides the moral compass for nursing practice and leadership (ANA, 2001; Bjarnason & LaSala, 2011).

Box 1-2 summarizes a contemporary list of 13 distinctive leadership styles, most of which match up to the eight theories just discussed.

Caring Leadership

Caring leadership in nursing comes from two primary sources: servant leadership and emotional intelligence in the management literature, and caring as a foundational value in nursing (Greenleaf, 2008; McMurry, 2012; Rhodes, Morris, & Lazenby, 2011; Spears, 2010). While it is uniquely suited to nursing leadership, it is hard to imagine any situation in which an uncaring leader would be preferred over a caring leader.

Servant-leaders choose to serve first and lead second, making sure that people's needs within the work setting are met (Greenleaf, 2008). Emotionally intelligent leaders are especially aware of not only their own feelings but others' feelings as well (see Box 1-1). Combining these leadership and management theories and the philosophy of caring in nursing, you can see that caring leadership is fundamentally people-oriented. The following are the characteristics and behaviors of caring leaders:

- They *respect* their coworkers as individuals.
- They *listen* to other people's opinions and preferences, giving them full consideration.
- They *maintain awareness* of their own and others' feelings.
- They *empathize* with others, understanding their needs and concerns.
- They *develop* their own and their team's capacities.
- They *are competent*, both in leadership and in clinical practice. This includes both knowledge and skill in leadership and clinical practice.

As you can see, caring leadership cuts across the leadership theories discussed so far and encompasses some of their best features. An authoritarian leader, for example, can be as caring as a democratic leader (Dorn, 2011). Caring leadership is attractive to many nurses because it applies many of the principles of working with patients and working with nursing staff to the interdisciplinary team.

Qualities of an Effective Leader

If leadership is seen as the ability to influence, what qualities must the leader possess in order to be able to do that? Integrity, courage, positive attitude, initiative, energy, optimism, perseverance, generosity, balance, ability to handle stress, and self-awareness are some of the qualities of effective leaders in nursing (Fig. 1.1):

- **Integrity.** Integrity is expected of health-care professionals. Patients, colleagues, and

---

box 1-2

Distinctive Styles of Leadership

1. Adaptive: flexible, willing to change and devise new approaches.
2. Emotionally Intelligent: aware of his/her own and others' feelings.
3. Charismatic: magnetic personalities who attract people to follow them.
4. Authentic: demonstrates integrity, character, and honesty in relating to others.
5. Level 5: ferociously pursues goals but gives credit to others and takes responsibility for his/her mistakes.
6. Mindful: thoughtful, analytic, and open to new ideas.
7. Narcissistic: doesn't listen to others and doesn't tolerate disagreement but may have a compelling vision.
8. No Excuse: mentally tough, emphasizes accountability and decisiveness.
9. Resonant: motivates others through their energy and enthusiasm.
10. Servant: "empathic, aware and healing," (p. 76) leads to serve others.
11. Storyteller: uses stories to convey messages in a memorable, motivating fashion.
12. Strength-Based: focuses and capitalizes on his/her own and others' talents.
13. Tribal: build a common culture with strong sharing of values and beliefs.

Adapted from Buchanan, L. (2012/June). 13 ways of looking at a leader. INC Magazine, 74–76.

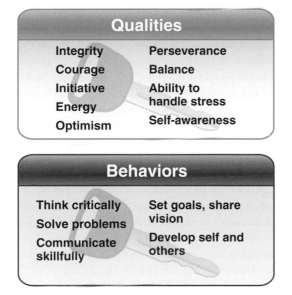

Qualities

Integrity   Perseverance

Courage   Balance

Initiative   Ability to
                   handle stress
Energy
                   Self-awareness
Optimism

Behaviors

Think critically   Set goals, share
                   vision
Solve problems
                   Develop self and
Communicate   others
skillfully

Figure 1.1 Keys to effective leadership.

employers all expect nurses to be honest, law-abiding, and trustworthy. Adherence to both a code of personal ethics and a code of professional ethics (Appendix 1, American Nurses Association Code of Ethics for Nurses) is expected of every nurse. Would-be leaders who do not exhibit these characteristics cannot expect them of their followers. This is an essential component of moral leadership.

■ **Courage.** Sometimes, being a leader means taking some risks. In the story of Billie Thomas, for example, Billie needed some courage to speak to her nurse manager about a problem she had observed.

■ **Positive attitude.** A positive attitude goes a long way in making a good leader. In fact, many outstanding leaders cite negative attitude as the single most important reason for not hiring someone (Maxwell, 1993, p. 98). Sometimes a leader's attitude is noticed by followers more quickly than are the leader's actions.

■ **Initiative.** Good ideas are not enough. To be a leader, you must act on those good ideas. No one will make you do this; this requires initiative on your part.

■ **Energy.** Leadership requires energy. Both leadership and followership are hard but satisfying endeavors that require effort. It

is also important that the energy be used wisely.

■ **Optimism.** When the work is difficult and one crisis seems to follow another in rapid succession, it is easy to become discouraged. It is important not to let discouragement keep you and your coworkers from seeking ways to resolve the problems. In fact, the ability to see a problem as an opportunity is part of the optimism that makes a person an effective leader. Like energy, optimism is "catching." Holman (1995) called this being a *winner* instead of a *whiner* (Table 1-3).

■ **Perseverance.** Effective leaders do not give up easily. Instead, they persist, continuing their efforts when others are tempted to stop trying. This persistence often pays off.

■ **Generosity.** Freely sharing your time, interest, and assistance with your colleagues is a trait of a generous leader. Sharing credit for successes and support when needed are other ways to be a generous leader (Buchanan, 2013; Disch, 2013).

■ **Balance.** In the effort to become the best nurses they can be, some nurses may forget that other aspects of life are equally important. As important as patients and colleagues are, family and friends are important, too. Although school and work are meaningful activities, cultural, social, recreational, and spiritual activities also have meaning. You need to find a balance between work and play.

■ **Ability to handle stress.** There is some stress in almost every job. Coping with stress in as positive and healthy a manner as possible helps to conserve energy and can be a model for

table 1-3	
Winner or Whiner—Which Are You?	
A winner says:	A whiner says:
"We have a real challenge here."	"This is really a problem."
"I'll give it my best."	"Do I have to?"
"That's great!"	"That's nice, I guess."
"We can do it!"	"That will never succeed."
"Yes!"	"Maybe . . ."

Source: Adapted from Holman, L. (1995). Eleven lessons in self-leadership: Insights for personal and professional success. Lexington, Ky.: A Lesson in Leadership Book.

others. Maintaining balance and handling stress are reviewed in Chapter 11.

- **Self-awareness.** How sharp is your emotional intelligence? People who do not understand themselves are limited in their ability to understand people with whom they are working. They are far more likely to fool themselves than are self-aware people. For example, it is much easier to be fair with a coworker you like than with one you do not like. Recognizing that you like some people more than others is the first step in avoiding unfair treatment based on personal likes and dislikes.

Behaviors of an Effective Leader

Leadership requires action. The effective leader chooses the action carefully. Important leadership behaviors include setting priorities, thinking critically, solving problems, respecting people, communicating skillfully, communicating a vision for the future, and developing oneself and others.

- **Setting priorities.** Whether planning care for a group of patients or creating a strategic plan for an organization, priorities continually shift and demand your attention. As a leader you will need to remember the three *E*'s of prioritization: evaluate, eliminate, and estimate. Continually evaluate what you need to do, eliminate tasks that someone else can do, and estimate how long your top priorities will take you to complete.
- **Thinking critically.** Critical thinking is the careful, deliberate use of reasoned analysis to reach a decision about what to believe or what to do (Feldman, 2002). The essence of critical thinking is a willingness to ask questions and to be open to new ideas or new ways to do things. To avoid falling prey to assumptions and biases of your own or others, ask yourself frequently, "Do I have the information I need? Is it accurate? Am I prejudging a situation?" (Jackson, Ignatavicius, & Case, 2004).
- **Solving problems.** Patient problems, paperwork problems, staff problems: these and others occur frequently and need to be solved. The effective leader helps people identify problems and work through the problem-solving process to find a reasonable solution.

- **Respecting and valuing the individual.** Although people have much in common, each individual has different wants and needs and has had different life experiences. For example, some people really value the psychological rewards of helping others; other people are more concerned about earning a decent salary. There is nothing wrong with either of these points of view; they are simply different. The effective leader recognizes these differences in people and helps them find the rewards in their work that mean the most to them.
- **Skillful communication.** This includes listening to others, encouraging exchange of information, and providing feedback:
  1. *Listening to others.* Listening is separate from talking with other people; listening involves both giving and receiving information. The only way to find out people's individual wants and needs is to watch what they do and to listen to what they say. It is amazing how often leaders fail simply because they did not listen to what other people were trying to tell them.
  2. *Encouraging exchange of information.* Many misunderstandings and mistakes occur because people fail to share enough information with each other. The leader's role is to make sure that the channels of communication remain open and that people use them.
  3. *Providing feedback.* Everyone needs some information about the effectiveness of their performance. Frequent feedback, both positive and negative, is needed so people can continually improve their performance. Some nurse leaders find it difficult to give negative feedback because they fear that they will upset the other person. How else can the person know where improvement is needed? Negative feedback can be given in a manner that is neither hurtful nor resented by the individual receiving it. In fact, it is often appreciated. Other nurse leaders, however, fail to give positive feedback, assuming that coworkers will know when they are doing a good job. This is also a mistake because everyone appreciates positive feedback. In fact, for some people, it is the most important reward they get from their jobs.

- **Communicating a vision for the future.** The effective leader has a vision for the future. Communicating this vision to the group and involving everyone in working toward that vision generate the inspiration that keeps people going when things become difficult. Even better, involving people in creating the vision is not only more satisfying for employees but also has the potential to produce the most creative and innovative outcomes (Kerfott, 2000). It is this vision that helps make work meaningful.
- **Developing oneself and others.** Learning does not end upon leaving school. In fact, experienced nurses say that school is just the beginning, that school only prepares you to continue learning throughout your career. As new and better ways to care for patients are developed, it is your responsibility as a professional to critically analyze them and decide whether they would be better for your patients than current ones. Effective leaders not only continue to learn but also encourage others to do the same. Sometimes, leaders function as teachers. At other times, their role is primarily to encourage others to seek more knowledge.

Anderson, Manno, O'Connor, and Gallagher (2010) invited five nurse managers from Penn Presbyterian Medical Center who had received top ratings in leadership from their staff to participate in a focus group on successful leadership. They reported that visibility, communication, and the values of respect and empathy were the key elements of successful leadership. The authors quoted participants to illustrate each of these elements (p. 186):

> Visibility: "I try to come in on the off shifts even for an hour or two just to have them see you."
> Communication: "Candid feedback" "A lot of rounding." (Note: this could also be visibility.)
> Respect and Empathy: "Do I expect you to take seven patients? No, because I wouldn't be able to do it." (punctuation adjusted).

These three key elements draw on components from several leadership qualities and behaviors: skillful communication, respecting and valuing the individual, and energy. Visibility is not as prominent in many of the leadership theories but deserves a place in the description of what effective leaders do.

Followership

Followership and leadership are separate but complementary roles. The roles are also reciprocal: without followers, one cannot be a leader. One also cannot be a follower without having a leader (Lyons, 2002).

It is as important to be an effective follower as it is to be an effective leader. In fact, most of us are followers: members of a team, attendees at a meeting, staff of a nursing care unit, and so forth.

Followership Defined

Followership is not a passive role. On the contrary, the most valuable follower is a skilled, self-directed professional, one who participates actively in determining the group's direction, invests his or her time and energy in the work of the group, thinks critically, and advocates for new ideas (Grossman & Valiga, 2000).

Imagine working on a patient care unit where all staff members, from the unit secretary to the assistant nurse manager, willingly take on extra tasks without being asked (Spreitzer & Quinn, 2001), come back early from coffee breaks if they are needed, complete their charting on time, support ways to improve patient care, and are proud of the high-quality care they provide. Wouldn't it be wonderful to be a part of that team?

Becoming a Better Follower

There are a number of things you can do to become a better follower:

- If you discover a problem, inform your team leader or manager right away.
- Even better, include a suggestion for solving the problem in your report.
- Freely invest your interest and energy in your work.
- Be supportive of new ideas and new directions suggested by others.
- When you disagree, explain why.
- Listen carefully and reflect on what your leader or manager says.
- Continue to learn as much as you can about your specialty area.
- Share what you learn.

Being an effective follower not only will make you a more valuable employee but will also increase the meaning and satisfaction that you get from your work.

Managing Up

Most team leaders and nurse managers respond positively to having staff who are good followers. Occasionally, you will encounter a poor leader or manager who can confuse, frustrate, and even distress you. Here are a few suggestions for handling this:

- Avoid adopting the ineffective behaviors of this individual.
- Continue to do your best work and to contribute leadership to the group.
- If the situation worsens, enlist the support of others on your team to seek a remedy; do not try to do this alone as a new graduate.
- If the situation becomes intolerable, consider the option of transferring to another unit or seeking another position (Deutschman, 2005; Korn, 2004).

There is still more a good follower can do. This is called *managing up*. Managing up is defined as "the process of consciously working with your boss to obtain the best possible results for you, your boss, and your organization" (Zuber & James quoted by Turk, 2007, p. 21). This is not a scheme to manipulate your manager or to get more rewards than you have earned. Instead, it is a guide for better understanding your manager, what he or she expects of you, and what your manager's own needs might be.

Every manager has areas of strength and weakness. A good follower recognizes these and helps the manager capitalize on areas of strength and compensate for areas of weakness. For example, if your nurse manager is slow completing quality improvement reports, you can offer to help get them done. On the other hand, if your nurse manager seems to be especially skilled in defusing conflicts between attending physicians and nursing staff, you can observe how he handles these situations and ask him how he does it. Remember that your manager is human, a person with as many needs, concerns, distractions, and ambitions as anyone else. This will help you keep your expectations of your manager realistic and reduce the distance between you and your manager.

There are several other ways in which to manage up. U.S. Army General and former Secretary of State Colin Powell said, "You can't make good decisions unless you have good information" (Powell, 2012, p. 42). Keep your manager informed. No one likes to be surprised, least of all a manager who finds that you have known about a problem (a nursing assistant who is spending too much time in the staff lounge, for example) and not brought it to her attention until it became critical. When you do bring a problem to your manager's attention, try to have a solution to offer. This is not always possible, but when it is, it will be very much appreciated.

Finally, show your appreciation whenever possible (Bing, 2010). Show respect for your manager's authority and appreciation for what your manager does for the staff of your unit. Let others know of your appreciation, particularly those to whom your manager must answer.

Conclusion

To be an effective nurse, you need to be an effective leader. Your patients, peers, and employer are depending on you to lead. Successful leaders never stop learning and growing. John Maxwell (1998), an expert on leadership, wrote, "Who we are is who we attract" (p. xi). To attract leaders, people need to start leading and never stop learning to lead.

The key elements of leadership and followership have been discussed in this chapter. Many of the leadership and followership qualities and behaviors mentioned here are discussed in more detail in later chapters.

Study Questions

1. Why is it important for nurses to be good leaders? What qualities have you observed from nurses that exemplify effective leadership in action? How do you think these behaviors might have improved the outcomes of their patients?

2. Why are effective followers as important as effective leaders?

3. Review the various leadership theories discussed in the chapter. Which ones especially apply to leading in today's health-care environment? Support your answer with specific examples.

4. Select an individual whose leadership skills you particularly admire. What are some qualities and behaviors that this individual displays? How do these relate to the leadership theories discussed in this chapter? In what ways could you emulate this person?

5. As a new graduate, what leadership and followership skills will you work on developing during the first 3 months of your first nursing position? Why?

Case Study to Promote Critical Reasoning

Two new associate-degree graduate nurses were hired for the pediatric unit. Both worked three 12-hour shifts a week, Jan on the day-to-evening shift and Ronnie at night. Whenever their shifts overlapped, they would compare notes on their experience. Jan felt she was learning rapidly, gaining clinical skills, and beginning to feel at ease with her colleagues.

Ronnie, however, still felt unsure of herself and often isolated. "There have been times," she told Jan, "that I am the only registered nurse on the unit all night. The aides and LPNs are really experienced, but that's not enough. I wish I could work with an experienced nurse as you are doing."

"Ronnie, you are not even finished with your 3-month orientation program," said Jan. "You should never be left alone with all these sick children. Neither of us is ready for that kind of responsibility. And how will you get the experience you need with no experienced nurses to help you? You must speak to our nurse manager about this."

"I know I should, but she's so hard to reach. I've called several times, and she's never available. She leaves all the shift assignments to her assistant. I'm not sure she even reviews the schedule before it's posted."

"You will have to try harder to reach her. Maybe you could stay past the end of your shift one morning and meet with her," suggested Jan. "If something happens when you are the only nurse on the unit, you will be held responsible."

1. In your own words, summarize the problem that Jan and Ronnie are discussing. To what extent is this problem due to a failure to lead? Who has failed to act?

2. What style of leadership was displayed by Jan, Ronnie, and the nurse manager? How effective was their leadership? Did Jan's leadership differ from that of Ronnie and the nurse manager? In what way?

3. In what ways has Ronnie been an effective follower? In what ways has Ronnie not been so effective as a follower?

4. If an emergency occurred and was not handled well while Ronnie was the only nurse on the unit, who would be responsible? Explain why this person or persons would be responsible.

5. If you found yourself in Ronnie's situation, what steps would you take to resolve the problem? Show how the leader characteristics and behaviors found in this chapter support your solution to the problem.

References

American Nurses Association (ANA). (2001). Code of Ethics for Nurses. Retrieved from www.nursingworld.org/MainMenuCategories/EthicsStandards/CodeofEthicsforNurses

Anderson, B.J., Manno, M., O'Connor, P., & Gallagher, E. (2010). Listening to nursing leaders. *Journal of Nursing Administration, 40*(4), 182–187.

Baggett, M.M., & Baggett, F.B. (2005). Move from management to high-level leadership. *Nursing Management, 36*(7), 12.

Barker, A.M. (1992). *Transformational nursing leadership: A vision for the future.* New York: National League for Nursing Press.

Bass, B.M., & Avolio, B.J. (1993). Transformational leadership: A response to critiques. In Chemers, M.M., & Ayman, R. (eds.). *Leadership Theory and Research: Perspectives and Direction.* San Diego: Academic Press.

Bennis, W. (1984). The four competencies of leadership. *Training and Development Journal,* August 1984, 15–19.

Bennis, W., Spreitzer, G.M., & Cummings, T.G. (2001). *The Future of Leadership.* San Francisco: Jossey-Bass.

Bing, S. (2010). Stanley Bing's top 10 strategies for managing up. *CBS News.* Retrieved from www.cbsnews.com

Bjarnason, D., & LaSala, C.A. (2011/March). Moral Leadership in Nursing. *Journal of Radiology Nursing, 30*(1), 18–24.

Blake, R.R., Mouton, J.S., & Tapper, M., et al. (1981). *Grid Approaches for Managerial Leadership in Nursing.* St. Louis: C.V. Mosby.

Blanchard, K., & Miller, M. (2007/September 11). The higher plane of leadership. *Leader to Leader Journal, 46,* 25–30.

Buchanan, L. (2012). The world needs big ideas. *INC Magazine, 34*(9), 57–58.

Buchanan, L. (2012/June). 13 ways of looking at a leader. *INC Magazine,* 74–76.

Buchanan, L. (2011/June). Care values. *INC Magazine,* 60–61.

Buchanan, L. (2013, June). Between Venus and Mars: 7 traits of true leaders. *INC Magazine, 35*(5), 64. Retrieved from http://www.inc.com/magazine/201306/leigh-buchanan/traits-of-true-leaders.html

Chrispeels, J.H. (2004). *Learning to Lead Together.* Thousand Oaks, Calif.: Sage Publications.

Code of Ethics for Nurses. (2001). *Nursing World.* Retrieved from www.nursingworld.org/MainMenuCategories/EthicsStandards/CodeofEthicsforNurses.

Dantley, M.E. (2005). Moral leadership: Shifting the management paradigm. In English, F.W., *The Sage Handbook of Educational Leadership* (pp. 34–46). Thousand Oaks, Calif.: Sage Publications.

Deutschman, A. (2005). Is your boss a psychopath? *Making Change. Fast Company, 96,* 43–51.

Disch, J. (2013). President's Message: Professional Generosity. *Nursing Outlook, 61,* 196–204.

Dorn, M. (2011). Characteristics of caring leadership. Retrieved from www.thecareguys.com Feldman, D.A. (2002). *Critical Thinking: Strategies for Decision Making.* Menlo Park, Calif.: Crisp Publications.

Feldman, D. (2002). *Critical thinking: Strategies for decision making.* Crisp Learning.

Goleman, D., Boyatzes, R., & McKee, A. (2002). *Primal Leadership: Realizing the Power of Emotional Intelligence.* Boston: Harvard Business School Press.

Greenleaf, R.K. (2008). Nine characteristics of effective, caring leaders. Greenleaf Center for Servant Leadership. Retrieved from www.greenleaf.org

Grossman, S., & Valiga, T.M. (2000). *The New Leadership Challenge: Creating the Future of Nursing.* Philadelphia: F.A. Davis.

Hersey, P., & Campbell, R. (2004). *Leadership: A Behavioral Science Approach.* Calif.: Leadership Studies Publishing.

Herzberg, F. (1966). *Work and the nature of man.* Cleveland: World Publishing.

Herzberg, F., Mausner, B., & Snyderman, B. (1959). *The motivation to work* (2nd ed.). New York: John Wiley & Sons.

Holman, L. (1995). *Eleven Lessons in Self-Leadership: Insights for Personal and Professional Success.* Lexington, Ky.: A Lesson in Leadership Book.

Jackson, M., Ignatavicius, D., & Case, B. (eds.). (2004). *Conversations in Critical Thinking and Clinical Judgement.* Pensacola, Fla.: Pohl.

Kerfott, K. (2000). Leadership: Creating a shared destiny. *Dermatological Nursing, 12*(5), 363–364.

Korn, M. (2004). Toxic Cleanup: How to Deal with a Dangerous Leader. *Fast Company, 88,* 17.

Leach, L.S. (2005). Nurse executive transformational leadership and organizational commitment. *Journal of Nursing Administration, 35*(5), 228–237.

Lyons, M.F. (2002). Leadership and followership. *The Physician Executive,* Jan/Feb, 91–93.

Maslow, A.H. (1970). *Motivation and personality* (2nd ed.). New York: Harper & Row.

Maxwell, J.C. (1993). *Developing the Leader Within You.* Tenn.: Thomas Nelson Inc.

Maxwell, J.C. (1998). *The 21 Irrefutable Laws of Leadership.* Tenn.: Thomas Nelson Inc.

McClelland, D. (1961). *The Achieving Society.* Princeton, NJ: D. Van Nostrand.

McMurry (2012). *Be a caring leader.* Managing People at Work. Retrieved from www.managingpeopleatwork.com/article.php?art_num=3982

McNichol, E. (2000). How to be a model leader. *Nursing Standard, 14*(45), 24.

Pavitt, C. (1999). Theorizing about the group communication-leadership relationship. In Frey, L.R. (Ed.), *The Handbook of Group Communication Theory and Research.* Thousand Oaks, Calif.: Sage Publications.

Porter-O'Grady, T. (2003). A different age for leadership, Part II. *Journal of Nursing Administration, 33*(2), 105–110.

Powell, C. (2012/May 21). The general's orders. (Features) (Excerpts) from book, *It worked for me: In life and leadership.* Harper Collins Pub. *Newsweek,* 40–44.

Rhodes, M.K., Morris, A.H., & Lazenby, R.B. (2011). Nursing at its best: Competent and caring. *Online Journal of Issues in Nursing, 16*(2), 10.

Scott, E., & Miles, J. (2013) Advancing Leadership Capacity in Nursing. *Nursing Administration Quarterly, 37*(1), 77–82.

Spears, L.C. (2010). Character and servant leadership: Ten characteristics of effective, caring leaders. *Journal of Virtues & Leadership, 1*(1), 25–30.

Spears, L.C., & Lawrence, M. (2004). *Practicing Servant-Leadership.* New York: Jossey-Bass.

Spreitzer, G.M., & Quinn, R.E. (2001). *A Company of Leaders: Five Disciplines for Unleashing the Power in Your Workforce.* San Francisco: Jossey-Bass.

Stewart, L., Holmes, C., & Usher, K. (2012). Reclaiming Caring in Nursing Leadership: A Deconstruction of

Leadership Using a Habermasian Lens. *Collegian, 19,* 223–229.

Tappen, R.M. (2001). *Nursing Leadership and Management: Concepts and Practice.* Philadelphia: F.A. Davis.

Trofino, J. (1995). Transformational leadership in health care. *Nursing Management, 26*(8), 42–47.

Turk, W. (2007, March/April). The art of managing up. *Defense AT&L,* 21–23.

White, R.K., & Lippitt, R. (1960). *Autocracy and democracy: An experimental inquiry.* New York: Harper & Row.

Wiseman, L., & McKeown, G. (2010/May). Managing yourself: Bringing out the best in your people. *Harvard Business Review.* Retrieved from http://hbr.org/2010/05/managing-yourself-bringing-out-the-best-in-your-people/ar/1

Every nurse needs to be a good leader and a good follower. In Chapter 1 we defined leadership and followership, and showed that even as a new nurse, you can be an effective leader. Not everyone needs to be a manager, however. New graduates are not ready to take on management responsibilities. Once you have had time to develop your clinical and leadership skills, then you can begin to think about taking on management responsibilities (Table 2-1).

Management

Are You Ready to Be a Manager?

For most new nurses, the answer is *no*, you should not accept managerial responsibility. Your clinical skills are still underdeveloped. You need to direct your energies to building your own skills, including your leadership skills, before you begin supervising other people.

What Is Management?

The essence of management is getting work done through others. The classic definition of management was Henri Fayol's 1916 list of managerial tasks: planning, organizing, commanding, coordinating, and controlling the work of a group of employees (Wren, 1972). But Mintzberg (1989) argued that managers really do whatever is needed

to make sure that employees do their work and do it well. Lombardi (2001) added that two-thirds of a manager's time is spent on people problems. The rest is taken up by budget work, going to meetings, preparing reports, and other administrative tasks.

Management Theories

There are two major but opposing schools of thought in management: scientific management and the human relations–based approach. As its name implies, the human-relations approach emphasizes the interpersonal aspects of managing people, whereas scientific management emphasizes the task aspects.

Scientific Management

Almost 100 years ago, Frederick Taylor argued that most jobs could be done more efficiently if they were analyzed thoroughly (Lee, 1980; Locke, 1982). Given a well-designed task and enough incentive to get the work done, workers will be more productive. For example, Taylor promoted the concept of paying people by the piece instead of by the hour. In health care, the equivalent of what Taylor recommended would be paying by the number of patients bathed or visited at home rather than by the number of hours worked. This creates an incentive to get

table 2-1

Differences Between Leadership and Management

Leadership	Management
Based on influence and shared meaning	Based on authority
An informal role	A formally designated role
An achieved position	As assigned position
Part of every nurse's responsibility	Usually responsible for budgets, appraising, hiring, and firing people
Requires initiative and independent thinking	Improved by the use of effective leadership skills

the most work done in the least amount of time. Taylorism stresses that there is a best way to do a job, which is usually the fastest way to do the job as well (Dantley, 2005).

Work is analyzed to improve efficiency. In health care, for example, there has been much discussion about the time and effort it takes to bring a disabled patient to physical therapy versus sending the therapist to the patient's home or inpatient unit. Reducing staff or increasing the productivity of existing employees to save money is also based on this kind of thinking.

Nurse managers who use the principles of scientific management will pay particular attention to the types of assessments and treatments done on the unit, the equipment needed to do them efficiently, and the strategies that would facilitate more efficient accomplishment of these tasks. Typically, these nurse managers keep careful records of the amount of work accomplished and reward those who accomplish the most.

Human Relations–Based Management

McGregor's theories X and Y provide a good contrast between scientific management and human relations–based management. Like Taylorism, Theory X reflects a common attitude among managers that most people do not want to work very hard and that the manager's job is to make sure that they do work hard (McGregor, 1960). To accomplish this, according to Theory X, a manager needs to employ strict rules, constant supervision, and the threat of punishment (reprimands, withheld raises, and threats of job loss) to create industrious, conscientious workers.

Theory Y, which McGregor preferred, is the opposite viewpoint. Theory Y managers believe that the work itself can be motivating and that people will work hard if their managers provide a supportive environment. A Theory Y manager

emphasizes guidance rather than control, development rather than close supervision, and reward rather than punishment (Fig. 2.1). A Theory Y nurse manager is concerned with keeping employee morale as high as possible, assuming that satisfied, motivated employees will do the best work. Employees' attitudes, opinions, hopes, and fears are important to this type of nurse manager. Considerable effort is expended to work out conflicts and promote mutual understanding to provide an environment in which people can do their best work.

Servant Leadership

The emphasis on people and interpersonal relationships is taken one step further by Greenleaf (2004), who wrote an essay in 1970 that began the servant leadership movement. Like transformational and caring leadership, servant leadership has a special appeal to nurses and other health-care

THEORY X

Work is something to be avoided

People want to do as little as possible

Use control-supervision-punishment

THEORY Y

The work itself can be motivating

People really want to do their job well

Use guidance-development-reward

Figure 2.1 Theory X versus Theory Y.

professionals. Despite its name, servant leadership applies more to people in supervisory or administrative positions than to people in staff positions.

The servant leader–style manager believes that people have value as people, not just as workers (Spears & Lawrence, 2004). The manager is committed to improving the way each employee is treated at work. The attitude is "employee first," not "manager first." So the manager sees himself or herself as being there for the employee. Here is an example:

Hope Marshall is a relatively new staff nurse at Jefferson County Hospital. When she was invited to be the staff nurse representative on the search committee for a new chief nursing officer, she was very excited about being on a committee with so many managerial and administrative people. As the interviews of candidates began, she focused on what they had to say. All the candidates had impressive résumés and spoke confidently about their accomplishments. Hope was impressed but did not yet prefer one over the other. Then the final candidate spoke to the committee. "My primary job," he said, "is to make it possible for each nurse to do the very best job he or she can do. I am here to make their work easier, to remove barriers, and to provide them with whatever they need to provide the best patient care possible." Hope had never heard the term servant leadership, but she knew immediately that this candidate, who articulated the essence of servant leadership, was the one she would support for this important position.

Qualities of an Effective Manager

Two-thirds of people who leave their jobs say the main reason was an ineffective or incompetent manager (Hunter, 2004). A survey of 3,266 newly licensed nurses found that lack of support from their manager was the nurses' primary reason for leaving their position, followed by a stressful work environment. Following are some of the indicators of their stressful work environment:

- 25% reported at least one needle stick in their first year.
- 39% reported at least one strain or sprain.
- 62% reported experiencing verbal abuse.
- 25% reported a shortage of supplies needed to do their work.

These results underscore the importance of having effective nurse managers who can create an environment in which new nurses thrive (Kovner, Brewer, Fairchild, et al., 2007).

Nurse managers hold pivotal positions in hospitals, nursing homes, and other health-care facilities. They report to the administration of these facilities, coordinate with a myriad of departments (the lab, dietary, pharmacy, and so forth) and care providers (physicians, nurse practitioners, therapists, and so forth), and supervise a staff that provides care around the clock. You can see why their effectiveness has considerable influence on the quality of the care provided under their direction (Trossman, 2011).

Consider for a moment the knowledge and skills needed by a nurse manager:

- Leadership, especially relationship building, teamwork, and mentoring skills
- Professionalism, including advocacy for nursing staff and support of nursing roles and ethical practice
- Advanced clinical expertise including quality improvement and evidence-based practice
- Human resource management expertise including staff development, and performance appraisals
- Financial management
- Coordination of patient care, including scheduling, work flow, work assignments, monitoring the quality of care provided, and documentation of that care (Jones, 2010; Fennimore & Wolf, 2011)

The effective nurse manager possesses a combination of qualities: leadership, clinical expertise, and business sense. None of these alone is enough; it is the combination that prepares an individual for the complex task of managing a unit or team of health-care providers. Consider each of these briefly:

- **Leadership.** All of the people skills of the leader are essential to the effective manager.
- **Clinical expertise.** Without possessing clinical expertise oneself, it is very difficult to help others develop their skills and evaluate how well they have done. It is probably not necessary (or even possible) to know everything all other professionals on the team know, but it is important to be able to assess

the effectiveness of their work in terms of patient outcomes.

- **Business sense.** Nurse managers also need to be concerned with the "bottom line," with the cost of providing the care that is given, especially in comparison with the benefit received from that care and the funding available to pay for it, whether from private insurance, Medicare, Medicaid, or out of the patient's own pocket. This is a complex task that requires knowledge of budgeting, staffing, and measurement of patient outcomes.

There is some controversy over the amount of clinical expertise versus business sense that is needed to be an effective nurse manager. Some argue that a person can be a "generic" manager, that the job of managing people is the same no matter what tasks he or she performs. Others argue that managers must understand the tasks themselves, better than anyone else in the work group. Our position is that both clinical skill and business acumen are needed, along with excellent leadership skills.

Behaviors of an Effective Manager

Mintzberg (1989) divided a manager's activities into three categories: interpersonal, decisional, and informational. We use these categories and have added some activities suggested by other authors (Dunham-Taylor, 1995; Montebello, 1994) and from our own observations of nurse managers (Fig. 2.2).

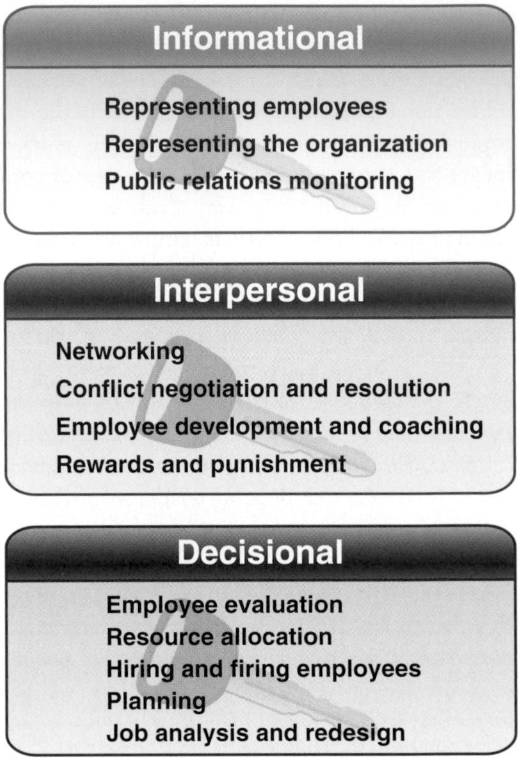

Interpersonal Activities

The interpersonal category is one in which leaders and managers have overlapping concerns. However, the manager has some additional responsibilities that are seldom given to leaders. These include the following:

- **Networking.** As we mentioned earlier, nurse managers are in pivotal positions, especially in inpatient settings where they have contact with virtually every service of the institution as well as with most people above and below them in the organizational hierarchy. This provides them with many opportunities to influence the status and treatment of staff nurses and the quality of the care provided to their patients. It is important that they "maintain the line of

Figure 2.2 Keys to effective management.

sight," or connection, between what they do as managers, patient care, and the mission of the organization (Mackoff & Triolo, 2008, p. 123). In other words, they need to keep in mind how their interactions with both their staff members and with administration affects the care provided to the patients for whom they are responsible.

- **Conflict negotiation and resolution.** Managers often find themselves resolving conflicts among employees, patients, and administration. Ineffective managers often ignore people's emotional side or mismanage feelings in the workplace (Welch & Welch, 2008).
- **Employee development.** Managers are responsible for providing for the continuing learning and upgrading of the skills of their employees.
- **Coaching.** It is often said that employees are the organization's most valuable asset (Shirey, 2007). Coaching is one way in which nurse managers can share their experience and expertise with the rest of the staff. The goal is to nurture the growth and development of the

employee (the "coachee") to do a better job through learning (McCauley & Van Velson, 2004; Shirey, 2007).

Some managers use a directive approach: "This is how it's done. Watch me." or "Let me show you how to do this." Others prefer a problem-solving approach: "Let's try to figure out what's wrong here" (Hart & Waisman, 2005). "How do you think we can improve our outcomes?"

You can probably see the parallel with democratic and autocratic leadership styles described in Chapter 1. The decision whether to be directive (e.g., in an emergency) or mutual problem-solving (e.g., when developing a long-term plan to improve infection control) will depend on the situation.

■ **Rewards and punishments.** Managers are in a position to provide specific rewards (e.g., salary increases, time off) and general rewards (e.g., praise, recognition) as well as punishments (withhold pay raises, deny promotions).

Decisional Activities

Nurse managers are responsible for making many decisions:

■ **Employee evaluation.** Managers are responsible for conducting formal performance appraisals of their staff members. Traditionally, formal reviews have been conducted once a year, but people need to know much sooner than that if they are doing well or need to improve. Effective managers are like coaches, regularly giving their staff feedback (Suddath, 2013).
■ **Resource allocation.** In decentralized organizations, nurse managers are often given an annual budget for their units and must allocate these resources wisely. This can be difficult when resources are very limited.
■ **Hiring and firing employees.** Nurse managers either make the hiring and firing decisions or participate in employment and termination decisions for their units.
■ **Planning for the future.** Not only is the day-to-day operation of most units complex and time-consuming, nurse managers must also look ahead to prepare themselves and their units for future changes in budgets, organizational priorities, and patient populations. They need to look beyond the four walls of their own organization to become aware of what is happening to their competition and to the health-care system (Kelly & Nadler, 2007).
■ **Job analysis and redesign.** In a time of extreme cost sensitivity, nurse managers are often required to analyze and redesign the work of their units to make them as efficient as possible.

Informational Activities

Nurse managers often find themselves in positions within the organizational hierarchy in which they acquire much information that is not available to their staff. They also have much information about their staff that is not readily available to the administration, placing them in a strategic position within the information web of any organization. The effective manager uses this knowledge for the benefit of both the staff and the organization. The following are some examples:

■ **Spokesperson.** Nurse managers often speak for administration when relaying information to their staff members. Likewise, they often speak for staff members when relaying information to administration. You could think of them as central information clearinghouses, acting as gatherers and disseminators of information to people above and below them in the organizational hierarchy (Shirey, Ebright, & McDaniel, 2008, p. 126).
■ **Monitoring.** Nurse managers are also expert "sensors," picking up early signs (information) of problems before they grow too big (Shirey, Ebright, & McDaniel, 2008). They are expected to monitor the many and various activities of their units or departments, including the number of patients seen, average length of stay, and important patient outcomes such as infection rates, fall rates, and so forth. They also monitor the staff (e.g., absentee rates, tardiness, unproductive time), the budget (e.g., money spent, money left in comparison with money needed to operate the unit), and the costs of procedures and services provided, especially those that are variable such as overtime or disposable vs. nondisposable medical supplies (Dowless, 2007).
■ **Reporting.** Nurse managers share information with their patients, staff members, and

table 2-2	
Bad Management Styles	
These are the types of managers you do not want to be and for whom you do not want to work:	
Know-it-all	Self-appointed experts on everything, these managers do not listen to anyone else.
Emotionally remote	Isolated from the staff and the work going on, these managers do not know what is going on in the workplace and cannot inspire others.
Purely mean	Mean, nasty, and dictatorial, these managers look for problems and reasons to criticize. They diminish people instead of developing them.
Overly nice	Desperate to please everyone, these managers agree to every idea and request, causing confusion and spending too much money on useless projects.
Afraid to decide	Indecisive managers may announce goals for their unit but fail to be clear about their expectations, assign responsibility, or set deadlines for accomplishment. In the name of fairness, these managers may not distinguish between competent and incompetent, or hardworking and unproductive employees, thus creating an unfair reward system.

Source: Based on Welch, J. & Welch, S. (2007, July 23). Bosses who get it all wrong. Bloomberg Businessweek, 88; Schaffer, R.H. (2010/September). Mistakes leaders keep making. Harvard Business Review, 87–91; Wiseman, L., & McKeown, A. (2010/May). Bringing out the best in your people. Harvard Business Review, Reprint R1005K, 1–5.

employers. This information may be related to the results of their monitoring efforts, new developments in health care, policy changes, and so forth.

Review Table 2-2, Bad Management Styles, to compare what you have just read about effective nurse managers with descriptions of some of the most common ineffective approaches to being a manager.

Conclusion

Nurse managers have complex, responsible positions in health-care organizations. Ineffective managers may do harm to their employees, their patients, and to the organization, while effective managers can help their staff members grow and develop as health-care professionals providing the highest quality care to their patients.

If you have wondered why there are so many conflicting and overlapping theories of leadership and management, it is because management theory is still at an immature (not fully developed) stage as well as being prone to fads (Micklethwait in Wooldridge, 2011). Even so, there is still much that is useful in the theories and much to be learned from them.

Study Questions

1. Why should new graduates decline nursing management positions? At what point do you think a nurse is ready to assume managerial responsibilities?

2. Which theory, scientific management or human relations, do you believe is most useful to nurse managers? Explain your choice.

3. Compare servant leadership with scientific management. Which approach do you prefer? Why?

4. Describe your ideal nurse manager in terms of the person for whom you would most like to work. Then describe the worst nurse manager you can imagine, and explain why this person would be very difficult to work with.

5. List 10 behaviors of nurse managers and then rank them from least to most important. What rationale(s) did you use in ranking them?

Case Studies to Promote Critical Reasoning

Case I

Joe Garcia has been an operating room nurse for 5 years. He is often on call on Saturdays and Sundays, but he enjoys his work and knows that he is good at it.

Joe was called to come in on a busy Saturday afternoon just as his 5-year-old daughter's birthday party was about to begin. "Can you find someone else just this once?" he asked the nurse manager who called him. "I should have let you know in advance that we have an important family event today, but I just forgot. If you can't find someone else, call me back, and I'll come right in." Joe's manager was furious. She said, "I don't have time to make a dozen calls. If you knew that you wouldn't want to come in today, you should not have accepted on-call duty. We pay you to be on call, and I expect you to be here in 30 minutes, not 1 minute later, or there will be consequences."

Joe decided that he no longer wanted to work in that institution. With his 5 years of operating room experience, he quickly found another position in an organization that was more supportive of its staff.

1. What style of leadership and school of management seemed to be preferred by Joe Garcia's manager?

2. What style of leadership and school of management were preferred by Joe?

3. Which of the listed qualities of leaders and managers did the nurse manager display? Which behaviors? Which ones did the nurse manager not display?

4. If you were Joe, what would you have done? If you were the nurse manager, what would you have done? Why?

5. Who do you think was right, Joe or the nurse manager? Why?

Case II

Sung Lee completed her 2-year associate degree in nursing right after high school. Upon graduation, she was offered a staff position at Harbordale nursing home and rehabilitation center where she had volunteered during high school. Most of her classmates accepted positions in local hospitals, but Sung Lee felt comfortable at Harbordale and had loved her volunteer work there. She thought it would be an advantage to already know many of the staff at Harbordale.

The director of nursing thought it would be best to place Sung Lee on a short-term unit. Most of the patients in the unit were recently discharged from the hospital and still recovering from an acute event such as stroke, injury, or extensive surgery. Sung Lee found her assignment challenging but satisfying. She admired her nurse manager, an experienced clinical nurse leader who became her mentor.

Six months later, the director of nursing called Sung Lee into her office. "Sung Lee," she said, "we are very pleased with your work. You have been a quick learner and very caring nurse. Your colleagues, patients, and physicians all speak well of you."

"Thank you," replied Sung Lee. "I know there's still a lot for me to learn, but I really love my work here."

"You may not be aware of this," continued the director of nursing, "but your nurse manager will be retiring next month. Our policy at Harbordale is to promote from within whenever possible, and I'd like to offer you her position. It's a little soon after graduation, but I'm sure you can handle it."

Sung Lee gasped. "I'm honored that you would consider me for this position. May I have a few days to think it over?"

1. Why did the director of nursing at Harbordale offer the nurse manager position to Sung Lee? If you had been in the director's position, would you have selected Sung Lee for the nurse manager position? Why or why not?

2. If Sung Lee does accept the nurse manager position, what do you think her first month will be like? Write a scenario that describes her first month as a nurse manager.

3. If Sung Lee declines this offer, how do you think the director of nursing will respond?

4. Write a list of typical nurse manager roles and responsibilities. For each one indicate how prepared you are to assume each role or responsibility and what you would need to prepare yourself to assume this responsibility.

References

Dantley, M.E. (2005). Moral leadership: Shifting the management paradigm. In English, F.W., *The sage handbook of educational leadership* (pp. 34–46). Thousand Oaks, Calif.: Sage Publications.

Dowless, R.M. (2007). Your guide to costing methods and terminology. *Nursing Management, 38*(4), 52–57.

Dunham-Taylor, J. (1995). Identifying the best in nurse executive leadership. *Journal of Nursing Administration, 25*(7/8), 24–31.

Fennimore, L., & Wolf, G. (2011). Nurse manager leadership development, *Journal of Nursing Administration, 41*(5), 204–210.

Greenleaf, R.K. (2004). Who is the servant-leader? In Spears, L.C., & Lawrence, M., *Practicing servant-leadership*. New York: Jossey-Bass.

Hart, L.B., & Waisman, C.S. (2005). *The leadership training activity book*. New York: AMACOM.

Hunter, J.C. (2004). *The world's most powerful leadership principle*. New York: Crown Business.

Jones, R.A. (2010). Preparing tomorrow's leaders. *Journal of Nursing Administration, 40*(4), 154–157.

Kelly, J., & Nadler, S. (2007, March 3-4). Leading from below. *Wall Street Journal*, R4.

Kovner, C.T., Brewer, C.S., Fairchild, S., et al. (2007). Newly licensed RNs' characteristics, work attitudes, and intentions to work. *American Journal of Nursing, 107*(9), 58–70.

Leo, J.A. (1990). *The gold and the garbage in management theories and prescriptions*. Athens, Ohio: Ohio University Press.

Locke, E.A. (1982). The ideas of Frederick Taylor. An evaluation. *Academy of Management Review, 7*(1), 14.

Lombardi, D.N. (2001). *Handbook for the new health care manager*. San Francisco: Jossey-Bass/AHA Press.

Mackoff, B.L., & Triolo, P.K. (2008). Why do nurse managers stay? Building a model engagement. Part I: Dimensions of engagement. *Journal of Nursing Administration, 38*(3), 118–124.

McCauley, C.D., & Van Velson, E. (eds.) (2004). *The center for creative leadership handbook of leadership development*. New York: Jossey-Bass.

McGregor, D. (1960). *The Human Side of Enterprise*. New York: McGraw-Hill.

Micklethwait, J. (2011). Foreword in Wooldridge, A. *Masters of management*, NY: Harper Collins.

Mintzberg, H. (1989). *Mintzberg on management: Inside our strange world of organizations*. New York: Free Press.

Montebello, A. (1994). *Work teams that work*. Minneapolis. Best Sellers Publishing.

Schaffer, R.H. (2010/September). Mistakes leaders keep making. *Harvard Business Review*, 87–91.

Shirey, M.R. (2007). Competencies and tips for effective leadership. *Journal of Nursing Administration, 37*(4), 167–170.

Shirey, M.R., Ebright, P.R., & McDaniel, A.M. (2008). Sleepless in America: Nurse managers cope with stress and complexity. *Journal of Nursing Administration, 38*(3), 125–131.

Spears, L.C., & Lawrence, M. (2004). *Practicing servant-leadership*. New York: Jossey-Bass.

Suddath, C. (2013, November 11–17). You get a D+ in teamwork. *Bloomberg Businessweek*, 91.

Trossman, S. (2011). Complex role in complex times. *The American Nurse, 43*(4), 1, 6, 7.

Welch, J., & Welch, S. (2007, July 23). Bosses who get it all wrong. *Bloomberg Businessweek*, 88.

Welch, J., & Welch, S. (2008, July 28). Emotional mismanagement. *Bloomberg Businessweek*, 84.

Wiseman, L., & McKeown, G. (2010/May). Bringing out the best in your people. *Harvard Business Review*, Reprint R1005k, 1–5.

Wren, D.A. (1972). *The evolution of management thought*. New York: Ronald Press.

chapter 3

Nursing Practice and the Law

OBJECTIVES

After reading this chapter, the student should be able to:

- Identify three major sources of laws.
- Explain the differences between various types of laws.
- Differentiate between negligence and malpractice.
- Explain the difference between an intentional and an unintentional tort.
- Explain how standards of care are used in determining negligence and malpractice.
- Describe how nurse practice acts guide nursing practice.
- Explain the purpose of licensure.
- Discuss issues of licensure.
- Explain the difference between internal standards and external standards.
- Discuss advance directives and how they pertain to clients' rights.
- Discuss the legal implications of the Health Insurance Portability and Accountability Act (HIPAA).

OUTLINE

The courtroom seemed cold and sterile. Scanning her surroundings with nervous eyes, Lialla decided she knew how Alice must have felt when the Queen of Hearts screamed for her head. The image of the White Rabbit running through the woods, looking at his watch, yelling, "I'm late! I'm late!" flashed before her eyes. For a few moments, she indulged herself in thoughts of being able to turn back the clock and rewrite the past. The future certainly

looked grim at that moment. The calling of her name broke her reverie. Mr. Marsh, the attorney for the plaintiff, wanted her undivided attention regarding the auspicious day when she committed a fatal medication error. That day, the client died following a cardiac arrest because Lialla failed to check the appropriate dosage and route for the medication. Although she thought she should question the order, Lialla "followed the health-care provider's order" and administered 40 mEq of potassium chloride by intravenous push. Her 15 years of nursing experience meant little to the court. Because she had not followed hospital protocol and had violated an important standard of practice, Lialla stood alone. She was being sued for malpractice with the possibility of criminal charges should she be found guilty of contributing to the client's death.

As client advocates, nurses have a responsibility to deliver safe care to their clients. This expectation requires that nurses have professional knowledge at their expected level of practice and be proficient in technological skills. A working knowledge of the legal system, client rights, and behaviors that may result in lawsuits helps nurses to act as client advocates. As long as nurses practice according to established standards of care, they may be able to avoid the kind of day in court that Lialla experienced.

General Principles

Meaning of Law

The word *law* has several meanings. For the purposes of this chapter, *law* refers to any system of regulations that govern the conduct of individuals within a community and/or society, in response to the need for regularity, consistency, and justice (Hill & Hill, 2009). In other words, *law* means those rules that prescribe and control social conduct in a formal and legally binding manner. Laws are created in one of three ways:

1. *Statutory laws* are created by various legislative bodies, such as state legislatures or Congress. Some examples of federal statutes include the Patient Self-Determination Act of 1990 and the Americans With Disabilities Act. State statutes include the state nurse practice acts, the state boards of nursing, and the Good Samaritan Act. Laws that govern nursing practice are statutory laws.
2. *Common law* is the traditional unwritten law of England, based on custom and usage, which began to develop over a thousand years before the founding of the United States (Hill & Hill, 2009). It develops within the court system as judicial decisions are made in various cases and precedents for future cases are set. In this way, a decision made in one case can affect decisions made in later cases of a similar nature. Many

times a judge in a subsequent case will follow the reasoning of a judge in a previous case. Therefore, one case sets a precedent for another.
3. *Administrative law* includes the procedures created by administrative agencies (governmental bodies of the city, county, state, or federal government) involving rules, regulations, applications, licenses, permits, available information, hearings, appeals, and decision making (Hill & Hill, 2009). These laws are established through the authority given to government agencies, such as state boards of nursing, by a legislative body. These governing boards have the duty to meet the intent of laws or statutes.

Sources of Law

The Constitution

The U.S. Constitution is the foundation of American law. The Bill of Rights, comprising the first 10 amendments to the Constitution, is the basis for protection of individual rights. These laws define and limit the power of the government and protect citizens' freedom of speech, assembly, religion, and the press, and freedom from unwarranted intrusion by government into personal choices. State constitutions can expand individual rights but cannot deprive people of rights guaranteed by the U.S. Constitution.

Constitutional law evolves. As individuals or groups bring suit to challenge interpretations of the Constitution, decisions are made concerning application of the law to that particular event. An example is the protection of freedom of speech. Are obscenities protected? Can one person threaten or criticize another person? The freedom to criticize is protected; threats are not protected. The definition of what constitutes obscenity is often debated and has not been fully clarified by the courts.

Statutes

Statutes are written laws created by a government or accepted governing body. Localities, state legislatures, and the U.S. Congress create statutes. Local statutes are usually referred to as ordinances. An example of a local ordinance might be a requirement that all garbage dumpsters must be covered at all times.

At the federal level, conference committees comprising representatives of both houses of Congress negotiate the resolution of any differences on wording of a bill before it is voted upon by both Houses of Congress and sent to the president to be signed into law. If the bill does not meet with the approval of the executive branch of government, the president can veto it. If that occurs, the legislative branch must have enough votes to override the veto or the bill will not become law.

Nurses have an opportunity to influence the development of statutory law both as citizens and as health-care providers. Writing to or meeting with state legislators or members of Congress is a way to demonstrate interest in such issues and their outcomes in terms of the laws passed. Passage of a new law is often a long process that includes some compromise of all interested individuals.

Administrative Law

The Department of Health and Human Services, the Department of Labor, and the Department of Education are the federal agencies that administer health-care–related laws. At the state level are departments of health and mental health and licensing boards.

Administrative agencies are staffed with professionals who develop the specific rules and regulations that direct the implementation of statutory law. These rules must be reasonable and consistent with existing statutory law and the intent of the legislature. Usually, the rules go into effect only after review and comment by affected persons or groups. For example, specific statutory laws give state nursing boards the authority to issue and revoke licenses, which means that each board of nursing has the responsibility to oversee the professional nurse's competence.

Types of Laws

Another way to look at the legal system is to divide laws into two categories: criminal law and civil law.

Criminal Law

Criminal laws were developed to protect society from actions that threaten its existence. Criminal acts, although directed toward individuals, are considered offenses against the state. The perpetrator of the act is punished, and the victim receives no compensation for injury or damages. There are three categories of criminal law:

1. *Felony:* the most serious category, including such acts as homicide, grand larceny, and nurse practice act violation
2. *Misdemeanor:* includes lesser offenses such as traffic violations or shoplifting of a small dollar amount
3. *Juvenile:* crimes carried out by individuals younger than 18 years; specific age varies by state and crime

There are occasions when a nurse breaks a law and is tried in criminal court. A nurse who obtains and/or distributes controlled substances illegally, either for personal use or for the use of others, is violating the law. Falsification of records of controlled substances is a criminal action. In some states, altering a patient record may lead to both civil and criminal action depending upon the treatment outcome. For example:

> *In New Jersey State v. Winter V, Nurse needed to administer a blood transfusion. Because she was in a hurry, she did not check the paperwork properly and therefore did not follow the standard of practice established for blood administration. The client was transfused with incompatible blood, suffered from a transfusion reaction, and died. Nurse V then intentionally attempted to conceal her conduct. She falsified the records, disposed of the blood and administration equipment, and failed to notify the patient's health-care provider of the error. The jury found Nurse V guilty of simple manslaughter and sentenced her to 5 years in prison (Sanbar, 2007).*

Civil Law

Civil laws usually involve the violation of one person's rights by another person. Areas of civil law that particularly affect nurses are tort law, contract law, antitrust law, employment discrimination, and labor laws.

Tort

The remainder of this chapter focuses primarily on tort law. By definition, tort law consists of a body of rights, obligations, and remedies that is applied by courts in civil proceedings for the purpose of providing relief for persons who have suffered harm from the wrongful acts of others. Simply put, a tort is a legal or civil wrong carried out by one person against the person or property of another. The person who sustains injury or suffers financial damage as the result of the conduct is known as the plaintiff, and the person who is responsible for causing the injury and incurs liability for the damage is known as the defendant (Loiacono, 2005). Tort law recognizes that individuals in their relationships with each other have a general duty not to harm each other. For example, as drivers of automobiles, everyone has a duty to drive safely so that others will not be harmed. A roofer has a duty to install a roof properly so that it will not collapse and injure individuals inside the structure. Nurses have a duty to deliver care in such a manner that the consumers of care are not harmed. These legal duties of care may be violated intentionally or unintentionally.

Quasi-Intentional Tort

A quasi-intentional tort has its basis in speech. These are voluntary acts that directly cause injury or anguish without meaning to harm or to cause distress. The elements of cause and desire are present, but the element of intent is missing. Quasi-intentional torts usually involve problems in communication that result in damage to a person's reputation, violation of personal privacy, or infringement of an individual's civil rights. These include defamation of character, invasion of privacy, and breach of confidentiality (Aiken, 2004, p. 139).

Negligence

Negligence is the unintentional tort of acting or failing to act as an ordinary, reasonable, prudent person, resulting in harm to the person to whom the duty of care is owed (Black, 2009). The legal elements of negligence consist of duty, breach of duty, causation, and harm or injury (Gic, 2009). All four elements must be present in the determination. For example, if a nurse administers the wrong medication to a client but the client is not injured, then the element of harm has not been met. However, if a nurse administers appropriate pain medication but fails to put up the side rails of the patient's bed, and the client falls and breaks a hip, all four elements have been satisfied. The duty of care is the standard of care. The law defines standard of care as that which a reasonable, prudent practitioner with similar education and experience would do or not do in similar circumstances (Gic, 2009).

Malpractice

Malpractice is the term used for professional negligence. When fulfillment of duties requires specialized education, the term *malpractice* is used. In most malpractice suits, the facilities employing the nurses who cared for a client are named as defendants in the suit. Vicarious liability is the legal principle cited in these cases. Three doctrines, *respondeat superior,* the borrowed servant doctrine, and the captain of the ship doctrine fall under vicarious liability. The captain of the ship doctrine, which is an adaptation from the "borrowed servant" rules came about in a case known as *McConnell v Williams* and refers to medical malpractice. The ruling declared that the person in charge is held accountable for all those falling under his or her supervision, regardless of whether the "captain" is directly responsible for an alleged error or act of alleged negligence, and despite the others' positions as hospital employees.

An important principle in understanding negligence is *respondeat superior* ("let the master answer") (Aiken, 2004, p. 279). This doctrine holds employers liable for any negligence by their employees when the employees were acting within the realm of employment and when the alleged negligent acts happened during employment (Aiken, 2004). The borrowed servant doctrine comes into play when an employee may be subject to the control and direction of an entity other than the primary employer. In this situation someone other than an individual's primary employer is responsible for his or her actions. For example, an anesthesiologist supervising a resident may be held liable for the resident's error.

Consider the following scenario:

A nursing instructor on a clinical unit in a busy metropolitan hospital instructed his students not to administer any medications unless he was present. Marcos, a second-level student, was unable to find his instructor, so he decided to administer digoxin to his client without supervision. The ordered dose was 0.125 mg. The unit dose came as digoxin 0.5 mg/mL. Marcos administered the entire amount without checking the digoxin dose or the client's blood digoxin and potassium levels. The client became toxic, developed a dysrhythmia, and was transferred to the intensive care unit. The family sued the hospital and the nursing school for malpractice. The nursing instructor was also sued under the principle of respondeat superior, even though specific instructions had been given to the students regarding administering medications without direct supervision.

Other Laws Relevant to Nursing Practice

Good Samaritan Laws

Fear of being sued has often prevented trained professionals from assisting during an emergency. To encourage physicians and nurses to respond to emergencies, many states developed what are now known as the Good Samaritan laws. When administering emergency care, nurses and physicians are protected from civil liability by Good Samaritan laws as long as they behave in the same manner as an ordinary, reasonable, and prudent professional in the same or similar circumstances (Glannon, 2005). In other words, when assisting during an emergency, nurses must still observe professional standards of care. However, if a payment is received for the care given, the Good Samaritan laws do not hold.

Confidentiality

It is possible for nurses to be involved in lawsuits other than those involving negligence. For example, clients have the right to confidentiality, and it is the duty of the professional nurse to ensure this right. This assures the client that information obtained by a nurse while providing care will not be communicated to anyone who does not have a need to know. This includes giving information by telephone to individuals claiming to be related to a client, giving information without a client's signed release, or removing documents from a health-care provider with a client's name or other information.

The Health Insurance Portability and Accountability Act (HIPAA) of 1996 was passed as an effort to preserve confidentiality, protect the privacy of health information, and improve the portability and continuation of health-care coverage. The HIPAA gave Congress until August 1999 to pass this legislation. Congress failed to act, and the Department of Health and Human Services took over developing the appropriate regulations (Charters, 2003). The latest version of this privacy act was published in the *Federal Register* in 2002 (Charters, 2003).

The increased use of electronic sources of documentation and transfer of client information presents many confidentiality issues. It is important for nurses to be aware of the guidelines protecting the sharing and transfer of information through electronic sources. Most health-care institutions have internal procedures to protect client confidentiality.

Consider the following example:

Bill was admitted to the hospital for pneumonia. With Bill's permission, an HIV test was performed, and the result was positive. This information was available on the computerized laboratory result printout. A nurse inadvertently left the laboratory results on the computer screen, which was partially facing the hallway. One of Bill's coworkers, who had come to visit him, saw the report on the screen. This individual reported the test results to Bill's supervisor. When Bill returned to work, he was fired for "poor job performance," although he had had superior job evaluations. In the process of filing a discrimination suit against his employer, Bill discovered that the information on his health status had come from this source. A lawsuit was filed against the hospital and the nurse involved based on a breach of confidentiality.

Social Networking

Another issue affecting confidentiality involves social networking. The increased use of smartphones has led to increased violations of confidentiality. These infractions often occur without intent yet pose a risk to clients and health-care personnel. Posting pictures and information on social networking sites that involve clinical experiences and/or work experiences can present a risk to patient confidentiality and violate HIPAA regulations. Many institutions have implemented policies that affect employees and student affiliations. These policies may result in employee termination and/or cancelling agreements with outside agencies using the health-care institution. Take the following example:

Several nursing students who received scholarships from an affiliating health-care institution were working their required shift in the emergency department. The staff brought in a birthday cake for one of the emergency department physicians. One of the students snapped a picture of the staff with the physician and posted it on her social network page. The computer screen with the names and information of the clients in the emergency department at the time was clearly visible behind the physician and the staff. Another staff member discovered this and notified the chief nursing officer of the hospital. The nursing student lost her scholarship, was terminated from her job, and was required to return all monies back to the institution. Disciplinary actions were taken against the staff involved in the incident.

Slander and Libel

Slander and libel are categorized as quasi-intentional torts. The term *slander* refers to the spoken word, and *libel* refers to the written word. Nurses rarely think of themselves as being guilty of slander or libel, but making a false verbal statement about a client's condition that may result in an injury to that client is considered slander. Making a false written statement is libel. For example, verbally stating that a client who had blood drawn for drug testing has a substance abuse problem, when in fact the client does not carry that diagnosis, could be considered a slanderous statement.

Slander and libel also refer to statements made about coworkers or other individuals whom you may encounter in both your professional and educational life. Think before you speak and write. Sometimes what may appear to be harmless to you, such as a complaint, may contain statements that damage another person's credibility personally and professionally. Consider this example:

Several nurses on a unit were having difficulty with the nurse manager. Rather than approach the manager or follow the chain of command, they decided to send a written statement to the chief executive officer (CEO) of the hospital. In this letter, they embellished some of the incidents that occurred and took out of context statements that the nurse manager had made, changing the meanings of the remarks. The nurse manager was called to the CEO's office and reprimanded for these events and statements, which in fact had not occurred. The nurse manager sued the nurses for slander and libel based on the premise that her personal and professional reputation had been tainted.

False Imprisonment

False imprisonment is confining an individual against his or her will by either physical (restraining) or verbal (detaining) means. The following are examples:

- Using restraints on individuals without the appropriate written consent
- Restraining mentally challenged individuals who do not represent a threat to themselves or others
- Detaining unwilling clients in an institution when they desire to leave
- Keeping persons who are medically cleared for discharge for an unreasonable amount of time
- Removing clients' clothing to prevent them from leaving the institution
- Threatening clients with some form of physical, emotional, or legal action if they insist on leaving

Sometimes clients are a danger to themselves and to others. Nurses need to decide on the appropriateness of restraints as a protective measure. Nurses should try to obtain the cooperation of the client before applying any type of restraint. The first step is to attempt to identify a reason for the risky or threatening behavior and resolve the problem. If this fails, document the need for restraints, consult with the physician, and carefully follow the institution's policies and standards of practice. Systematic documentation and continual assessment are of highest importance when caring for clients who have restraints. Any changes in client status must be reported and documented. Failure to follow these guidelines may result in greater harm to the client and possibly a lawsuit for the staff. Consider the following:

Mr. Harrison, who is 87 years old, was admitted to the hospital through the emergency department with severe lower abdominal pain of 3 days' duration. Physical assessment revealed severe dehydration and acute distress. A surgeon was called, and an abdominal laparotomy was performed, revealing a ruptured appendix. Surgery was successful, and the client was sent to the intensive care unit for 24 hours. On transfer to the surgical floor the next day, Mr. Harrison was in stable condition. Later that night, he became confused, irritable, and anxious.

He attempted to climb out of bed and pulled out his indwelling urinary catheter. The nurse restrained him. The next day, his irritability and confusion continued. Mr. Harrison's nurse placed him in a chair, tying him in and restraining his hands. Three hours later he was found in cardiopulmonary arrest. A lawsuit of wrongful death and false imprisonment was brought against the nurse manager, the nurses caring for Mr. Harrison, and the institution. During discovery, it was determined that the primary cause of Mr. Harrison's behavior was hypoxemia. A violation of law occurred with the failure of the nursing staff to notify the physician of the client's condition and to follow the institution's standard of practice on the use of restraints.

To protect themselves against charges of negligence or false imprisonment in such cases, nurses should discuss safety needs with clients, their families, or other members of the health-care team. Careful assessment and documentation of client status are imperative and also components of good nursing practice. Confusion, irritability, and anxiety often have metabolic causes that need correction, not restraint.

There are statutes and case laws specific to the admission of clients to psychiatric institutions. Most states have guidelines for emergency involuntary hospitalization for a specific period of time. Involuntary admission is considered necessary when clients demonstrate a danger to themselves or others. Specific procedures and legal guidelines must be followed. A determination by a judge or administrative agency and/or certification by a specified number of health-care providers that a person's mental health justifies his or her detention and treatment may be required. Once admitted, these clients may not be restrained unless the guidelines established by state law and the institution's policies provide for this possibility. Clients who voluntarily admit themselves to psychiatric institutions are also protected against false imprisonment. Nurses working in areas such as emergency departments, mental health facilities, and so forth need to be cognizant of these issues and find out the policies of their state and employing institution.

Assault and Battery

Assault is threatening to do harm. Battery is touching another person without his or her consent. The significance of an assault lies in the threat:

"If you don't stop pushing that call bell, I'll give you this injection with the biggest needle I can find" is considered an assaultive statement. Battery would occur if the injection were given when it was refused, even if medical personnel deemed it was for the "client's good." With few exceptions, clients have a right to refuse treatment. Holding down a violent client against his or her will and injecting a sedative is battery. Most medical treatments, particularly surgery, would be considered battery if clients failed to provide informed consent.

Standards of Practice

Avedis Donabedian (1988) said, "Standards are professionally developed expressions of the range of acceptable variations from a norm or criterion." Concern for the quality of care is a major part of nursing's responsibility to the public. Therefore, the nursing profession is accountable to the consumer for the quality of its services.

One of the defining characteristics of a profession is the ability to set its own standards. Nursing standards were established as guidelines for the profession to ensure acceptable quality of care (Beckman, 1995). Standards of practice are also used as criteria to determine whether appropriate care has been delivered. In practice, they represent the minimum acceptable level of care. Nurses are judged on generally accepted standards of practice for their level of education, experience, position, and specialty area. Standards take many forms. Some are written and appear as criteria of professional organizations, job descriptions, agency policies and procedures, and textbooks. Others, which may be intrinsic to the custom of practice, are not found in writing (Beckman, 1995).

State boards of nursing and professional organizations vary by role and responsibility in relation to standards of development and implementation (ANA, 1998; 2011). Statutes written by the government, professional organizations, and health-care institutions establish standards of practice. The nurse practice acts of individual states define the boundaries of nursing practice within the state. In Canada, the provincial and territorial associations define practice.

The courts have upheld the authority of boards of nursing to regulate standards. The boards accomplish this through direct or delegated statutory language (ANA, 1998; 2004; 2011). The American

Nurses Association (ANA) also has specific standards of practice in general and in several clinical areas (ANA, 2010) (see Appendix 2). In Canada, the colleges of registered nurses and the registered nurses associations of the various provinces and territories have published practice standards. These may be found at www.cna-aiic.ca.

Institutions develop internal standards of practice. The standards are usually explained in a specific institutional policy (for example, guidelines for the appropriate administration of a specific chemotherapeutic agent), and the institution includes these standards in its policy and procedure manuals. The guidelines are based on current literature and research. It is the nurse's responsibility to meet the institution's standards of practice. It is the institution's responsibility to notify the health-care personnel of any changes and instruct the personnel about the changes. Institutions may accomplish this task through written memos or meetings and in-service education.

With the expansion of advanced nursing practice, it has become particularly important to clarify the legal distinction between nursing and medical practice. It is important to be aware of the boundaries between these professional domains because crossing them can result in legal consequences and disciplinary action. The nurse practice act and related regulations developed by most state legislatures and state boards of nursing help to clarify nursing roles at the various levels of practice.

Use of Standards in Nursing Negligence Malpractice Actions

When omission of prudent care or acts committed by a nurse or those under his or her supervision cause harm to a client, standards of nursing practice are among the elements used to determine whether malpractice or negligence exists. Other criteria may include but are not limited to (ANA, 1998; 2011):

- State, local, or national standards
- Institutional policies that alter or adhere to the nursing standards of care
- Expert opinions on the appropriate standard of care at the time
- Available literature and research that substantiates a standard of care or changes in the standard

Patient's Bill of Rights

In 1973 the American Hospital Association approved a statement called the Patient's Bill of Rights. It was revised in October 1992. Patient rights were developed with the belief that hospitals and health-care institutions would support these rights with the goal of delivering effective client care. In 2003 the Patient's Bill of Rights was replaced by the Patient Care Partnership. These standards were derived from the ethical principle of autonomy. This document may be found at www.aha.org/advocacy-issues/communicatingpts/pt-care-partnership.shtml.

Informed Consent

Informed consent is a legal document in all 50 states. It requires physicians to divulge the benefits, risks, and alternatives to a suggested treatment, nontreatment, or procedure. It allows for fully informed, rational persons to be involved in choices about their health care (Marr, 2003).

Without consent, many of the procedures performed on clients in a health-care setting may be considered battery or unwarranted touching. When clients consent to treatment, they give health-care personnel the right to deliver care and perform specific treatments without fear of prosecution. Although physicians are responsible for obtaining informed consent, nurses often find themselves involved in the process.

It is the physician's responsibility to give information to a client about a specific treatment or medical intervention (*Giese v. Stice,* 1997). While the nurse may witness the signature of a patient for a procedure, or surgery, the nurse should not be providing the details such as the benefits, risk, or possible outcomes. The individual institution is not responsible for obtaining the informed consent unless (1) the physician or practitioner is employed by the institution or (2) the institution was aware or should have been aware of the lack of informed consent and did not act on this fact (Guido, 2001). Some institutions require the physician or independent practitioner to obtain his or her own informed consent by obtaining the client's signature at the time the explanation for treatment is given.

Although some nurses may believe that they only need to obtain the client's signature on the informed consent document, nursing professionals have a larger responsibility in evaluating a client's ability to give informed consent. The nurse's role is to: (a) act as the patient's advocate, (b) protect the patient's dignity, (c) identify any fears, and (d) determine the patient's level of understanding and approval of the proposed care.

Every client brings a different and unique response depending on his or her personality, level of education, emotions, and cognitive status. A good practice is to ask a client to restate the information offered. This helps confirm that the client has received an appropriate amount of information and has understood it. The nurse is obliged to report any concerns about the client's understanding regarding what he or she has been told, or any concerns about the client's ability to make decisions.

The informed consent form should contain all the possible negative outcomes as well as the positive ones. The following are some criteria to help ensure that a client has given an informed consent (Berman & Snyder, 2012):

■ A mentally competent adult has voluntarily given the consent.
■ The client understands exactly to what he or she is consenting.
■ The consent includes the risks involved in the procedure, alternative treatments that may be available, and the possible result if the treatment is refused.
■ The consent is written.
■ A minor's parent or guardian usually gives consent for treatment.

Ideally, a nurse should be present when the health-care provider who is performing the treatment, surgery, or procedure is explaining the benefits and risks to the client.

To be able to give informed consent, the client must be fully informed. Clients have the right to refuse treatment, and nurses must respect this right. If a client refuses the recommended treatment, he or she must be informed of the possible consequences of this decision.

Implied consent occurs when consent is assumed. This may be an issue in an emergency when an individual is unable to give consent, as in the following scenario:

An elderly woman is involved in a car accident on a major highway. The paramedics called to the scene find her unresponsive and in acute respiratory distress; her vital signs are unstable. The paramedics immediately intubate her and begin treating her cardiac dysrhythmias. Because she is unconscious and unable to give verbal consent, there is an implied consent for treatment.

Staying Out of Court

Prevention

Unfortunately, the public's trust in the medical profession has declined over recent years. Consumers are better informed and more assertive in their approach to health care. They demand good and responsible care. If clients and their families perceive that behaviors are uncaring or that attitudes are impersonal, they are more likely to sue for what they view as errors in treatment.

The same applies to nurses. If nurses demonstrate an interest in clients and their families and display caring behaviors toward clients, a relationship develops. Individuals usually do not initiate lawsuits against those they view as "caring friends." The potential to change the attitudes of health-care consumers is within the power of health-care personnel. Demonstrating care and concern and making clients and families aware of choices and methods help decrease liability. Nurses who involve clients and their families in decisions about care reduce the likelihood of a lawsuit. Tips to prevent legal problems are listed in Box 3-1.

All health-care personnel are accountable for their own actions and adherence to the accepted

---

box 3-1

Tips for Avoiding Legal Problems

- Keep yourself informed regarding new research related to your area of practice.
- Insist that the health-care institution keep personnel apprised of all changes in policies and procedures and in the management of new technological equipment.
- Always follow the standards of care or practice for the institution.
- Delegate tasks and procedures only to appropriate personnel.
- Identify clients at risk for problems, such as falls or the development of decubiti.
- Establish and maintain a safe environment.
- Document precisely and carefully.
- Write detailed incident reports, and file them with the appropriate personnel or department.
- Recognize certain client behaviors that may indicate the possibility of a lawsuit.

standards of health care. Most negligence and malpractice cases arise from a violation of the accepted standards of practice and the policies of the employing institution. Common causes of negligence are listed in Table 3-1. Expert witnesses are called to cite the accepted standards and assist attorneys in formulating the legal strategies pertaining to those standards. For example, most medication errors can be traced to a violation of the accepted standard of medication administration, originally referred to as the Five Rights (Kozier et al., 1995; Taylor, Lillis, & LeMone, 2008). These were later amended to Seven Rights (Balas, Scott, & Rogers, 2004). In 2011, one more criterion was added, now making Eight Rights (Eisenhauer et al., 2007).

More recently Elliot and Liu (2010) proposed Nine Rights.

1. Right drug
2. Right dose
3. Right route
4. Right time
5. Right client
6. Right reason
7. Right documentation
8. Right form
9. Right response

Marcos, the nursing student described earlier in this chapter, violated the right-dose principle and therefore made a medication error.

Appropriate Documentation

The adage "not documented, not done" holds true in nursing. According to the law, if something has not been documented, then the responsible party did not do whatever needed to be done. If a nurse did not "do" something, he or she will be left open to negligence or malpractice charges.

Nursing documentation needs to be legally credible. Legally credible documentation is an accurate accounting of the care the client received. It also indicates the competence of the individual who delivered the care.

Charting by exception creates defense difficulties. When this method of documentation is used, investigators need to review the entire patient record in an attempt to reconstruct the care given to the client. Clear, concise, and accurate documentation helps nurses when they are named in lawsuits. Often, this documentation clears the individual of any negligence or malpractice. Documentation is credible when it is:

- **Contemporaneous** (documenting at the time care was provided)
- **Accurate** (documenting exactly what was done)
- **Truthful** (documenting only what was done)
- **Appropriate** (documenting only what could be discussed comfortably in a public setting)

Box 3-2 lists some documentation tips.

table 3-1	
Common Causes of Negligence	
Problem	**Prevention**
Client falls	Identify clients at risk. Place notices about fall precautions. Follow institutional policies on the use of restraints. Always be sure beds are in their lowest positions. Use side rails appropriately.
Equipment injuries	Check thermostats and temperature in equipment used for heat or cold application. Check wiring on all electrical equipment.
Failure to monitor	Observe IV infusion sites as directed by institutional policy. Obtain and record vital signs, urinary output, cardiac status, etc., as directed by institutional policy and more often if client condition dictates. Check pertinent laboratory values.
Failure to communicate	Report pertinent changes in client status. Document changes accurately. Document communication with appropriate source.
Medication errors	Follow the Seven Rights. Monitor client responses. Check client medications for multiple drugs for the same actions.

box 3-2

Some Documentation Guidelines

Medications
- Always chart the time, route, dose, and response.
- Always chart PRN medications and the client response.
- Always chart when a medication was not given, the reason (e.g., client in Radiology, Physical Therapy; do not chart that the medication was not on the floor), and the nursing intervention.
- Chart all medication refusals, and report them.

Physician Communication
- Document each time a call is made to a physician, even if he or she is not reached. Include the exact time of the call. If the physician is reached, document the details of the message and the physician's response.
- Read verbal orders back to the physician, and confirm the client's identity as written on the chart. Chart only verbal orders that you have heard from the source, not those told to you by another nurse or unit personnel.

Formal Issues in Charting
- Before writing on the chart, check to be sure you have the correct patient record.
- Check to make sure each page has the client's name and the current date stamped in the appropriate area.
- If you forgot to make an entry, chart "late entry," and place the date and time at the entry.
- Correct all charting mistakes according to the policy and procedures of your institution.
- Chart in an organized fashion, following the nursing process.
- Write legibly and concisely, and avoid subjective statements.
- Write specific and accurate descriptions.
- When charting a symptom or situation, chart the interventions taken and the client response.
- Document your own observations, not those that were told to you by another party.
- Chart frequently to demonstrate ongoing care, and chart routine activities.
- Chart client and family teaching and their response.

It is not good practice to sign off on medications for all patients for a shift before the medications are administered. Doing so is considered a fraudulent act and may leave a nurse open to charges of negligence in the form of a medication error if the medications are then not administered as documented. If injury occurs because the patient never received a medication, and the nurse documented that the patient received it, the nurse can be charged with criminal negligence.

Nursing units are busy and often understaffed. These realities exist but should not be allowed to interfere with the safe delivery of health care. Clients have a right to safe and effective health care, and nurses have an obligation to deliver this care.

Common Actions Leading to Malpractice Suits

- Failure to assess a client appropriately
- Failure to report changes in client status to the appropriate personnel
- Failure to document in the patient record
- Altering or falsifying a patient record
- Failure to obtain informed consent
- Failure to report a coworker's negligence or poor practice
- Failure to provide appropriate education to a client and/or family members
- Violation of internal or external standards of practice

In the case *Tovar v. Methodist Healthcare* (2005), a 75-year-old female client came to the emergency department complaining of a headache and weakness in the right arm. Although an order for admission to the neurological care unit was written, the client was not transported until 3 hours later. After the client was in the unit, the nurses called one physician regarding the client's status. Another physician returned the call 90 minutes later. Three hours later, the nurses called to report a change in the client's neurological status. A STAT computed tomography scan was ordered, which revealed a massive brain hemorrhage. The nurses were cited for the following:

1. Delay in transferring the client to the neurological unit
2. Failure to advocate for the client

The client presented with an acute neurological problem requiring admission to an intensive care unit where appropriate observation and interventions were available. A delay in transfer may lead to delay in appropriate treatment. According to the American Association of Neuroscience Nursing standards of practice (2012), nurses need to accurately assess the client's changing neurological status and advocate for the client. In this instance, the court stated that the nurses should have been more assertive in attempting to reach the physician and request a prompt medical evaluation. The court sided with the family, agreeing with the plaintiff's medical expert's conclusion that the client's death was related to improper management by the nursing staff.

If a Problem Arises

When served with a summons or complaint, people often panic, allowing fear to overcome reason.

First, simply answer the complaint. Failure to do this may result in a default judgment, causing greater distress and difficulties.

Second, many things can be done to protect oneself if named in a lawsuit. Legal representation can be obtained to protect personal property. Never sign any documents without consulting the malpractice insurance carrier or a legal representative. If you are personally covered by malpractice insurance, notify the company immediately and follow its instructions carefully.

Institutions usually have lawyers to defend themselves and their employees. Whether or not you are personally insured, contact the legal department of the institution where the act took place. Maintain a file of all papers, proceedings, meetings, and telephone conversations about the case. Do not withhold any information from your attorneys, even if that information can be harmful to you. A pending or ongoing legal case should not be discussed with coworkers or friends.

Let the attorneys and the insurance company help decide how to handle the difficult situation. They are in charge of damage control. Concealing information usually causes more damage than disclosing it.

Sometimes, nurses believe they are not being adequately protected or represented by the attorneys from their employing institution. If this happens, consider hiring a personal attorney who is experienced in malpractice law. This information can be obtained through either the state bar association or the local trial lawyers association.

Anyone has the right to sue; however, that does not mean that there is a case. Many negligence and malpractice cases find in favor of the health-care providers, not the client or the client's family. The following case demonstrates this situation:

The Supreme Court of Arkansas heard a case that originated from the Court of Appeals in Arkansas. A client died in a single-car motor vehicle accident shortly after undergoing an outpatient colonoscopy performed under conscious sedation. The family sued the center for performing the procedure and permitting the client to drive home. The court agreed that sedation should not be administered without the confirmation of a designated driver for later. It also agreed that an outpatient facility needs to have directives stating that nurses and physicians may not administer sedation unless transportation is available for later. However, the court ruled physicians and nurses may rely on information from the client. If the client states that someone will be available for transportation after the procedure, sedation may be administered. The second aspect of the case revolved around the client's insistence on leaving the facility and driving himself. When a client leaves against medical advice, the health-care personnel have a legal duty to warn and strongly advise the client against the highly dangerous action. However, nurses and physicians do not have a legal right to restrain the client physically, keep his clothes, or take away car keys. Nurses are not obligated to call a taxi, call the police, admit the client to the hospital, or personally escort the client home if the client insists on leaving. Clients have some responsibility for their own safety (Young v GastroIntestinal Center, Inc., 2005). In this case, the nurses acted appropriately. They adhered to the standard of practice, documented that the client stated that someone would be available to transport him home, and fulfilled the duty to warn.

Professional Liability Insurance

We live in a litigious society. Although there are a variety of opinions on the issue, in today's world nurses need to consider obtaining professional liability insurance (Aiken, 2004). Various forms of professional liability insurance are available. These policies have been developed to protect nurses against personal financial losses if they are involved in a medical malpractice suit. If a nurse is charged with malpractice and found guilty, the employing institution has the right to sue the nurse to reclaim damages. Professional malpractice insurance protects the nurse in these situations.

End-of-Life Decisions and the Law

When a heart ceases to beat, a client is in a state of cardiac arrest. In health-care institutions and in the community, it is common to begin cardiopulmonary resuscitation (CPR) when cardiac arrest occurs. In health-care institutions, an elaborate mechanism is put into action when a client "codes." Much controversy exists concerning when these mechanisms should be used and whether individuals who have no chance of regaining full viability should be resuscitated.

Do Not Resuscitate Orders

A do not resuscitate (DNR) order is a specific directive to health-care personnel not to initiate CPR measures. Only a physician can write a DNR order, usually after consulting with the client or family. Other members of the health-care team are expected to comply with the order. Clients have the right to request a DNR order. However, they may make this request without a full understanding of what it really means. Consider the following example:

> When Mrs. Vincent, 58 years old, was admitted to the hospital for a hysterectomy, she stated, "I want to be made a DNR." The nurse, concerned by the statement, questioned Mrs. Vincent's understanding of a DNR order. The nurse asked her, "Do you mean that if you are walking down the hall after your surgery and your heart stops beating, you do not want the nurses or physicians to do anything? You want us to just let you die?" Mrs. Vincent responded with a resounding, "No, that is not what I mean. I mean if something happens to me and I won't be able to be the way I am now, I want to be a DNR!" The nurse then explained the concept of a DNR order.

New York state has one of the most complete laws regarding DNR orders for acute and long-term care facilities. The New York law sets up a hierarchy of surrogates who may ask for a DNR status for incompetent clients. The state has also ordered that all health-care facilities ask clients their wishes regarding resuscitation (www.ny.gov). The ANA advocated that every facility have a written policy regarding the initiation of such orders (ANA, 1992). The client, or if the client is unable to speak for himself or herself, a family member or guardian should make clear the client's preference for either having as much as possible done or withholding treatment (see the next section, Advance Directives). After the Terri Schiavo case the ANA reconfirmed its stance on this issue (ANA, 2005).

box 3-3

Elements to Include in a DNR Order

- Statement of the institution's policy that resuscitation will be initiated unless there is a specific order to withhold resuscitative measures
- Statement from the client regarding specific desires
- Description of the client's medical condition to justify a DNR order
- Statement about the role of family members or significant others
- Definition of the scope of the DNR order
- Delineation of the roles of various caregivers

American Nurses Association. (1992). Position statement on nursing care and do not resuscitate decisions. Washington, DC: ANA.

Elements to include in a DNR order are listed in Box 3-3.

Advance Directives

The legal dilemmas that may arise in relation to DNR orders often require court decisions. For this reason, in 1990, Senator John Danforth of Missouri and Senator Daniel Moynihan of New York introduced the Patient Self-Determination Act to address questions regarding life-sustaining treatment. The act was created to allow people the opportunity to make decisions about treatment in advance of a time when they might become unable to participate in the decision-making process. Through this mechanism, families can be spared the burden of having to decide what the family member would have wanted.

Federal law requires that health-care institutions that receive federal money (from Medicare, for example) inform clients of their right to create advance directives. The Patient Self-Determination Act (S.R. 13566) provides guidelines for developing advance directives concerning what will be done for individuals if they are no longer able to participate actively in making decisions about care options. The act states that institutions must:

- **Provide information to every client.** On admission, all clients must be informed in writing of their rights under state law to accept or refuse medical treatment while they are competent to make decisions about their care. This includes the right to execute advance directives.
- **Document.** All clients must be asked whether they have a living will or have chosen a durable power of attorney for health care (also

known as a health-care surrogate). The response must be indicated on the medical record, and a copy of the documents, if available, should be placed on the client's chart.

- **Educate.** Nurses, other health-care personnel, and the community need to understand what the Patient Self-Determination Act and state laws regarding advance directives require.
- **Be respectful of clients' rights.** All clients are to be treated with respectful care regardless of their decision regarding life-prolonging treatments.
- **Have cultural humility.** Recognize that culture affects clients' decisions regarding end-of-life care. Nurses should familiarize themselves with the cultural and spiritual beliefs of their clients in order to deliver culturally sensitive care.

Living Will and Durable Power of Attorney for Health Care (Health–Care Surrogate)

The two most common forms of advance directives are living wills and durable power of attorney for health care (health-care surrogate). Living wills and other advance directives describe individual preferences regarding treatment in the event of a serious accident or illness. These legal documents indicate an individual's wishes regarding care decisions (www.mayoclinic.com/health/living-wills/HA00014).

A living will is a legally executed document that states an individual's wishes regarding the use of life-prolonging medical treatment in the event that he or she is no longer competent to make informed treatment decisions on his or her own behalf and is suffering from a terminal condition (Catalano, 2000; Flarey, 1991). A condition is considered terminal when, to a reasonable degree of medical certainty, there is little likelihood of recovery or the condition is expected to cause death. A terminal condition may also refer to a persistent vegetative state characterized by a permanent and irreversible condition of unconsciousness in which there is (1) absence of voluntary action or cognitive behavior of any kind and (2) an inability to communicate or interact purposefully with the environment (Hickey, 2008).

Another function of an advance directive is to designate a health-care surrogate. The role of the health-care surrogate is to make the client's wishes known to medical and nursing personnel. Chosen by the client, the health-care surrogate is usually a family member or close friend. Imperative in the designation of a health-care surrogate is a clear understanding of the client's wishes should the need arise to know them.

In some situations, clients are unable to express themselves adequately or competently, although they are not terminally ill. For example, clients with advanced Alzheimer's disease or other forms of dementia cannot communicate their wishes; clients under anesthesia are temporarily unable to communicate; and the condition of comatose clients does not allow for expression of health-care wishes. In these situations, the health-care surrogate can make treatment decisions on behalf of the client. However, when a client regains the ability to make his or her own decisions and is capable of expressing them effectively, he or she resumes control of all decision making pertaining to medical treatment (Reigle, 1992). Nurses and physicians may be held accountable when they go against a client's wishes regarding DNR orders and advance directives.

In the case of *Wendland v. Sparks* (1998), the physician and nurses were sued for "not initiating CPR." In this case, the client had been in the hospital for more than 2 months for lung disease and multiple myeloma. Although improving at the time, during the hospitalization the client had experienced three cardiac arrests. Even after this, she had not requested a DNR order. Her family had not discussed this either. After one of the arrests, the client's husband had told the physician that he wanted his wife placed on artificial life support if it was necessary (Guido, 2001). The client had a fourth cardiac arrest. One nurse went to obtain the crash cart, and another went to get the physician who happened to be in the area. The physician checked the client's heart rate, pupils, and respirations and stated, "I just cannot do it to her." (Guido, 2001, p. 158). She ordered the nurses to stop the resuscitation, and the physician pronounced the death of the client. The nurses stated that if they had not been given a direct order they would have continued their attempts at resuscitation. "The court ruled that the physician's judgment was faulty and that the family had the right to sue the physician for wrongful death" (Guido, 2001, p. 158). The nurses were cleared in this case because they were following a physician's order.

Nursing Implications

The Patient Self-Determination Act does not specify who should discuss treatment decisions or advance directives with clients. Because directives are often implemented on nursing units, however, nurses must be knowledgeable about living wills and health-care surrogates and be prepared to answer questions that clients may have about directives and the forms used by the health-care institution.

The responsibility for creating an awareness of individual rights often falls on nurses because they are client advocates. It is the responsibility of the health-care institution to educate personnel about its policies so that nurses and others involved in client care can inform health-care consumers of their choices. Nurses who are unsure of the policies in their health-care institution should contact the appropriate department.

Legal Implications of Mandatory Overtime

Although mostly a workplace and safety issue, there are legal implications to mandatory overtime. Due to nursing shortages, hospitals have increasingly forced nurses to work overtime (ANA, 2011). The ANA conducted a survey of almost 220,000 RNs from 13,000 nursing units in over 550 hospitals. The survey produced a 70% report rate and the results indicated that:

- 54% of nurses in adult medical units and emergency rooms revealed that they do not have sufficient time with patients;
- The amount of overtime has increased during the past year with 43% of all RNs working extra hours because the unit is short staffed or busy; and
- Inadequate staffing affected unit admissions, transfers, and discharges more than 20% of the time (ANA, 2011).

Overtime causes physical and mental fatigue, increased stress, and decreased concentration. Subsequently, these conditions lead to medical errors such as failure to assess appropriately, report, document, and administer medications safely. This practice of overtime ignores other responsibilities nurses have outside of their professional lives, which affects their mood, motivation, and productivity (Bae, Brewer, & Kovner, 2011).

Forced overtime causes already fatigued nurses to deliver nursing care that may be less than optimum, which in turn may lead to negligence and malpractice. This can result in the nurse losing his or her license and perhaps even facing a wrongful death suit due to an error in judgment. Needleman, Buerhaus, Pankratz, Liebson, Stevens, and Harris (2011) found that patient mortality increased by 2% on nursing units that had nurses working shifts 8 hours or more over their scheduled time due to registered nurse short staffing issues. Many states have implemented legislation restricting mandatory overtime for nurses. It is important for nurses to know and understand the laws of their particular state dealing with this issue.

Nurses practice under state or provincial (Canada) nurse practice acts, which state that nurses are held accountable for the safety and welfare of their clients. Once a nurse accepts an assignment for the client, that nurse becomes liable under his or her license.

Licensure

Licensure is defined by the National Council of State Boards of Nursing as "the process by which boards of nursing grant permission to an individual to engage in nursing practice after determining that the applicant has attained the competency necessary to perform a unique scope of practice. Licensure is necessary when the regulated activities are complex, require specialized knowledge and skill and independent decision making." (NCSBN, 2012). Licenses are given by a government agency to allow an individual to engage in a professional practice and use a specific title. State boards of nursing issue nursing licenses, thus limiting practice to a specific jurisdiction (Blais & Hayes, 2011).

Licensure can be mandatory or permissive. Permissive licensure is a voluntary arrangement whereby an individual chooses to become licensed to demonstrate competence. However, the license is not required to practice. Mandatory licensure requires a nurse to be licensed in order to practice. In the United States and Canada, licensure is mandatory.

Qualifications for Licensure

The basic qualification for licensure requires graduation from an approved nursing program. In the United States, states may add additional requirements, such as disclosures regarding health or medications that could affect practice. Most states require disclosure of criminal conviction.

Licensure by Examination

A major accomplishment in the history of nursing licensure was the creation of the Bureau of State Boards of Nurse Examiners. The formation of this agency led to the development of an identical examination in all states. The original examination, called the State Board Test Pool Examination, was created by the testing department of the National League for Nursing. This was done through a collaborating contract with the state boards. Initially, each state determined its own passing score; however, the states did adopt a common passing score. The examination is called the NCLEX-RN and is used in all states and territories of the United States. This test is prepared and administered through a testing company, Pearson Professional Testing of Minnesota (Ellis & Hartley, 2004).

NCLEX-RN

The NCLEX-RN is administered through computerized adaptive testing (CAT). Candidates must register to take the examination at an approved testing center in their area. Because of a large test bank, CAT permits a variety of questions to be administered to a group of candidates. Candidates taking the examination at the same time may not necessarily receive the same questions. Once a candidate answers a question, the computer analyzes the response and then chooses an appropriate question to ask next. If the question was answered correctly, the following question may be more difficult; if the question was answered incorrectly, the next question may be easier.

In April 2013 the new test plan was implemented. Changes in the test plan were based on the *Findings from the 2011 RN Practice Analysis: Linking the NCLEX Examination to Practice* (NCSBN, 2012). The minimum number of questions any candidate may receive is 75, and the maximum is 265. Although the maximum amount of time for taking the examination is 6 hours, candidates who do well or those who are not performing well may finish as soon as 1 hour. The test ends once the analysis of the examination clearly determines that the candidate has successfully passed, has undoubtedly failed, has answered the maximum number of questions, or has reached the time limit (NCSBN, 2012). The computer scores the test at the time it is taken; however, candidates are not notified of their status at the time of completion. The information first goes to the testing service, which in turn notifies the appropriate state board. The state board notifies the candidate of the examination results.

Nursing practice requires the application of knowledge, skills, and abilities (NCSBN, 2012). The items are written to reflect the levels of Bloom's taxonomy and are organized around client needs to reflect the candidates' ability to make nursing decisions regarding client care through application and analysis of information. The examination is organized into four major client need categories. Two of these categories, safe and effective care and physiological needs, include subdivisions (NCSBN, 2012). Integrated processes incorporate "nursing process, caring, communication and documentation and teaching/learning" (NCSBN, 2012, p. 3). Table 3-2 summarizes the categories and subcategories.

table 3-2	
Major Categories and Subcategories of Client Needs	
Category	**Subcategories**
Safe Effective Care Environment	Management of Care Safety and Infection Control
Health Promotion and Maintenance	Basic Care and Comfort
Psychosocial Integrity	Pharmacological and Parenteral Therapies
Physiological Integrity	Reduction of Risk Potential
	Physiological Adaptation

Source: Adapted from NCSBN NCLEX-RN test plan (NCSBN, 2007, pp. 3–4.)

Earlier, all questions were written in a multiple-choice format. In 2003, alternative formats were introduced. These alternative-format questions include fill-in-the-blank; multiple-response answers; audio and video type; "hot spots" that require the candidate to identify an area on a picture, graph, or chart; and drag-and-drop (NCSBN, 2012). More information on alternative formats can be found on the NCSBN Web site: www.ncsbn.org.

Preparing for the NCLEX-RN

There are several ways to prepare for the NCLEX-RN. Some candidates attend review courses, others view videos and DVDs, and others review books. These methods assist in reviewing information that was learned during the classroom education. Each individual needs to decide what works best for him or her. It is helpful to take practice tests, because it familiarizes one with the computer and the examination format. The NCSBN offers an online NCLEX-RN study program.

To prepare for the NCLEX, take time to look at the test blueprint provided by the NCSBN. This gives candidates a comprehensive overview of the types of questions to expect on the examination. Candidates can review alternative test formats by accessing www.pearsonvue.com/nclex/. Some test-taking tips follow.

- Be positive. Remind yourself that you worked hard to reach this milestone and how prepared you are to take the licensure examination.
- Turn negative thoughts into positive ones. Rather than saying, "I hope I pass," tell yourself, "I know I will do well."
- Acknowledge your feelings regarding the NCLEX. It is fine to admit that you are anxious; however, use your positive thoughts to control the anxiety.
- Also use diaphragmatic breathing (deep breathing) to control anxiety. Deep breathing augments the relaxation response of the body. Use this method at the beginning of the test or if you encounter a question that you find confusing.
- Control the situation by making a list of the items you may need to take the test. Pack them in a bag several days before, and keep them in a place where you will remember to take them.

- Eat well and get a good night's sleep before the test. Avoid foods high in sugar and caffeine. Contrary to popular belief, caffeine interferes with your ability to concentrate. Eat complex carbohydrates and protein to maintain your blood glucose level.
- Several days before you are scheduled to take the test, travel to the test site along the same route at the time you plan to go. Have an alternate itinerary in case there is a disruption in your route. This will alleviate any unnecessary stress in arriving at the examination site.
- Leave early and give yourself plenty of time to get to your destination. Arriving early also gives you a sense of control.
- Finally, remember your own basic needs. Testing centers tend to be cold. Pack a jacket or sweater. Check with the testing center to see if you are allowed to bring water or snacks.

Licensure Through Endorsement

Nurses licensed in one state may obtain a license in another state through the process of endorsement. Each application is considered independently and is granted a license based on the rules and regulations of the state.

States differ in the number of continuing education credits required, legal requirements, and other educational requirements. Some states require that nurses meet the current criteria for licensure at the time of application, whereas others may grant the license based on the criteria in effect at the time of the original licensure (Ellis & Hartley, 2004). When applying for a license through endorsement, a nurse should always contact the board of nursing for the state and find out the exact requirements for licensure. This information can usually be found on the board of nursing Web site for that particular state.

Multistate Licensure

The concept of multistate licensure allows a nurse licensed in one state to practice in additional states without obtaining additional licenses. NCSBN created a Multistate Licensure Compact, now referred to as the Nurse Licensure Compact, that permits this practice. States that belong to the compact have passed legislation adopting the terms of this agreement and are known as party states (https://www.ncsbn.org/nlc.htm). The nurse's home state is the state where he or she lives and received his or her original license. Renewal of the license is completed in the home state.

A nurse can hold only one home-state license. If the nurse moves to another state that belongs to the compact, the nurse applies for licensure within that state based on residency. The nurse is expected to follow the guidelines for nursing practice for that new state. The multistate licensure applies only to a basic registered nurse license, not to advanced practice. More information on multistate licensure can be found on the NCSBN Web site.

Disciplinary Action

State boards of nursing maintain rules and regulations for the practice of nursing. These may be found in the state's nurse practice acts. Violation of these regulations results in disciplinary actions as delineated by these boards. Issues of primary concern include but are not limited to the following:

- Falsifying documents to obtain a license
- Being convicted of a felony
- Practicing while under the influence of drugs or alcohol
- Functioning outside the scope of practice
- Engaging in child or elder abuse

Nurses convicted of a felony or found guilty in a malpractice action may find themselves before their state board of nursing or, in Canada, the provincial or territorial regulatory body.

Disciplinary action may include but is not limited to the suspension or revocation of a nursing license, mandatory fines, and mandatory continuing education. For more information regarding the regulations that guide nursing practice, consult the board of nursing in your state or, in Canada, your provincial or territorial regulatory body.

Conclusion

Nurses need to understand the legalities involved in the delivery of safe health care. It is important to know the standards of care established within your institution and the rules and regulations in the nurse practice acts of your state, province, or territory because these are the standards to which you will be held accountable. Health-care consumers have a right to quality care and the expectation that all information regarding diagnosis and treatment will remain confidential. Nurses have an obligation to deliver quality care and respect client confidentiality. Caring for clients safely and avoiding legal difficulties require nurses to adhere to the expected standards of care and document changes in client status carefully. Licensure helps to ensure that health-care consumers are receiving competent and safe care from their nurses.

Study Questions

1. How do federal laws, court decisions, and state boards of nursing affect nursing practice? Give an example of each.

2. Obtain a copy of the nurse practice act in your state. What are some of the penalties for violation of the rules and regulations?

3. Review the minutes and/or documents of a state board meeting. What were the most common issues for nurses to be called before the board of nursing? What were the resulting disciplinary actions?

4. The next time you are on your clinical unit, look at the nursing documentation done by several different staff members. Do you believe it is adequate? Explain your rationale.

5. How does your clinical institution handle medication errors?

6. If a nurse is found to be less than proficient in the delivery of safe care, how should the nurse manager remedy the situation?

7. Discuss where appropriate standards of care may be found. Explain whether each is an example of an internal or external standard of care.

8. Explain the importance of federal agencies in setting standards of care in health-care institutions.

9. What is the difference between consent and informed consent?

10. Look at the forms for advance directives and DNR policies in your institution. Do they follow the guidelines of the Patient Self-Determination Act?

11. What are the most common errors nurses commit that lead to negligence and/or malpractice?

12. What impact would a law that prevents mandatory overtime have on nurses, nursing care, and the health-care industry? Find out if your state has mandatory overtime legislation.

Case Study to Promote Critical Reasoning

Mr. Evans, 40 years old, was admitted to the hospital's medical-surgical unit from the emergency department with a diagnosis of acute abdomen. He had a 20-year history of Crohn's disease and had been on prednisone, 20 mg, every day for the past year. Three months ago he was started on the new biological agent etanercept, 50 mg, subcutaneously every week. His last dose was 4 days ago. Because he was allowed nothing by mouth (NPO), total parenteral nutrition was started through a triple-lumen central venous catheter line, and his steroids were changed to Solu-Medrol, 60 mg, by intravenous (IV) push every 6 hours. He was also receiving several IV antibiotics and medication for pain and nausea.

Over the next 3 days, his condition worsened. He was in severe pain and needed more analgesics. One evening at 9 p.m., it was discovered that his central venous catheter line was out. The registered nurse notified the physician, who stated that a surgeon would come in the morning to replace it. The nurse failed to ask the physician what to do about the IV steroids, antibiotics, and fluid replacement; the client was still NPO. She also failed to ask about the etanercept. At 7 a.m., the night nurse noticed that the client had had no urinary output since 11 p.m. the night before. She documented that the client had no urinary output but forgot to report this information to the nurse assuming care responsibilities on the day shift.

The client's physician made rounds at 9 a.m. The nurse for Mr. Evans did not discuss the fact that the client had not voided since 11 p.m., did not request orders for alternative delivery of the steroids and antibiotics, and did not ask about administering the etanercept. At 5 p.m. that evening, while Mr. Evans was having a computed tomography scan, his blood pressure dropped to 70 mm Hg, and because no one was in the scan room with him, he coded. He was transported to the ICU and intubated. He developed severe sepsis and acute respiratory distress syndrome.

1. List all the problems you can find with the nursing care in this case.

2. What were the nursing responsibilities in reporting information?

3. What do you think was the possible cause of the drop in Mr. Evans' blood pressure and his subsequent code?

4. If you worked in risk management, how would you discuss this situation with the nurse manager and the staff?

Case Study on Mandatory Overtime

Juan was completing his charting on his three babies in the neonatal intensive care unit. He had just finished orientation and this was his third day working. He was very tired and looking forward to his time off the next several days. Usually the nurse-to-baby ratio in the NICU was 1:2; however, the unit had been running short staffed and each nurse assumed additional patient responsibilities. Prior to him giving report, Juan's nurse manager came to him and stated, "Ada called in sick. We do not have anyone else to cover the unit and we are under our nurse-to-patient ratio. I need you to stay and work today." When Juan protested that he had already worked three 12-hour shifts and one 8-hour shift, the nurse manager told him that if he refused, she could "fire him" and report him for patient abandonment.

1. If you were Juan, how would you respond to the nurse manager?

2. What options does Juan have in this situation?

3. What information should Juan find out regarding "mandatory overtime"?

4. If Juan makes an error that results in harm to a patient, can he be held accountable?

References

Aiken, T.D. (2004). *Legal, Ethical and political issues in nursing,* 2nd ed. Philadelphia: F.A. Davis.

American Association of Neuroscience Nurses, (2012). Neuroscience nursing scope and standards of practice. Washington, DC: ANA.

American Nurses Association (ANA). (1992). Position statement on nursing care and do not resuscitate decisions. Washington, DC: ANA.

American Nurses Association (ANA). (1998). Legal aspects of standards and guidelines for clinical nursing practice. Washington, DC: ANA.

American Nurses Association (ANA). (2005). American Nurses Association Statement on the Terri Schiavo Case. Retrieved on October 2, 2012, from http://nursingworld.org/FunctionalMenuCategories/MediaResources/PressReleases/2005/pr03238523.aspx

American Nurses Association (ANA). (2010). Nursing: scope and standards of practice. Pub 03SSNP. Washington, DC: ANA.

American Nurses Association (ANA). (2011). Nurse staffing plans and ratios. Retrieved on September 28, 2012, from www.nursingworld.org/MainMenuCategories/Policy-Advocacy/State/Legislative-Agenda-Reports/State-StaffingPlansRatios

Bae, S.H., Brewer, C.S., & Kovner, C.T. (2011). State mandatory overtime regulations and newly licensed nurses' mandatory and voluntary overtime and total work hours. *Nursing Outlook* (doi:10.1016/j), pp. 1–12. Retrieved on October 2, 2012, from www.nursingoutlook.org

Balas, M., Scott, L., & Rogers, A. (2004). The prevalence and nature of errors and near errors reported by hospital staff nurses. *Applied Nursing Research, 17*(4), 224–230.

Beckman, J.P. (1995). *Nursing malpractice: Implications for clinical practice and nursing education.* Seattle: Washington University Press.

Berman, A.J., & Snyder, S. (2012). *Kozier and Erb's fundamentals of nursing: Concepts, process and practice* (9th ed.). Upper Saddle River, N.J.: Prentice-Hall.

Black, H.C. (2009). In Gardner, B.A. (ed.), *Black's Law dictionary* (9th ed.). St. Paul: West Publishing.

Blais, K.K., & Hayes, J.S. (2011). *Professional nursing practice: Concepts and perspectives* (6th ed.). Upper Saddle River, N.J.: Prentice-Hall.

Catalano, J.T. (2000). *Nursing now! Today's issue, tomorrow's trends,* 2nd ed. Philadelphia: F.A. Davis.

Charters, K.G (2003). HIPAA's latest privacy rule. *Policy, Politics & Nursing Practice, 4*(1), 75–78.

Donabedian, A. (1988). The quality of care: How can it be assessed? *Journal of the American Medical Association, 260*(12), 1743–1748.

Eisenhauer, L.A., Hurley, A.C., & Dolan, N. (2007). Nurses' reported thinking during medication administration. *Journal of Nursing Scholarship, 39*(1), 82–87.

Elliott, M., & Liu, Y. (2010). The nine rights of medication administration: An overview. *British Journal of Nursing, 19*(5), 300.

Ellis, J.R., & Hartley, C.L. (2004). *Nursing in today's world: trends, issues and management,* 8th ed. Philadelphia: Lippincott, Williams & Wilkins.

Flarey, D. (1991). Advanced directives: In search of self-determination. *Journal of Nursing Administration, 21*(11), 17.

Gic, J. (2009). Nursing and the Law. In Shafeek, S., *Legal medicine.* Philadelphia: Mosby Elsevier.

Giese v. Stice. 567 N.W. 2d 156 (Nebraska, 1997).

Glannon, J.W. (2005). *The law of torts: Examples and explanations* (3rd ed.). Frederick, MD: Aspen Publishers.

Guido, G.W. (2001). *Legal and ethical issues in nursing,* 3rd ed. Upper Saddle River, N.J.: Prentice-Hall.

Hickey, J. (2008). *Clinical practice of neurological and neurosurgical nursing,* 6th ed. Philadelphia: Lippincott, Williams and Wilkins.

Hill, G.N., & Hill, K.T. (2009). The people's law dictionary: Taking the mystery out of legal language. Retrieved on September 28, 2012, from http://dictionary.law.com/Default.aspx?searched=common%20law&type=1

Kozier, B., Erb, G., Blais, K., et al. (1995). *Fundamentals of nursing: Concepts, process and practice,* 15th ed. Menlo Park, Calif.: Addison-Wesley.

Loiacono, K. (2005). A good fight in the house over medical malpractice 'reform.' *Trial, 11.* Retrieved June 18, 2014, from http://www.thefreelibrary.com/A+good+fight+in+the+House+over+medical+malpractice+'reform'.-a0115404605

Marr, S. (2003). Protect your practice: Informed consent. *Plastic Surgical Nursing, 22*(4), pp. 180–197.

Mayo Clinic. Living wills and advance directives. Available from www.mayoclinic.com/health/living-wills/HA00014

National Council of State Boards of Nursing. (2012). *Fast facts about alternative item formats and the NCLEX examination.* Retrieved on October 2, 2012, from www.ncsbn.org

National Council of State Boards of Nursing. (2012). *Nursing regulation.* Retrieved on October 1, 2012, from www.ncsbn.org.

National Council of State Boards of Nursing. (2012). *2013 NCLEX-RN test plan.* Retrieved on October 2, 2012, from www.ncsbn.org.

National Council of State Boards of Nursing (2012). Nurse licensure compact. Retrieved on October 4, 2012, from https://www.ncsbn.org/nlc.htm.

Needleman, J., Buerhaus, P., Pankratz, S., Liebson, C.L., Stevens, S.R., and Harris, M. (2011). Nurse staffing and inpatient hospital mortality. *New England Journal of Medicine, 364*(11), 1037–1045.

New York state end-of-life laws (2012). Retrieved October 3, 2012, from www.nyc.gov/html/doh/html/hca/advance-directives.shtml

Reigle, J. (1992). Preserving patient self-determination through advance directives. *Heart Lung, 21*(2), 196–198.

Sanbar, S.S. (2007). *Legal medicine* (7th ed.). Philadelphia: Mosby Elsevier.

Taylor, C., Lillis, C., & LeMone, P. (2008). *Fundamentals of nursing: The art and science of nursing care.* Philadelphia: Lippincott, Williams & Wilkins.

Tovar v. Methodist Healthcare. (2005). S.W. 3d WL 3079074 (Texas App., 2005).

Wendland v. Sparks. (1998). 574 N.W. 2d 327 (Iowa, 1998).

Young v. Gastrolntestinal Center, Inc. (2005). S.W. 3d WL 675751 (Arkansas, 2005).

Questions of Values and Ethics

It is 1961. In a large metropolitan hospital, a group is meeting to consider the cases of three individuals. Ironically, the cases have something in common. Martin Curtin, age 76; Irina Kresnick, age 31; and Lucretia Singleton, age 5, are all suffering from chronic renal failure and need hemodialysis. Equipment is scarce, the cost of the treatment is prohibitive, and it is doubtful that treatment will be covered by health insurance. The hospital is able to provide this treatment to only one of these individuals. Who shall live, and who shall die? In a novel of the same name, Noah Gordon called this decision-making group The Death Committee (Gordon, 1963). Today, such groups are referred to as ethics committees.

In previous centuries, health-care practitioners had neither the knowledge nor the technology to prolong life. The main function of nurses and physicians was to support patients through times of illness, help them toward recovery, or keep them comfortable until death. There were few "who shall live, and who shall die?" decisions. Over the last 20 years, technological advances such as multiple organ transplantation, use of stem cells, and sophisticated life support systems created unique situations stimulating serious conversations and debates over the use of such techniques.

Health care saw its first technological advances during 1947 and 1948 as the polio epidemic raged through Europe and the United States. This devastating disease initiated the development of units for patients who required manual ventilation (the "iron lung"). During this period, Danish physicians invented a method of manual ventilation by using a tube placed in the trachea of polio patients. This was the beginning of mechanical ventilation as we know it today. The development of mechanical ventilation required more intensive nursing care and patient observation. The care and monitoring of patients proved to be more efficient when they were kept in a single care area; hence the term *intensive care.*

The late 1960s brought greater technological advances. Open heart surgery, in its infancy at the time, became available for patients seriously ill with cardiovascular disease. These patients required specialized nursing care and nurses specifically educated in the use of advancing technology. These new therapies and monitoring methods provided the impetus for the development of intensive care units and the emerging critical care nursing specialty (AACN.org, 2006).

In the past, a vast majority of individuals receiving critical care services would have died. However, the development of new drugs and advances in biomechanical technology permit physicians and nurses to challenge nature. These advances have enabled health-care professionals to provide patients with treatments that in many cases increase their life expectancy and enhance their quality of life. However, this progress is not without its drawbacks as it also brings new, perplexing questions.

The ability to prolong life has created some heartbreaking situations for families and complex ethical dilemmas for health-care professionals. Decisions regarding terminating life support on a teenager involved in a motor vehicle accident, instituting life support on a 65-year-old active productive father, or providing stem cell transplants to a terminally ill child are a few examples. At what point do new parents say good-bye to their neonate who was born far too early to survive outside of the womb? Families and professionals face some of the most difficult ethical decisions at times like this. How is death defined? When does it occur? Perhaps these questions need to be asked: What is life? Is there a difference between life and living?

To help find answers to some of these questions, health-care professionals have looked to philosophy, especially the branch that deals with human behavior. Over time, to assist in dealing with these issues, the field of biomedical ethics (or, simply, bioethics), a subdiscipline of ethics—the philosophical study of morality—has evolved. In essence, bioethics is the study of medical morality, which concerns the moral and social implications of health care and science in human life (DeGrazia, Mappes, & Brand-Ballard, 2010).

In order to understand biomedical ethics, it is important to appreciate the basic concepts of values, belief systems, ethical theories, and morality. The following sections will define these concepts and then discuss ways nurses can help the interprofessional team and families resolve ethical dilemmas.

Values

Individuals talk about *value* and *values* all the time. The term *value* refers to the worth of an object or thing. However, the term *values* refers to how individuals feel about ideas, situations, concepts. *Merriam-Webster's Collegiate Dictionary* defines *value* as the "estimated or appraised worth of something, or that quality of a thing that makes it more or less desirable, useful" (http://www.merriam-webster.com/dictionary/value). Values, then, are judgments about the importance or unimportance of objects, ideas, attitudes, and attributes. Values become a part of a person's conscience and worldview. They provide a frame of reference and act as pilots to guide behaviors and assist people in making choices.

Morals

Morals arise from an individual's conscience. They act as a guide for individual behavior and are learned through family systems, instruction, and socialization. Morals find their basis within individual values. Morals have a larger social component than values and focus more on good versus bad behaviors (Kirschenbaum, 2000). For example, if you value fairness and integrity, then your morals include those values and you judge others based on your concept of morality.

Values and Moral Reasoning

Reasoning is the process of making inferences from a body of information and entails forming conclusions, making judgments, or making inferences from knowledge for the purpose of answering questions, solving problems, and formulating a plan that determines actions (Butts & Rich, 2012). Reasoning allows individuals to think for themselves and not to take the beliefs and judgments of others at face value. Moral reasoning relates to the process of forming conclusions and creating action plans centered around moral and/or ethical issues.

Values, viewpoints, and methods of moral reasoning have developed over time. Older worldviews have now emerged in modern history, such as the emphasis on virtue ethics or a focus on what type of person one would like to become (Butts & Rich, 2012). Virtue ethics are discussed later in this chapter.

Value Systems

A value system is a set of related values. For example, one person may value (believe to be important) societal aspects of life, such as money, objects, and status. Another person may value more abstract concepts, such as kindness, charity, and caring. Values may vary significantly, based on an individual's culture, family teachings, and religious upbringing. An individual's system of values frequently affects how he or she makes decisions. For example, one person may base a decision on cost, and another person placed in the same situation may base the decision on a more abstract quality, such as kindness. There are different categories of values:

■ *Intrinsic values* are those related to sustaining life, such as food and water (Zimmerman, 2010).
■ *Extrinsic values* are not essential to life. They include the value of objects, both physical and abstract. Extrinsic values are not an end in themselves but offer a means of achieving something else. Things, people, and material items are extrinsically valuable (Zimmerman, 2010).
■ *Personal values* are qualities that people consider important in their private lives. Concepts such as strong family ties and acceptance by others are personal values.
■ *Professional values* are qualities considered important by a professional group. Autonomy, integrity, and commitment are examples of professional values.

People's behaviors are motivated by values. Individuals take risks, relinquish their own comfort and security, and generate extraordinary efforts because of their values (Edge & Groves, 2005). Patients with traumatic brain injury may overcome tremendous barriers because they value independence. Race-car drivers may risk death or other serious injury because they value competition and winning.

Values also generate the standards by which people judge others. For example, someone who values work over leisure activities will look unfavorably on the coworker who refuses to work throughout the weekend. A person who believes that health is more important than wealth would approve of spending money on a relaxing vacation or perhaps joining a health club rather than putting the money in the bank.

Often people adopt the values of individuals they admire. For example, a nursing student may begin to value humor after observing it used effectively with patients. Values provide a guide for decision making and give additional meaning to life. Individuals develop a sense of satisfaction when they work toward achieving values that they believe are important.

How Values Are Developed

Values are learned (Csongradi, 2012). Ethicists attribute the basic question of whether values are taught, inherited, or passed on by some other mechanism to Plato, who lived more than 2,000 years ago. A recent theory suggests that values and moral knowledge are acquired much in the same manner as other forms of knowledge, through real-world experience.

Values can be taught directly, incorporated through societal norms, and modeled through behavior. Children learn by watching their parents, friends, teachers, and religious leaders. Through continuous reinforcement, children eventually learn about and then adopt values as their own. Because of the values they hold dear, people often make great demands on themselves and others, ignoring the personal cost. For example:

Lora grew up in a family in which educational achievement was highly valued. Not surprisingly, she adopted this as one of her own values. Lora became a physician, married, and had a son named Davis. She placed a great deal of effort on teaching her son educational skills in order to get him into "the best private school" in the area. As he moved through the program, his grades did not reflect his mother's great effort, and he felt as though he had disappointed his mother as well as himself. By the time David reached the age of nine, he had developed many somatic complaints such as stomachaches and headaches.

Values change with experience and maturity. For example, young children often value objects, such as a favorite blanket or stuffed animal. Older children are more likely to value a particular event, such as a family trip. As they enter adolescence, they may value peer opinion over the opinions of their parents. Young adults often value certain ideals, such as beauty and heroism. The values of adults are formed from all of these experiences as well as from learning and thought.

The number of values that people hold is not as important as what values they consider important. Choices are influenced by values. The way people use their own time and money, choose friends, and pursue a career are all influenced by values.

Values Clarification

Values clarification is deciding what one believes is important. It is the process that helps people become aware of their values. Values play an important role in everyday decision making. For this reason, nurses need to be aware of what they do and do not value. This process helps them to behave in a manner that is consistent with their values.

Both personal and professional values influence nurses' decisions. Understanding one's own values simplifies solving problems, making decisions, and developing better relationships with others when one begins to realize how others develop their values. Kirschenbaum (2000) suggested using a three-step model of choosing, prizing, and acting, with seven substeps, to identify one's own values (Box 4-1).

You may have used this method when making the decision to go to nursing school. For some people, nursing is a first career; for others, it is a second career. Using the model in Box 4-1, the valuing process is analyzed:

1. **Choosing.** After researching alternative career options, you freely chose nursing school. This choice was most likely influenced by such factors as educational achievement and abilities, finances, support and encouragement from others, time, and feelings about people.
2. **Prizing.** Once the choice was made, you were satisfied with it and told your friends about it.

box 4-1
Values Clarification

Choosing
1. Choosing freely
2. Choosing from alternatives
3. Deciding after giving consideration to the consequences of each alternative

Prizing
4. Being satisfied about the choice
5. Being willing to declare the choice to others

Acting
6. Making the choice a part of one's worldview and incorporating it into behavior
7. Repeating the choice

Adapted from Raths, L.E., Harmon, M., & Simmons, S.B. (1979). Values and teaching. New York: Charles E. Merrill.

3. **Acting.** You have entered school and begun the journey to your new career. Later in your career, you may decide to return to school for a bachelor's or master's degree in nursing.

As you progressed through school, you probably started to develop a new set of values—your professional values. Professional values are those established as being important in your practice. These values include caring, quality of care, and ethical behaviors.

Belief Systems

Belief systems are an organized way of thinking about why people exist in the universe. The purpose of belief systems is to explain such issues as life and death, good and evil, and health and illness. Usually these systems include an ethical code that specifies appropriate behavior. People may have a personal belief system, participate in a religion that provides such a system, or follow a combination of the two.

Members of primitive societies worshipped events in nature. Unable to understand the science of weather, for example, early civilizations believed these events to be under the control of someone or something that needed to be appeased, and they developed rituals and ceremonies to appease these unknown entities. They called these entities gods and believed that certain behaviors either pleased or angered the gods. Because these societies associated certain behaviors with specific outcomes, they created a belief system that enabled them to function as a group.

As higher civilizations evolved, belief systems became more complex. Archeology has provided evidence of the religious practices of ancient civilizations that support the evolution of belief systems (Wack, 1992). The Aztec, Mayan, Incan, and Polynesian cultures each had a religious belief system composed of many gods and goddesses for the same functions. The Greek, Roman, Egyptian, and Scandinavian societies believed in a hierarchy of gods and goddesses. Although given different names by different cultures, it is very interesting that most of the deities had similar purposes. For example, the Greeks looked to Zeus as the king of the gods, and Thor represented the king of the Norse gods. Both used a thunderbolt as their symbol. Sociologists believe that these religions developed to explain what was then unexplainable. Human beings have a deep need to create order from chaos and to have logical explanations for events. Religion offers theological explanations to answer questions which cannot be explained by "pure" science.

Along with the creation of rites and rituals, religions also developed codes of behaviors, or ethical codes. These codes contribute to the social order and provide rules regarding how to treat family members, neighbors, the young, and the old. Many religions also developed rules regarding marriage, sexual practices, business practices, property ownership, and inheritance.

For some individuals, the advancement of science has minimized the need for belief systems, as science can now provide explanations for many previously unexplainable phenomena. In fact, the technology explosion has created an even greater need for these belief systems. Technological advances often place people in situations where they may welcome rather than oppose religious convictions to guide difficult decisions. Many religions, particularly Christianity, focus on the will of a supreme being, and technology, for example, is considered a gift that allows health-care personnel to maintain the life of a loved one. Other religions, such as certain branches of Judaism, focus on free choice or free will, leaving such decisions in the hands of humankind. For example, many Jewish leaders believe that if genetic testing indicates that an infant will be born with a disease such as Tay-Sachs that causes severe suffering and ultimately death, terminating the pregnancy may be an acceptable option.

Belief systems often help survivors in making decisions and living with them afterward. So far, technological advances have created more questions than answers. As science explains more and more previously unexplainable phenomena, people need beliefs and values to guide their use of this new knowledge.

Ethics and Morals

Although the terms *morals* and *ethics* are often used interchangeably, *ethics* usually refers to a standardized code as a guide to behaviors, whereas *morals* usually refers to an individual's own code for acceptable behavior.

Ethics

Ethics is the part of philosophy that deals with the rightness or wrongness of human behavior. It is also concerned with the motives behind behaviors. *Bioethics,* specifically, is the application of ethics to issues that pertain to life and death. The implication is that judgments can be made about the rightness or goodness of health-care practices.

Ethical Theories

Several ethical theories have emerged to justify moral principles (Guido, 2001). *Deontological theories* take their norms and rules from the duties that individuals owe each other by the goodness of the commitments they make and the roles they take upon themselves. The term *deontological* comes from the Greek word *deon* (duty). This theory is attributed to the 18th-century philosopher Immanuel Kant (Kant, 1949). Deontological ethics considers the intention of the action, not the consequences of the action. In other words, it is the individual's good intentions or goodwill (Kant, 1949) that determines the worthiness or goodness of the action.

Teleological theories take their norms or rules for behaviors from the consequences of the action. This theory is also called *utilitarianism*. According to this concept, what makes an action right or wrong is its utility, or usefulness. Usefulness is considered to be the amount of happiness the action carries. "Right" encompasses actions that have good outcomes, whereas "wrong" is composed of actions that result in bad outcomes. This theory had its origins with David Hume, a Scottish philosopher. According to Hume, "Reason is and ought to be the slave of the passions" (Hume, 1978, p. 212). Based on this idea, ethics depends on what people want and desire. The passions determine what is right or wrong. However, individuals who follow teleological theory disagree on how to decide on the "rightness" or "wrongness" of an action (Guido, 2001) because individual passions differ.

Principalism is an arising theory receiving a great deal of attention in the biomedical ethics community. This theory integrates existing ethical principles and tries to resolve conflicts by relating one or more of these principles to a given situation. Ethical principles actually influence professional decision making more than ethical theories.

Ethical Principles

Ethical codes are based on principles that can be used to judge behavior. Ethical principles assist decision making because they are a standard for measuring actions. They may be the basis for laws, but they themselves are not laws. Laws are rules created by a governing body. Laws can operate because the government has the power to enforce them. They are usually quite specific, as are the punishments for disobeying them. Ethical principles are not confined to specific behaviors. They act as guides for appropriate behaviors. They also take into account the situation in which a decision must be made. Ethical principles speak to the essence or fundamentals of the law rather than to the exactness of the law (Macklin, 1987). Here is an example:

Mrs. Van Gruen, 82 years old, was admitted to the hospital in acute respiratory distress. She was diagnosed with aspiration pneumonia and soon became septic, developing acute respiratory distress syndrome. She had a living will, and her attorney was her designated health-care surrogate. Her competence to make decisions was uncertain because of her illness. The physician presented the situation to the attorney, indicating that without a feeding tube and tracheostomy, Mrs. Van Gruen would die. According to the laws governing living wills and health-care surrogates, the attorney could have made the decision to withhold all treatments. However, he believed he had an ethical obligation to discuss the situation with his client. The client requested that the tracheostomy and the feeding tube be inserted, which was done.

Following are several of the ethical principles that are most important to nursing practice: autonomy, nonmaleficence, beneficence, justice, fidelity, confidentiality, veracity, and accountability. In some situations, two or more principles may conflict with each other, leading to an ethical dilemma. Making a decision under these circumstances is very difficult.

Autonomy

Autonomy is the freedom to make decisions for oneself. This ethical principle requires that nurses respect patients' rights to make their own choices about treatment. Informed consent before treatment, surgery, or participation in research is an example. To be able to make an autonomous choice, individuals need to be informed of the purpose, benefits, and risks of the procedures to which they are agreeing. Nurses accomplish this by providing information and supporting patients' choices.

Closely linked to the ethical principle of autonomy is the legal issue of competence. A patient needs to be deemed competent in order to make a decision regarding treatment options. When patients refuse treatment, health-care personnel and family members who think differently often question the patient's "competence" to make a decision. Of note is the fact that when patients agree with health-care treatment decisions, rarely is their competence questioned (AACN News, 2006).

Nurses are often in a position to protect a patient's autonomy. They do this by ensuring that others do not interfere with the patient's right to proceed with a decision. If a nurse observes that a patient has insufficient information to make an appropriate choice, is being forced into a decision, or is unable to understand the consequences of the choice, then the nurse may act as a patient advocate to ensure the principle of autonomy.

Sometimes nurses have difficulty with the principle of autonomy because it also requires respecting another's choice, even if the nurse disagrees with it. According to the principle of autonomy, a nurse cannot replace a patient's decision with his or her own, even when the nurse honestly believes that the patient has made the wrong choice. A nurse can, however, discuss concerns with patients and make sure patients have thought about the consequences of the decision they are about to make.

Nonmaleficence

The ethical principle of nonmaleficence requires that no harm be done, either deliberately or unintentionally. This rather complicated word comes from Latin roots: *non,* which means not; *male* (pronounced mah-leh), which means bad; and *facere,* which means to do.

The principle of nonmaleficence also requires that nurses protect from danger individuals who are unable to protect themselves because of their physical or mental condition. An infant, a person under anesthesia, and a person with Alzheimer's disease are examples of people with limited ability to protect themselves. Nurses are ethically obligated to protect their patients when the patients are unable to protect themselves.

Often, treatments meant to improve patient health lead to harm. This is not the intention of the nurse or of other health-care personnel, but it is a direct result of treatment. Nosocomial infections as a result of hospitalization are harmful to patients. The nurses did not deliberately cause the infection. The side effects of chemotherapy or radiation therapy may result in harm. Chemotherapeutic agents cause a decrease in immunity that may result in a severe infection, whereas radiation may burn or damage the skin. For this reason, many patients opt not to pursue treatments.

The obligation to do no harm extends to the nurse who for some reason is not functioning at an optimal level. For example, a nurse who is impaired by alcohol or drugs is knowingly placing patients at risk. Other nurses who observe such behavior have an ethical obligation to protect patients according to the principle of nonmaleficence.

Beneficence

The word *beneficence* also comes from Latin: *bene,* which means well, and *facere,* which means to do.

The principle of beneficence demands that good be done for the benefit of others. For nurses, this means more than delivering competent physical or technical care. It requires helping patients meet all their needs, whether physical, social, or emotional. Beneficence is caring in the truest sense, and caring fuses thought, feeling, and action. It requires knowing and being truly understanding of the situation and the thoughts and ideas of the individual (Benner & Wrubel, 1989).

Sometimes physicians, nurses, and families withhold information from patients for the sake of beneficence. The problem with doing this is that it does not allow competent individuals to make their own decisions based on all available information. In an attempt to be beneficent, the principle of autonomy is violated. This is just one of many examples of the ethical dilemmas encountered in nursing practice. For instance:

Mrs. Liu has just been admitted to the oncology unit with ovarian cancer. She is scheduled to begin chemotherapy treatment. Her two children and her husband have requested that the physician ensure that Mrs. Liu not be told her diagnosis because they believe she would not be able to cope with it. The information is communicated to the nursing staff. After the first treatment, Mrs. Liu becomes very ill. She refuses the next treatment, stating that she did not feel sick until she came to the hospital. She asks the nurse what could possibly be wrong with her that she needs a medicine that makes her sick when she does not feel sick. Only people who get cancer medicine get this sick! Mrs. Liu then asks the nurse, "Do I have cancer?"

As the nurse, you understand the order that the patient not be told her diagnosis. You also understand your role as a patient advocate.

1. To whom do you owe your duty: the family or the patient?
2. How do you think you may be able to be a patient advocate in this situation?
3. What information would you communicate to the family members, and how can you assist them in dealing with their mother's concerns?

Justice

The principle of justice obliges nurses and other health-care professionals to treat every person equally regardless of gender, sexual orientation, religion, ethnicity, disease, or social standing (Edge & Groves, 2005). This principle also applies in the work and educational setting. Everyone should be treated and judged by the same criteria according to this principle. Here is an example:

Mr. Johnson, found on the street by the police, was admitted through the emergency room to a medical unit. He was in deplorable condition: his clothes were dirty and ragged, he was unshaven, and he was covered with blood. His diagnosis was chronic alcoholism, complicated by esophageal varices and end-stage liver disease. Several nursing students overheard the staff discussing Mr. Johnson. The essence of the conversation was that no one wanted to care for him because he was dirty and smelly and brought this condition on himself. The students, upset by what they heard, went to their instructor about the situation. The instructor explained that every individual has a right to good care despite his or her economic or social position. This is the principle of justice.

The concept of *distributive justice* necessitates the fair allocation of responsibilities and advantages, especially in a society where resources may be limited. Considered as an ethical principle, distributive justice refers to what society or a larger group feels indebted to its individual members regarding: (1) individual needs, contribution, and responsibility; (2) the resources available to the society or organization; and (3) the society's or organization's responsibility to the common good (www .ascensionhealth.org/; Davis, Arokar, Liaschenko, & Drought, 1997). Health-care costs have increased tremendously over the years, and access to care has become a social and political issue. In order to understand distributive justice, certain concepts need to be addressed: need, individual effort, ability to pay, contribution to society, and age.

Age has become an extremely controversial issue as it leads to quality-of-life questions, particularly technological care at the end of life (Ensign, 2012). The other issue regarding age revolves around technology in neonatal care. How do health-care providers place value on one person's quality of life over that of another? Should millions of dollars be spent preserving the life of an 80-year-old man who volunteers in his community, plays golf twice a week, and teaches reading to underprivileged children, or should that money be spent on a 26-week-old fetus that will most likely require intensive therapies and treatments for a lifetime, adding up to more millions of health-care dollars? In the social and business world, welfare payments are based on need, and jobs and promotions are usually distributed on the basis of an individual's contributions and achievements. Is it possible to apply these measures to health-care allocations?

Philosopher John Rawls addressed the issues of justice as fairness and justice as the foundation of social structures (Nussbaum, 2002). According to Rawls, the idea of the original position should be used to negotiate the principles of justice. The original position based on Kant's social contract theory presents a hypothetical situation in which individuals act as a trustee for the interests of all individuals. The individuals, known as negotiators, are knowledgeable in the areas of sociology, political science, and economics. However, they are placed under certain limitations referred to as the *veil of ignorance*. These limitations represent the moral essentials of original position arguments.

The veil of ignorance eliminates information about age, gender, socioeconomic status, and religious convictions from the issues. Once this information is unavailable to the negotiators, the vested interests of involved parties disappear. According to Rawls, in a just society the rights protected by justice are not issues for political bargaining or subject to the calculations of social interests. Simply put, everyone has the same rights and liberties.

Fidelity

The principle of fidelity requires loyalty. It is a promise that the individual will fulfill all commitments made to himself or herself and to others. For nurses, fidelity includes the professional's loyalty to fulfill all responsibilities and agreements expected as part of professional practice. Fidelity is the basis for the concept of accountability—taking responsibility for one's own actions (Shirey, 2005).

Confidentiality

The principle of confidentiality states that anything said to nurses and other health-care providers by their patients must be held in the strictest confidence. Confidentiality presents both a legal and an ethical issue. Exceptions exist only when patients give permission for the release of information or when the law requires the release of specific information. Sometimes, just sharing information without revealing an individual's name can be a breach in confidentiality if the situation and the individual are identifiable. It is important to realize that what seems like a harmless statement can become harmful if other people can piece together bits of information and identify the patient.

Nurses come into contact with people from different walks of life. Within communities, people know other people who know other people, and so on. Individuals have lost families, jobs, and insurance coverage because nurses shared confidential information and others acted on that knowledge (AIDS Update Conference, 1995).

In today's electronic environment, the principle of confidentiality has become a major concern. Many health-care institutions, insurance companies, and businesses use electronic media to transfer information. These institutions store sensitive and confidential information in computer databases. These databases need to have security safeguards to prevent unauthorized access. Health-care institutions have addressed the situation through the use of limited access, authorization passwords, and security tracking systems. However, even the most secure system is vulnerable and can be accessed by an individual who understands the complexities of computer systems.

Veracity

Veracity requires nurses to be truthful. Truth is fundamental to building a trusting relationship. Intentionally deceiving or misleading a patient is a violation of this principle. Deliberately omitting a part of the truth is deception and violates the principle of veracity. This principle often creates ethical dilemmas. When is it permissible to lie? Some ethicists believe it is never appropriate to deceive another individual. Others think that if another ethical principle overrides veracity, then lying is permissible. Consider this situation:

Ms. Allen has just been told that her father has Alzheimer's disease. The nurse practitioner wants to come into the home to discuss treatment. Ms. Allen refuses, saying that the nurse practitioner should under no circumstances tell her father the diagnosis. She explains to the practitioner that she is sure he will kill himself if he learns that he has Alzheimer's disease. She bases this concern on statements he has made regarding this disease. The nurse practitioner replies that medication is available that might help her father. However, it is available only through a research study being conducted at a nearby university. To participate in the research, the patient must be informed of the purpose of the study, the medication to be given and its side effects, and follow-up procedures. Ms. Allen continues to refuse to allow her father to be told his diagnosis because she is certain he will commit suicide.

The nurse practitioner faces a dilemma: does he abide by Ms. Allen's wishes based on the principle of beneficence, or does he abide by the principle of veracity and inform his patient of the diagnosis. What would you do?

Accountability

Accountability is linked to fidelity and means accepting responsibility for one's actions. Nurses are accountable to their patients and to their colleagues. When providing care to patients, nurses are responsible for their actions, good and poor. If something was not done, do not chart or tell a colleague that it was. An example of violating accountability is the story of Anna:

Anna was a registered nurse who worked nights on an acute care unit. She was an excellent nurse, but as the acuity of the patients' conditions increased, she was unable to keep up with both patients' needs and the technology, particularly intravenous (IV) lines. She began to chart that all the IVs were infusing as they should, even when they were not. Each morning, the day shift would find that the actual infused amount did not agree with what the paperwork showed. One night, Anna allowed an entire liter to be infused in 2 hours into a patient who had congestive heart failure. When the day staff came on duty, they found the patient expired, the bag empty, and the tubing filled with blood. Anna's IV sheet showed 800 mL left in the bag. It was not until a lawsuit was filed that Anna took responsibility for her behavior.

The idea of a standard of care evolves from the principle of accountability. Standards of care provide a rule for measuring nursing actions. This action also involves safety issues. According to the Institute of Medicine, organizations also have accountability for patient care and the actions of personnel. The organization has a duty to ensure a safe environment and that the personnel receive appropriate training and education (Jerak-Zuident, 2012).

Ethical Codes

A code of ethics is a formal statement of the rules of ethical behavior for a particular group of individuals. A code of ethics is one of the hallmarks of a profession. This code makes clear the behavior expected of its members.

The Code of Ethics for Nurses with Interpretive Statements provides values, standards, and principles to help nursing function as a profession. The original code was developed in 1985. In 1995 the American Nurses Association Board of Directors and the Congress on Nursing Practice initiated the Code of Ethics Project (ANA, 2002). The code may be viewed online at www.nursingworld.org.

Ethical codes are subject to change. They reflect the values of the profession and the society for which they were developed. Changes occur as society and technology evolve. For example, years ago no thought was given to do not resuscitate (DNR) orders or withholding food and fluids. Technological advances have since made it possible to keep people in a kind of twilight life, comatose and unable to participate in living in any way, but nevertheless making DNR and withholding very important issues in health care. Technology has increased knowledge and skills, but the ability to make decisions regarding care is still guided by the principles of autonomy, nonmaleficence, beneficence, justice, confidentiality, fidelity, veracity, and accountability.

Virtue Ethics

Virtue ethics focuses on virtues, or moral character, rather than on duties or rules that emphasize the consequences of actions. Consider the following example:

Norman is driving along the road and finds a crying child sitting by a fallen bicycle. It is obvious that the child needs assistance. From one ethical standpoint (utilitarianism), helping the child will increase Norman's personal feelings of "doing good." The deontological stance states that by helping, Norman is behaving in accordance with a moral rule such as "Do unto others . . . ." Virtue ethics looks at the fact that helping the person would be charitable or benevolent.

Plato and Aristotle are considered the founders of virtue ethics. Its roots can be found in Chinese philosophy. During the 1800s, virtue ethics disappeared, but in the late 1950s it reemerged as an Anglo-American philosophy. Neither deontology nor utilitarianism considered the virtues of moral character and education and the question: "What type of person should I be, and how should I live" (Hooker, 2000; Driver, 2001). Virtues include such qualities as honesty, generosity, altruism, and reliability. They are concerned with many other elements as well, such as emotions and emotional reactions, choices, values, needs, insights, attitudes, interests, and expectations. To embrace a virtue means that you are a person with a certain complex way of thinking. Nursing has practiced virtue ethics for many years.

Nursing Ethics

Up to this point, the ethical principles discussed apply to ethics for nurses; however, nurses do not customarily find themselves enmeshed in the biomedical ethical decision-making processes that gain the attention of the news media. However, the ethical principles that guide nursing practice are rooted in the philosophy and science of health care and are considered a subcategory of bioethics (Butts & Rich, 2012).

Nursing ethics deals with the experiences and needs of nurses and nurses' perceptions of their experiences (Varcoe et al., 2007). It is viewed from the perspective of nursing theory and practice (Johnstone, 1999). Relationships are the center of nursing ethics. These relationships focus on ethical issues that impact nurses and their patients.

Organizational Ethics

Organizational ethics focus on the workplace and are aimed at the organizational level. Every organization, even one with hundreds of thousands of employees, consists of individuals. Each individual makes his and her own decisions about how to behave in the workplace. Each person has the opportunity to make the organization a more or less ethical place. These individual decisions can have a powerful effect on the lives of many others in the organization as well as in the surrounding community. Shirey (2005) explains that employees need to experience uniformity between what the organization states and what it practices.

Research conducted by the Ethics Research Center concluded the following:

■ If positive outcomes are desired, ethical culture is what makes the difference;
■ Leadership, especially senior leadership, is the most critical factor in promoting an ethical culture; and
■ In organizations that are trying to strengthen their culture, formal program elements can help to do that (Harned, 2005, p. 1).

When looking for a professional position, it is important to consider the organizational culture. What are the values and beliefs of the organization? Do they blend with yours, or are they in conflict with your value system? To find out this information, look at the organization's mission, vision, and value statements. Speak with other nurses who work in the organization. Do they see consistency between what the organization states and what it actually expects from the employees? For example, if an organization states that it collaborates with the nurses in decision making, do nurses sit on committees that have input into the decision-making process? Conflicts between a nurse's professional values and those of the organization result in moral distress for the nurse.

Ethical Issues on the Nursing Unit

Organizational ethics refer to the values and expected behaviors entrenched within the organizational culture. The nursing unit represents a sub-culture of the organization. Ideally, the nursing unit should mirror the ethical atmosphere and culture of the organization. This requires the individuals that comprise the unit to hold the same values and model the expected behaviors.

Conflicts of the values and ethics among individuals who work together on the unit often create issues that result in moral suffering for some nurses. Moral suffering occurs when nurses experience a feeling of uneasiness or concern regarding behaviors or circumstances that challenge their own moral beliefs and values. These situations may be the result of unit policies, physicians' orders that the nurse believes may not be beneficial for the patient, professional behaviors of colleagues, or family attitudes about the patient.

Perhaps one of the most disconcerting ethical issues nurses on the unit face is the one that challenges their professional values and ethics. Friendships often emerge from work relationships, and these friendships may interfere with judgments. Similarly, strong negative feelings may cloud a nurse's ability to view a situation fairly and without prejudice. Take the following example:

Addie and Jamie attended nursing school together and developed a strong friendship. They work together on the pediatric surgical unit of a large teaching hospital. Jamie made a medication error that caused a problem, resulting in a child having to be transferred to the intensive care unit. Addie realized what had happened and confronted Jamie. Jamie begged her not to say anything. Addie knew the error should be reported, but how would this affect her longtime friendship with Jamie? Taking this situation to the other extreme, if a friendship had not been involved, would Addie react the same way?

When working with others, it is important to hold true to your personal values and morals. Practicing virtue ethics, that is, "doing the right thing," may cause difficulty due to the possible consequences of the action. Nurses should support each other but not at the expense of patients or each other's professional duties. There are times when not acting virtuously may cause a colleague more harm.

Moral Distress in Nursing Practice

Moral distress occurs when nurses know the action they need to take, but for some reason are unable to act. Therefore, the action or actions they take cause conflict as the decision goes against their personal and professional values, morals, and beliefs. This challenges nurses' integrity and authenticity.

Moral distress presents a serious problem in nursing practice and adds to nurses feeling a loss of integrity and dissatisfaction within the work setting. It threatens the quality of care and may adversely affect costs.

Moral distress occurs when nurses know the action they need to take, but for some reason are unable to act. Therefore, the action or actions they take cause conflict as the decision goes against their personal and professional values, morals, and beliefs. This challenges nurses' integrity and authenticity.

Studies have shown that nurses exposed to moral distress suffer from emotional and physical problems and eventually leave the bedside and the profession (Redman & Fry, 2000). Sources of moral distress vary; however, contributing factors include end-of-life challenges, nurse-physician conflict, disrespectful interactions, and workplace violence. Nursing organizations such as the Association for Critical Care Nurses (AACN) have developed guidelines addressing the issue of moral distress.

Ethical Dilemmas

What is a dilemma? The word *dilemma* is of Greek derivation. A lemma was an animal resembling a ram and having two horns. Thus came the saying "stuck on the horns of a dilemma." The story of

Hugo illustrates a hypothetical dilemma, with a touch of humor:

One day, Hugo, dressed in a bright red cape, walked through his village into the countryside. The wind caught the corners of the cape, and it was whipped in all directions. As he walked down the dusty road, Hugo happened to pass by a lemma. Hugo's bright red cape caught the lemma's attention. Lowering its head, with its two horns poised in attack position, the animal began to chase Hugo down the road. Panting and exhausted, Hugo reached the end of the road, only to find himself blocked by a huge stone wall. He turned to face the lemma, which was ready to charge. A decision needed to be made, and Hugo's life depended on this decision. If he moved to the left, the lemma would gore his heart. If he moved to the right, the lemma would gore his liver. No matter what his decision, Hugo would be "stuck on the horns of the lemma."

Like Hugo, nurses are often faced with difficult dilemmas. Also, as Hugo found, an ethical dilemma can be a choice between two serious alternatives.

An ethical dilemma occurs when a problem exists that forces a choice between two or more ethical principles. Deciding in favor of one principle will violate the other. Both sides have goodness and badness to them, but neither decision satisfies all the criteria that apply. Ethical dilemmas also have the added burden of emotions. Feelings of anger, frustration, and fear often override rationality in the decision-making process. Consider the case of Mr. Sussman:

Mr. Sussman, 80 years old, was admitted to the neuroscience unit after suffering a left hemispheric bleed. He had a total right hemiplegia and was completely nonresponsive, with a Glasgow Coma Scale score of 8. He had been on IV fluids for 4 days, and the question was raised of placing a jejunostomy tube for enteral feedings. The older of his two children asked what were the chances of his recovery. The physician explained that Mr. Sussman's current state was probably the best he could attain but that "miracles happen every day" and stated that tests could help in determining the prognosis. The family asked that these tests be performed. After the results were available, the physician explained that the prognosis was grave and that IV fluids were insufficient to sustain life. The jejunostomy

tube would be a necessity if the family wished to continue with food and fluids. After the physician left, the family asked the nurse, Gail, who had been with Mr. Sussman during the previous 3 days, "If this was your father, what would you do?" This situation became an ethical dilemma for Gail as well.

If you were Gail, what would you say to the family? Depending on your answer, what would be the principles that you might violate?

Resolving Ethical Dilemmas Faced by Nurses

Ethical dilemmas can occur in any aspect of life, personal or professional. This section focuses on the resolution of professional dilemmas. The various models for resolving ethical dilemmas consist of 5 to 14 sequential steps. Each step begins with the complete understanding of the dilemma and concludes with the evaluation of the implemented decision.

The nursing process provides a helpful mechanism for finding solutions to ethical dilemmas. The first step is assessment, including identification of the problem. The simplest way to do this is to create a statement that summarizes the issue. The remainder of the process evolves from this statement (Box 4-2).

Assessment

Ask yourself, "Am I directly involved in this dilemma?" An issue is not an ethical dilemma for nurses unless they are directly involved in or have been asked for their opinion about a situation. Some nurses involve themselves in situations even when their opinion has not been solicited. This is generally unwarranted, unless the issue involves a violation of the professional code of ethics.

Nurses are frequently in the position of hearing both sides of an ethical dilemma. Often, all that is wanted is an empathetic listener. At other times,

---

box 4-2

Questions to Help Resolve Ethical Dilemmas

- What are the medical facts?
- What are the psychosocial facts?
- What are the patient's wishes?
- What values are in conflict?

when guidance is requested, nurses can help people work through the decision-making process (remember the principle of autonomy).

Collecting data from all the decision makers helps identify the reasoning process being used by these individuals as they struggle with the issue. The following questions assist in the information-gathering process:

- *What are the medical facts?* Find out how the physicians, physical and occupational therapists, dietitians, and nurses view the patient's condition and treatment options. Speak with the patient, if possible, and determine his or her understanding of the situation.
- *What are the psychosocial facts?* In what emotional state is the patient right now? The patient's family? What kind of relationship exists between the patient and his or her family? What are the patient's living conditions? Who are the individuals who form the patient's support system? How are they involved in the patient's care? What is the patient's ability to make medical decisions about his or her care? Do financial considerations need to be taken into account? What does the patient value? What does the patient's family value? The answers to these questions will provide a better understanding of the situation. Ask more questions, if necessary, to complete the picture. The social facts of a situation also include institutional policies, legal aspects, and economic factors. The personal belief systems of physicians and other health-care professionals also influence this aspect.
- *What are the cultural beliefs?* Cultural beliefs play a major role in ethical decisions. Some cultures do not allow surgical interventions as they fear that the "life force" may escape. Many cultures forbid organ donation. Other cultures focus on the sanctity of life, thereby requesting all methods for sustaining life be used regardless of the futility.
- *What are the patient's wishes?* Remember the ethical principle of autonomy. With very few exceptions, if the patient is competent, his or her decisions take precedence. Too often, the family's or physician's worldview and belief system overshadow those of the patient. Nurses can assist by maintaining the focus on the patient. If the patient is unable to communicate, try to discover whether the individual has discussed the issue in the past. If the patient has completed a living will or designated a health-care surrogate, this will help determine the patient's wishes. By interviewing family members, the nurse can often learn about conversations in which the patient has voiced his or her feelings about treatment decisions. Through guided interviewing, the nurse can encourage the family to tell anecdotes that provide relevant insights into the patient's values and beliefs.
- *What values are in conflict?* To assess values, begin by listing each person involved in the situation. Then identify the values represented by each person. Ask such questions as, "What do you feel is the most pressing issue here?" and "Tell me more about your feelings regarding this situation." In some cases, there may be little disagreement among the people involved, just a different way of expressing beliefs. In others, however, a serious value conflict may exist.

Planning

For planning to be successful, everyone involved in the decision must be included in the process. Thompson and Thompson (1992) listed three specific and integrated phases of this planning:

1. *Determine the goals of treatment.* Is cure a goal, or is the goal to keep the patient comfortable? Is life at any cost the goal, or is the goal a peaceful death at home? These goals need to be patient-focused, reality-centered, and attainable. They should be consistent with current medical treatment and, if possible, be measurable according to an established period.
2. *Identify the decision makers.* As mentioned earlier, nurses may or may not be decision makers in these health-related ethical dilemmas. It is important to know who the decision makers are and what their belief systems are. When the patient is a capable participant, this task is much easier. However, people who are ill are often too exhausted to speak for themselves or to ensure that their voices are heard. When this happens, the patient needs an advocate. Family, friends, spiritual advisers, and nurses often act as

advocates. A family member may need to be designated as the primary decision maker or *health-care surrogate.*

The creation of living wills, establishment of advance directives, and appointment of a health-care surrogate while a person is still healthy often ease the burden for the decision makers during a later crisis. Patients can exercise autonomy through these mechanisms, even though they may no longer be able to communicate their wishes directly. When these documents are not available, the information gathered during the assessment of social factors helps identify those individuals who may be able to act in the patient's best interest.

3. *List and rank all the options.* Performing this task involves all the decision makers. It is sometimes helpful to begin with the least desired choice and methodically work toward the preferred treatment choice that is most likely to lead to the desired outcome. Asking all participating parties to discuss what they believe are reasonable outcomes to be attained with the use of available medical treatment often helps in the decision process. By listening to others in a controlled situation, family members and health-care professionals discover that they actually want the same result as the patient but had different ideas about how to achieve their goal.

Implementation

During the implementation phase, the patient or the surrogate (substitute) decision maker(s) and members of the health-care team reach a mutually acceptable decision. This occurs through open discussion and sometimes negotiation. An example of negotiation follows:

Elena's mother has metastatic ovarian cancer. She and Elena have discussed treatment options. Her physician suggested the use of a new chemotherapeutic agent that has demonstrated success in many cases. But Elena's mother emphatically states that she has "had enough" and prefers to spend her remaining time doing whatever she chooses. Elena wants her mother to try the drug. To resolve the dilemma, the oncology nurse practitioner and the physician talk with Elena and her mother. Everyone reviews the facts and expresses their feelings about the situation. Seeing Elena's distress, Elena's

mother says, "OK, I will try the drug for a month. If there is no improvement after this time, I want to stop all treatment and live out the time I have with my daughter and her family." All agreed that this was a reasonable decision.

The role of the nurse during the implementation phase is to ensure that communication does not break down. Ethical dilemmas are often emotional issues, filled with guilt, sorrow, anger, and other strong emotions. These strong feelings can cause communication failures among decision makers. Remind yourself, "I am here to do what is best for this patient."

Keep in mind that an ethical dilemma is not always a choice between two attractive alternatives. Many are between two unattractive, even unpleasant, choices. Elena's mother's options did not include the choice she really wanted: good health and a long life.

Once an agreement is reached, the decision makers must accept it. Sometimes, an agreement is not reached because the parties cannot reconcile their conflicting belief systems or values. At other times, caregivers are unable to recognize the worth of the patient's point of view. Occasionally, the patient or the surrogate may make a request that is not institutionally or legally possible (Ensign, n.d.). In some cases, a different institution or physician may be able to honor the request. In other cases, the patient or surrogate may request information from the nurse regarding illegal acts. When this happens, the nurse should ask the patient and family to consider the consequences of their proposed actions. It may be necessary to bring other counselors into the discussion (with the patient's permission) to negotiate an agreement.

Evaluation

As in the nursing process, the purpose of evaluation in resolving ethical dilemmas is to determine whether the desired outcomes have occurred. In the case of Mr. Sussman, some of the questions that could be posed by Gail to the family are as follows:

- "I have noticed the amount of time you have been spending with your father. Have you observed any changes in his condition?"
- "I see Dr. Washburn spoke to you about the test results and your father's prognosis. How do you feel about the situation?"

box 4-3
The Moral Model

M: Massage the dilemma
O: Outline the option
R: Resolve the dilemma
A: Act by applying the chosen option
L: Look back and evaluate the complete process,
    including actions taken

■ "Now that Dr. Washburn has spoken to you about your father's condition, have you considered future alternatives?"

Changes in patient status, availability of medical treatment, and social facts may call for reevaluation of a situation. The course of treatment may need to be altered. Continued communication and cooperation among the decision makers are essential.

Another model, the MORAL model created by Thiroux (1977) and refined for nursing by Halloran (1982), is gaining popularity. The MORAL acronym reminds nurses of the sequential steps needed for resolving an ethical dilemma. This ethical decision-making model is easily implemented in all patient care settings (Box 4-3).

Current Ethical Issues

During fall 1998, Dr. Jack Kevorkian (sometimes called Dr. Death in the media) openly admitted that at the patient's request, he gave the patient a lethal dose of medication, causing death. His statement raised the consciousness of the American people and the health-care system about the issues of euthanasia and assisted suicide. Do individuals have the right to consciously end their own lives when they are suffering from terminal conditions? If they are unable to perform the act themselves, should others assist them in ending their lives? Should assisted suicide be legal? There are no answers to these difficult questions, and patients and their families face these same questions every day.

The Terri Schiavo case gained tremendous media attention, probably becoming the most important case of clinical ethics in more than a decade. Her illness and death created a major medical, legal, theological, ethical, political, and social controversy. The case brought to the forefront the deep divisions and fears that reside in society regarding life and death, the role of the government and courts in life decisions, and

the treatment of disabled persons (Hoffman & Schwartz, 2006). Many aspects of this case will never be clarified; however, many questions raised by this case need to be addressed for future ethical decision making. Some of these are:

1. What is the true definition of a persistent vegetative state?
2. How is cognitive recovery determined?
3. What role do the courts play when there is a family dispute? Who has the right to make decisions when an individual is married?
4. What are the duties of surrogate decision makers? (Hook & Mueller, 2005)

The primary goal of nursing and other health-care professions is to keep people alive and well or, if this cannot be done, to help them live with their problems and die peacefully. To accomplish this, health-care professionals struggle to improve their knowledge and skills so they can care for their patients, provide them with some quality of life, and help return them to wellness. The costs involved in achieving this goal can be astronomical.

Questions are being raised more and more often about who should receive the benefits of this technology. Managed care and the competition for resources are also creating ethical dilemmas. Other difficult questions, such as who should pay for care when the illness may have been due to poor health-care practices such as smoking or substance abuse, are also being debated.

Practice Issues Related to Technology

Genetics and the Limitations of Technology

In issues of technology, the principles of beneficence and nonmaleficence may be in conflict. A specific technology administered with the intention of "doing good" may result in enormous suffering. Causing this type of torment is in direct conflict with the idea of "do no harm" (Burkhardt & Nathaniel, 2007). At times, this is an accepted consequence, such as in the use of chemotherapy. However, the ultimate outcome in this case is that recovery is expected. In situations in which little or no improvement is expected, the issue of whether the good outweighs the bad prevails. Suffering induced by technology may include physical, spiritual, and emotional components for the patient and the families.

Today, many infants who have low birth weight or birth defects, who not so long ago would have been considered unable to live, are maintained on machines in highly sophisticated neonatal units. This process may keep babies alive only to die several months later or may leave them with severe chronic disabilities. Children with chronic disabilities require additional medical, educational, and social services. These services are expensive and often require families to travel long distances to obtain them (Urbano, 1992).

The use of ultrasound during pregnancy is an expected standard of care. In the past these pictures were mostly two-dimensional and were used mostly to determine the size of the fetus for development and in relationship to the mother's pelvic anatomy. Today, with the advanced technology, visualization of internal organs such as the heart, kidneys, and brain is possible. If a defect is found, parents now have additional options, which present further ethical decisions.

Genetic diagnosis and gene therapy present new ethical issues for nursing. *Genetic diagnosis* is a process that involves analyzing parents or an embryo for a genetic disorder. This is usually done before in vitro fertilization for couples who run a high risk of conceiving a child with a genetic disorder. The embryos are tested, and only those that are free of genetic flaws are implanted.

Genetic screening is used as a tool to determine whether couples hold the possibility of giving birth to a genetically impaired infant. Testing for the most common genetic disorders has become an expected standard of practice of health-care providers caring for women who are planning to become pregnant or who are pregnant. Couples are encouraged to seek out information regarding their genetic health history in order to identify the possibilities of having a child with a genetic disorder. If a couple has one child with a genetic disorder, genetic specialists test the parents and/or the fetus for the presence of the gene.

Genetic screening leads to issues pertaining to reproductive rights. It also opens new issues. What is a disability versus a disorder, and who decides this? Is a disability a disease, and does it need to be cured or prevented? The technology is also used to determine whether individuals are predisposed to certain diseases, such as breast cancer or Huntington's chorea. This has created additional ethical issues regarding genetic screening. For example:

Bianca, 33 years old, is diagnosed with breast cancer. She has two daughters, ages 6 and 4 years. Bianca's mother and grandmother had breast cancer. Neither survived more than 5 years post-treatment. Bianca undergoes a lumpectomy followed by radiation and chemotherapy. Her cancer is found to be nonhormonally dependent. Due to her age and family history, Bianca's oncologist recommends that she see a geneticist and have genetic testing for the BRCA-1 and BRCA-2 genes. Bianca makes an appointment to discuss the testing. She meets with the nurse who has additional education in genetics and discusses the following questions: "If I am positive for the genes, what are my options? Should I have a bilateral mastectomy with reconstruction?" "Will I be able to get health insurance coverage, or will the companies consider this to be a preexisting condition?" "What are the future implications for my daughters?"

If you were the nurse, how would you address these concerns?

Genetic engineering is the ability to change the genetic structure of an organism. Through this process, researchers have created disease-resistant fruits and vegetables and certain medications, such as insulin. This process theoretically allows for the genetic alteration of embryos, eliminating genetic flaws and creating healthier babies. This technology enables researchers to make a brown-haired individual blonde, to change brown eyes to blue, and to make a short person taller. Envision being able to "engineer" your child. Imagine, as Aldous Huxley did in *Brave New World* (1932), being able to create a society of perfect individuals: "We also predestine and condition. We decant our babies as socialized human beings, as Alphas or Epsilons, as future sewage workers or future . . . he was going to say future World controllers but correcting himself said future directors of Hatcheries, instead" (p. 12).

The ethical implications pertaining to genetic technology are profound. For example, some questions raised by the Human Genome Project relate to:

■ Fairness in the use of the genetic information.
■ Privacy and confidentiality of obtained genetic information.
■ Genetic testing of an individual for a specific condition due to family history. Should testing

be performed if no treatment is available? Should parents have the right to have minors tested for adult-onset diseases? Should parents have the right to use gene therapy for genetic enhancement?

The Human Genome Project (HGP) is dedicated to mapping and identifying the genetic composition of humans. Scientists hope to identify and eradicate many of the genetic disorders affecting individuals. Initiated in 1990, the Human Genome Project was projected to be a 13-year effort coordinated by the U.S. Department of Energy and the National Institutes of Health. However, because of swift technological advances, in February 2001 the scientists announced they had cracked the human genetic code and accomplished the following goals (Human Genome Project Information, 2002):

- Identified all of the genes in human DNA
- Determined the sequences of the three billion chemical bases that make up human DNA
- Stored this information in databases
- Developed tools for data analysis
- Addressed the ethical, legal, and social issues that may arise from the project

Rapid advances in the science of genetics and its applications present new and complex ethical and policy issues for individuals, health-care personnel, and society. Economics come into play because, currently, only those who can afford the technology have access to it. However, more recently many health insurance companies will cover certain types of prenatal genetic testing, particularly when a propensity for a disorder exists due to family history or ethnicity. Efforts need to be directed toward creating standards that identify the uses for genetic data and the protection of human rights and confidentiality. As of 2012, due to the amount of data collected, the HGP has developed a "universal storage area" so that this information is internationally accessible to scientists, geneticists, and researchers (www.genome.gov). This is truly the new frontier.

Stem Cell Use and Research

Over the last several years, issues regarding stem cell research and stem cell transplant technology have come to the forefront of ethical discussion.

Stem cell research shows promise in possibly curing neurological disorders such as Parkinson's disease, spinal cord injury, and dementia. Questions have been raised regarding the moral and ethical issues of using stem cells from fetal tissue for research and the treatment of disease. Stem cell transplants have demonstrated success in helping cancer patients recover and giving them a chance for survival when traditional treatments have failed.

A new business has emerged from this technology as companies now store fetal cord blood for future use if needed. This blood is collected at the time of delivery and may be used for the infant and possibly future siblings if necessary. The cost for this service is high, which limits its availability to only those who can afford the process.

When faced with the prospect of a child who is dying from a terminal illness, some parents have resorted to conceiving a sibling in order to obtain the stem cells for the purpose of using them to save the first child. Nurses who work in pediatrics and pediatric oncology units may find themselves dealing with this situation. It is important for nurses to examine their own feelings regarding these issues and understand that, regardless of their personal beliefs, the family is in need of sensitivity and the best nursing care.

A primary responsibility of nursing is to help patients and families cope with the purposes, benefits, and limitations of the new technologies. Hospice nurses and critical care nurses help patients and their families with end-of-life decisions. Nurses will need to have knowledge about the new genetic technologies because they will fill the roles of counselors and advisers in these areas. Many nurses now work in the areas of in vitro fertilization and genetic counseling.

Professional Dilemmas

Most of this chapter has dealt with patient issues, but ethical problems may involve leadership and management issues as well. What do you do about an impaired coworker? Personal loyalties often cause conflict with professional ethics, creating an ethical dilemma. For this reason, most nurse practice acts now address this problem and require the reporting of impaired professionals and providing rehabilitation for them.

Other professional dilemmas may involve working with incompetent personnel. This may be frustrating for both staff and management. Regulations created to protect individuals from unjustified loss of position and the enormous amounts of paperwork, remediation, and time that must be exercised to terminate an incompetent health-care worker often make management look the other way.

Employing institutions that provide nursing services have an obligation to establish a process for the reporting and handling of practices that jeopardize patient safety (ANA, 1994; IOM, 2007). The behaviors of incompetent staff place patients and other staff members in jeopardy; eventually, the incompetency may lead to legal action that may have been avoidable if a different approach had been taken.

Conclusion

Ethical dilemmas are becoming more common in the changing health-care environment. More questions are being raised, and fewer answers are available. New guidelines need to be developed to assist in finding viable solutions to these questions. Technology wields enormous power to alter the human organism and enable health-care providers to prolong human life, but economics may force the profession to rethink answers to questions such as, "What is life versus what is living?" and "When is it okay to terminate human life?" Will society become the brave new world of Aldous Huxley? Again and again the question is raised, "Who shall live, and who shall die?" What is *your* answer?

Study Questions

1. What is the difference between intrinsic and extrinsic values? Make a list of your intrinsic values.

2. Consider a decision you made recently that was based on your values. How did you make your choice?

3. Describe how you could use the valuing process of choosing, prizing, and acting in making the decision considered in Question 2.

4. Which of your personal values would be primary if you were assigned to care for an anacephalic infant whose parents have decided to donate the baby's organs?

5. The parents of the anacephalic infant in Question 4 confront you and ask, "What would you do if this were your baby?" What do you think would be most important for you to consider in responding to them?

6. Your friend is single and feels that her "biological clock is ticking." She decides to undergo in vitro fertilization using donor sperm. She tells you that she has researched the donor's background extensively and wants to show you the "template" for her child. She asks for your professional opinion about this situation. How would you respond? Identify the ethical principles involved.

7. Over the past several weeks, you have noticed that your closest friend, Jimmy, has been erratic and has been making poor patient-care decisions. On two separate occasions, you quietly intervened and "fixed" his errors. You have also noticed that he volunteers to give pain medications to other nurses' patients, and you see him standing very close to other nurses when they remove controlled substances from the medication distribution center. Today you watched him go to the center immediately after another colleague and then saw him go into the men's room. Within about 20 minutes his behavior had changed completely. You suspect that he may be taking controlled substances. You and Jimmy have been friends for more than 20 years. You grew up together and went to nursing school together. You realize that if you approach him, you may jeopardize this close friendship that means a great deal to you. Using the MORAL ethical decision-making model, devise a plan to resolve this dilemma.

Case Study to Promote Critical Reasoning

Andy is assigned to care for a 14-year-old girl, Amanda, admitted with a large tumor located in the left groin area. During an assessment, Amanda shares her personal feelings with Andy. She tells him that she feels "different" from her friends. She is ashamed of her physical development because all her girlfriends have "breasts" and boyfriends. She is very flat-chested and embarrassed. Andy listens attentively to Amanda and helps her focus on some of her positive attributes and talents.

A CT scan is ordered and reveals that the tumor extends to what appears to be the ovary. A gynecological surgeon is called in to evaluate the situation. An ultrasonic-guided biopsy is performed. It is discovered that the tumor is an enlarged lymph node and that the "ovary" is actually a testis. Amanda has both male and female gonads.

When this information is given to Amanda's parents, they do not want her to know. They feel that she was raised as "their daughter." They ask the surgeon to remove the male gonads and leave only the female gonads. That way, "Amanda will never need to know." The surgeon refuses to do this. Andy believes that the parents should discuss the situation with Amanda as they are denying her choices. The parents are adamant about Amanda not knowing anything. Andy returns to Amanda's room, and Amanda begins asking all types of questions regarding the tests and the treatments. In answering, Andy hesitates, and Amanda picks up on this, demanding that he tell her the truth.

1. How should Andy respond?

2. What are the ethical principles in conflict?

3. What are the long-term effects of Andy's decision?

References

AIDS Update Conference. (1995). Hollywood Memorial Hospital, Hollywood, Fla.

American Association of Critical Care Nurses (AACN). At loggerheads: Questioning patient autonomy. Retrieved on January 11, 2006, from www.aacn.org/AACN/aacnnews.nsf/GetArticle/ArticleThree184?

American Nurses Association (ANA). (1994). Guidelines on Reporting Incompetent, Unethical, or Illegal Practices. Washington, DC: ANA.

American Nurses Association (ANA). (2002). Code of Ethics Project. Washington, DC: ANA.

Benner, P., & Wrubel, J. (1989). *The Primacy of Caring: Stress and Coping in Health and Illness.* Menlo Park, Calif.: Addison Wesley.

Burkhardt, M.A., & Nathaniel, A.K. (2007). *Ethics and Issues in Contemporary Nursing.* Albany, N.Y.: Delmar.

Butts, J.B., & Rich, K.L. (2012). *Nursing Ethics: Across the Curriculum and Into Practice,* (3rd ed.). Boston: Jones & Bartlett.

Csongradi, C. (2012). *Why the Topic of Bioethics in Science Classes? A New Look at an Old Debate.* Retrieved on December 31, 2012, from www.actionbioscience.org/education/csongradi.html

Davis, A.J., Arokar, M.A., Liaschenko, J., & Drought, T.S. (1997). *Ethical Dilemmas and Nursing Practice,* 4th ed. Stamford, Conn.: Appleton & Lange.

DeGrazia, D., Mappes, T.A., & Brand-Ballard, J. (2010). *Biomedical Ethics,* 7th ed. St. Louis: McGraw-Hill.

Driver, J. (2001). *Uneasy Virtue.* New York: Cambridge University Press.

Edge, R.S., & Groves, J.R. (2005). *The Ethics of Healthcare: A Guide for Clinical Practice,* 3rd ed. Albany, N.Y.: Thomson–Delmar Learning.

Ensign, M.R. (n.d.). Ethical issues and the elderly: Guidance for elder care providers. Retrieved on December 31, 2012, from www.ensignlaw.com/Ethical%20Issues%20and%20Elderly.html#_ftn12

Gordon, N. (1963). *The Death Committee.* New York: Fawcett Crest.

Guido, G.W. (2001). *Legal and Ethical Issues in Nursing* (3rd ed.). Saddle River, N.J.: Prentice-Hall.

Halloran, M.C. (1982). Rational ethical judgments utilizing a decision-making tool. *Heart Lung, 11*(6), 566–570.

Harned, P. (2005). National business ethics survey, 2005. *Ethics Today Online, 4*(2). Retrieved on January 13, 2005, from www.ethics.org/today/et_current. html pres

Hoffman, D.E., & Schwartz, J. (2006). Who decides whether a patient lives or dies? *Trial, 42*(10), 30–37.

Hook, C.C., & Mueller, P.S. (2005). The Terri Schiavo saga: The making of a tragedy and lessons learned. Retrieved on April 20, 2006, from www.mayoclinicproceedings.com/inside.asp?AID=1054&UID=8934

Hooker, B. (2000). *Ideal Code, Real World.* Oxford, U.K.: Oxford University Press.

Human Genome Project. Retrieved on July 19, 2002, from www.ornl.gov/hgmis/about

Hume, D. (1978). A treatise of human nature. In Johnson, O.A, *Ethics,* 4th ed. New York: Holt, Rinehart, and Winston, 212.

Huxley, A. (1932). *Brave New World.* New York: Harper Row Publishers.

Jerak-Zuident, S. (2012). Certain uncertainties: Modes of patient safety in healthcare. *Social Studies of Science, 42*(5), 732–752.

Johnstone, M.J. (1999). *Bioethics: A nursing perspective,* 3rd ed. Sydney, Australia: Harcourt Saunders.

Kant, I. (1949). *Fundamental Principles of the Metaphysics of Morals.* New York: Liberal Arts.

Key Ethical Principles (2012). Retrieved on December 31, 2012, from www.ascensionhealth.org/

Kirschenbaum, H. (2000). From values clarification to character education: A personal journey. *Journal of Humanistic Counseling, Education and Development, 39*(1), 4–20.

Macklin, R. (1987). Mortal choices: Ethical dilemmas in modern medicine. *Annals in Internal Medicine, 11*(8), 695–698.

Merriam-Webster Dictionary, (2012). Retrieved on December 23, 2012, from www.merriam-webster.com/dictionary/values

National Human Genome Research Institute. (2012). 1000 genomes project data available on Amazon Cloud. Retrieved on December 31, 2012, from www. genome.gov

Nussbaum, M. (2002). The enduring significance of John Rawls. The Chronicle of Higher Education. Retrieved on December 31, 2012, from http://chronicle.com/article/The-Enduring-Significance-of/7360

Raths, L.E., Harmon, M., & Simmons, S.B. (1979). *Values and Teaching.* New York: Charles E. Merrill.

Redman, B., & Fry, S.T. (2000). Nurses' ethical conflicts: What is really known about them? *Journal of Nursing Ethics, 7*(4), 360–366.

Shirey, M.R. (2005). Ethical climate in nursing practice: The leader's role. *Journal of Nursing Administration, 7*(2), 59–67.

Thiroux, J. (1977). *Ethics: Theory and Practice.* Philadelphia: MacMillan.

Thompson, J., & Thompson, H. (1992). *Bioethical Decision Making for Nurses.* New York: Appleton-Century-Crofts.

Urbano, M.T. (1992). *Preschool Children with Special Health-Care Needs.* San Diego: Singular Publishing.

Varcoe, C., Doane, G., Pauly, B., Rodney, P., et al. (2007). Ethical practise in nursing: Working the in-betweens. *Journal of Advanced Nursing, 45*(3), 316–325.

Wack, J. (1992). *Sociology of Religion.* Chicago: University of Chicago Press.

Zimmerman, M.J. "Intrinsic vs. Extrinsic Value," *The Stanford Encyclopedia of Philosophy* (Winter 2010 Edition), Edward N. Zalta (ed.). Retrieved on December 30, 2012, from http:// plato.stanford.edu/archives/win2010/entries/value-intrinsic-extrinsic/

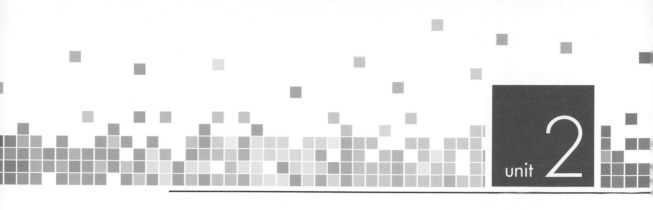

unit 2

Working Within an Organization

Organizations, Power, and Empowerment

The topics in this chapter—organizations, power, and empowerment—are not as remote from a nurse's everyday experience as you may first think. While it is difficult to focus on these "big picture" factors when caught up in the busy day-to-day work of a staff nurse, they have a significant effect on you and your practice, as you will see in this chapter. Consider two scenarios, which are analyzed in the scenarios.

Were the disappointments experienced by Hazel Rivera and the critical care department staff predictable? Could they have been avoided? Without a basic understanding of organizations and of the part that power plays in health-care institutions, people are doomed to be continually surprised by the response to their well-intentioned efforts. As you read this chapter, you will learn why Hazel Rivera and the staff of the critical care department were disappointed.

This chapter begins by looking at some of the characteristics of the organizations in which nurses work and how these organizations operate. Then it focuses on the subject of power within organizations: what it is, how it is obtained, and how nurses can be empowered.

Understanding Organizations

One of the attractive features of nursing as a career is the wide variety of settings in which nurses can work. From rural migrant health clinics to organ transplant units, nurses' skills are needed wherever there are concerns about people's health. Relationships with patients may extend for months or years, as they do in school health or in nursing homes, or they may be brief and never repeated, as often happens in doctors' offices, operating rooms, and emergency departments.

Types of Health-Care Organizations

Although some nurses work as independent practitioners, as consultants, or in the corporate world, most nurses are employed by health-care organizations. These organizations can be classified into three types on the basis of their sponsorship and financing:

1. **Private not-for-profit.** Many health-care organizations were founded by civic, charitable, or religious groups. Many of today's hospitals,

Scenario 1

In school, Hazel Rivera had always received high praise for the quality of her nursing care plans. "Thorough, comprehensive, systematic, holistic—beautiful!" was the comment she received on the last one she wrote before graduation.

Now Hazel is a staff nurse on a busy orthopedic unit. Although her time to write comprehensive care plans during the day is limited, Hazel often stays after work to complete them. Her friend Carla refuses to stay late with her. "If I can't complete my work during the shift, then they have given me too much to do," she said.

At the end of their 3-month probationary period, Hazel and Carla received written evaluations of their progress and comments about their value to the organization. To Hazel's surprise, her friend Carla received a higher rating than she did. Why? ■

Scenario 2

The nursing staff of the critical care department of a large urban hospital formed an evidence-based practice group about a year ago. They had made many changes in their practice based on reviews of the research on several different procedures, and they were quite pleased with the results.

"Let's look at the bigger picture next month," their nurse manager suggested. "We should consider the research on different models of patient care. We might get some good ideas for our unit." The staff nurses agreed. It would be a nice change to look at the way they organized patient care in their department.

The nurse manager found a wealth of information on different models for organizing nursing care. They finally decided that a separate geriatric intensive care unit made sense since a large proportion of their patient population was in their 70s, 80s, and 90s.

Several nurses volunteered to form an ad hoc committee to design a similar unit for older patients within their critical care department. When the plan was presented, both the nurse manager and the staff thought it was excellent. The nurse manager offered to present the plan to the vice president for nursing. The staff eagerly awaited the vice president's response.

The nurse manager returned with discouraging news. The vice president did not support their concept and said that, although they were free to continue developing the idea, they should not assume that it would ever be implemented. What happened? ■

long-term care facilities, home-care services, and community agencies began this way. Some have been in existence for generations. Although they need sufficient money to pay their staff and expenses, as not-for-profit organizations they do not have to generate a profit in addition to meeting expenses.

2. **Public.** Government-operated health service organizations range from county public health departments to complex medical centers, such as those operated by the Veterans Administration, a federal agency.

3. **Private for-profit.** Increasing numbers of health-care organizations are operated for profit like other businesses. These include large hospital and nursing home chains, health maintenance organizations, and many freestanding centers that provide special services, such as surgical and diagnostic centers.

The differences between these categories have become blurred for several reasons:

■ All compete for patients, especially for patients with health-care insurance or the ability to pay their own health-care bills.
■ All experience the effects of cost constraints.
■ All may provide services that are eligible for government reimbursement, particularly Medicaid and Medicare funding, if they meet government standards.

Organizational Characteristics

The size and complexity of many health-care organizations make them difficult to understand. One way to begin is to find a metaphor or image that describes their characteristics. Morgan (1997) suggested using animals or other familiar images to describe an organization. For example, an aggressive organization that crushes its competitors is like a bull elephant, whereas a timid organization in danger of being crushed by that bull elephant is like a mouse. Using a different kind of image, an organization adrift without a clear idea of its future in a time of crisis could be described as a rudderless boat on a stormy sea, whereas an organization with its sights set clearly on exterminating its competition could be described as a guided missile.

Organizational Culture

People seek stability, consistency, and meaning in their work. An organizational culture is an enduring set of shared values, beliefs, and assumptions (Cameron & Quinn, 2006). It is taught (often indirectly) to new employees as the "right way" or "our way" to provide care and relate to one another. As with the cultures of societies and communities, it is easy to observe the superficial aspects of an organization's culture, but much of it remains hidden from the casual observer. Perera and Peiro (2012) note that "the real values of an organization are those that actually govern its behavior and decision-making processes, whether they are formally stated or not" (2012, p. 752) Edgar Schein, a well-known scholar of organizational culture, identified three levels of organizational culture:

1. **Artifact level:** visible characteristics such as patient room layout, paint colors, lobby design, logo, directional signs, etc.
2. **Espoused beliefs:** written goals, philosophy of the organization
3. **Underlying assumptions:** unconscious but powerful beliefs and feelings, such as a commitment to cure every patient, no matter the cost (Schein, 2004)

Organizational cultures differ greatly. Some are very traditional, preserving their well-established ways of doing things even when these processes no longer work well. Others, in an attempt to be progressive, chase the newest management fad or buy the latest high-technology equipment. Some are warm, friendly, and open to new people and new ideas. Others are cold, defensive, and indifferent or even hostile to the outside world (Tappen, 2001). These very different organizational cultures have a powerful effect on employees and the people served by the organization. Organizational culture shapes people's behavior, especially their responses to each other, a particularly important factor in health care.

Culture of Safety

The way in which a health-care organization's operation affects patient safety has been a subject of much discussion. The shared values, attitudes, and behaviors that are directed to preventing or minimizing patient harm have been called the culture of safety (Vogus & Sutcliffe, 2007). The following are important aspects of an organization's culture of safety:

■ Willingness to acknowledge mistakes
■ Vigilance in detecting and eliminating error-prone situations
■ Openness to questioning existing systems and to changing them to prevent errors (Armstrong & Laschinger, 2006; Vogus & Sutcliffe, 2007).

It is not easy to change an organization's culture. In fact, Hinshaw (2008) points out we are trying to create a culture of safety at a particularly difficult time, given the shortages of nurses and other resources within the health-care system (Connaughton & Hassinger, 2007). Nurses who are not well prepared, not valued by their employer or colleagues, not involved in decisions about organizing patient care, and are fatigued due to excessive workloads are certainly more likely to be error-prone. Increased workload and stress have been found to increase adverse events by as much as 28% (Weissman et al., 2007; Redman, 2008). Clearly, organizational factors can contribute either to an increase in errors or to protecting patient safety.

Care Environments

There is also much concern about the environment in which care is provided, an issue that is closely related to patient safety. Patients face less risk of failure to rescue or death in better care environments (see Aiken et al., 2008). What constitutes a better care environment? Collegial relationships with physicians, skilled nurse managers with high levels of leadership ability, emphasis on staff development, and quality of care are important factors. Mackoff and Triolo (2008) offer a list of factors that contribute to excellence and longevity (low turnover) of nurse managers:

■ *Excellence:* always striving to be better, refusing to accept mediocrity

- *Meaningfulness:* being very clear about the purpose of the organization (serving the poor, healing the environment, protecting abused women, for example)
- *Regard:* understanding the work people do and valuing it
- *Learning and growth:* providing mentors, guidance, opportunities to grow and develop

Identifying an Organization's Culture

The culture of an organization is intangible; you cannot see it or touch it, but you will know if you violate one of its norms. To learn about the culture of an organization when you are applying for a new position or trying to familiarize yourself with your new workplace, you can ask several people who are familiar with the organization or work there to describe it in a few words. You could also ask about staff workloads, participation in decision making, or examples of nursing's role in ensuring patient safety.

Does it matter in what type of organization you work? The answer, emphatically, is yes. For example, the extreme value placed on "busyness" in hospitals, i.e., being seen doing something at all times, can lead to manager actions such as floating a staff member to a "busier" unit if she or he is found reading a new research study or looking up information on the Internet (Scott-Findley & Golden-Biddle, 2005). Even more important, a hospital or nursing home with a positive work environment is not only a better place for nurses to work but also safer for patients, while an organization that ignores threats to patient safety endangers both its staff and those who receive their care.

Once you have grasped the totality of an organization in terms of its overall culture, you are ready to analyze it in a little more detail, particularly its goals, structure, and processes.

Organizational Goals

Try answering the following question:

> *Question:* Every health-care organization has just one goal, which is to keep people healthy, restore them to health, or assist them in dying as comfortably as possible, correct?
> *Answer:* The statement is only partially correct. Most health-care organizations have a mission statement similar to this but also

have a number of other goals, not all of which are directed to providing excellent patient care.

Does this answer surprise you? What other goals might a health-care organization have? Following are some examples:

- **Survival.** Organizations have to maintain their own existence. Many health-care organizations are cash-strapped, causing them to limit hiring, streamline work, and reduce costs, putting enormous pressure on their staff (Roark, 2005). The survival goal is threatened when reimbursements are reduced, competition increases, the organization fails to meet standards, or patients are unable to pay their bills (Trinh & O'Connor, 2002).
- **Growth.** Chief executive officers (CEOs) typically want their organizations to grow by expanding into new territories, adding new services, and bringing in new patients.
- **Profit.** For-profit organizations are expected to return some profit to their owners. Not-for-profit organizations have to be able to pay their bills and to avoid falling into debt. This is sometimes difficult to accomplish.
- **Status.** Many CEOs also want their health-care organization to be known as the best in its field, for example, by having the best transplant unit, having the shortest wait time in the emergency room, having world renowned physicians, providing "the best nursing care in the community" (Frusti, Niesen, & Campion, 2003), providing gourmet meals, or having the most attractive birthing rooms in town.
- **Dominance.** Some organizations also want to drive others out of the health-care business or acquire them, surpassing the goal of survival and moving toward dominance of a particular market by driving out the competition.

Problems can arise if the mission statement of a health-care organization is not well aligned (i.e., in agreement) with day-to-day actions of its leaders. This disconnect can reduce morale, lead to gaps in the quality of care provided, and tarnish its image in the community (Nelson, 2013). The disconnect between these goals may have profound effects on every one of the organization's employees, nurses

---

box 5-1

What Is a Bureaucracy?

Although it seems as if everyone complains about "the bureaucracy," not everyone is clear about what a bureaucracy really is. Max Weber defined a *bureaucratic organization* as having the following characteristics:

- **Division of labor.** Specific parts of the job to be done are assigned to different individuals or groups. For example, nurses, physicians, therapists, dietitians, and social workers all provide portions of the health care needed by an individual.
- **Hierarchy.** All employees are organized and ranked according to their level of authority within the organization. For example, administrators and directors are at the top of most hospital hierarchies, whereas aides and maintenance workers are at the bottom.
- **Rules and regulations.** Acceptable and unacceptable behavior and the proper way to carry out various tasks are defined, often in writing. For example, procedure books, policy manuals, bylaws, statements, and memos prescribe many types of behavior, from acceptable isolation techniques to vacation policies.
- **Emphasis on technical competence.** People with certain skills and knowledge are hired to carry out specific parts of the total work of the organization. For example, a community mental health center has psychiatrists, social workers, and nurses to provide different kinds of therapies and clerical staff to do the typing and filing.

Some bureaucracy is characteristic of the formal operation of every organization, even the most deliberately informal, because it promotes smooth operations within a large and complex group of people.

Adapted from Weber, M. (1969). Bureaucratic organization. In Etzioni, A. (ed.). Readings on modern organizations. Englewood Cliffs, N.J.: Prentice-Hall.

---

included. For example, return to the story of Hazel Rivera. Why did she receive a less favorable rating than her friend Carla?

After comparing ratings with those of her friend Carla, Hazel asked for a meeting with her nurse manager to discuss her evaluation. The nurse manager explained the rating: Hazel's care plans were very well done, and the nurse manager genuinely appreciated Hazel's efforts to make them so. The problem was that Hazel had to be paid overtime for this work according to the union contract, and this reduced the amount of overtime pay the nurse manager had available when the patient care load was especially high. "The corporation is very strict about staying within the budget," she said. "In fact, my rating is higher when I don't use up all of my budgeted overtime hours." When Hazel asked what she could do to improve her rating, the nurse manager offered to help her streamline the care plans and manage her time better so that the care plans could be done during her shift.

Staff nurses can contribute to the accomplishment of organizational goals. This begins with recognition that there is a *connection* between the work they do and achievement of the organization's goals. An example would be to reduce rehospitalization of discharged patients. To contribute to achieving this goal, nurses can better prepare patients to care for themselves when they go home. This is a *specific action* to be taken, a change in practice that nurses can integrate into patient care. Monthly *reports* on changes in the rate of rehospi-

talization provide information about the progress made toward achieving the goal. *Recognition* of this progress motivates them to continue these efforts (Berkow et al., 2012).

Structure

The Traditional Approach

Almost all health-care organizations have a hierarchical structure of some kind (Box 5-1). In a traditional hierarchical structure, employees are ranked from the top to the bottom, as if they were on the steps of a ladder (Fig. 5.1). The number of people on the bottom rungs of the ladder is almost always much greater than the number at the top. The president or CEO is usually at the top of this ladder; the housekeeping and maintenance crews are usually at the bottom. Nurses fall somewhere in

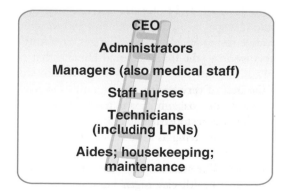

Figure 5.1 The organizational ladder.

the middle of most health-care organizations, higher than the cleaning people, aides, and technicians, parallel with therapists but lower than physicians and administrators. The organizational structure of a small ambulatory care center in a horizontal form is illustrated in Figure 5.2.

The people at the top of the ladder have authority to issue orders, spend the organization's money, and hire and fire people. Much of this authority is delegated to people below them, but they retain the right to reverse a decision or regain control of these activities whenever they deem necessary.

The people at the bottom have little authority but do have other sources of power. They usually play no part in deciding how money is spent or who will be hired or fired but are responsible for carrying out the directions issued by people above them on the ladder. Their primary source of power is the importance of the work they do: if there was no one at the bottom, most of the work would not get done.

Some amount of bureaucracy is characteristic of the formal operation of every organization, even the most deliberately informal, because it promotes smooth and consistent operations within a large and complex group of people.

More Innovative Structures

There is much interest in restructuring organizations, not only to save money but also to make the best use of a health-care organization's most valuable resource, its people. This begins with hiring the right people. It also involves providing them with the resources they need to function and the kind of leadership that can inspire the staff and unleash their creativity (Rosen, 1996).

Increasingly, people recognize that organizations need to be both efficient and adaptable. Organizations need to be prepared for uncertainty, for rapid changes in their environment, and for quick, creative responses to these challenges. In addition, they need to provide an internal climate that not only allows but also motivates employees to work to the best of their ability.

Innovative organizations have adapted an increasingly *organic* structure that is more dynamic, more flexible, and less centralized than the static traditional hierarchical structure (Yourstone & Smith, 2002). In these organically structured organizations, many decisions are made by the people who will implement them, not by their bosses.

The organic network emphasizes increased flexibility of the organizational structure (Fig. 5-3), decentralized decision making, and autonomy for working groups and teams. Rigid unit structures are reorganized into autonomous teams that consist of professionals from different departments and disciplines. Each team is given a specific task or function (e.g., intravenous team, a hospital infection control team, a child protection team in a community agency). The teams are responsible for their own self-correction and self-control, although they may also have a designated leader. Together, team members make decisions about work assignments and how to deal with problems that arise. In other words, the teams supervise and manage themselves.

Supervisors, administrators, and support staff have different functions in an organic network. Instead of spending their time directing and controlling other people's work, they become planners and resource people. They are responsible for providing the conditions required for the optimal functioning of the teams, and they are expected to ensure that the support, information, materials, and funds needed to do the job well are available to the teams. They also act as coordinators between the teams so that the teams are cooperating rather than blocking each other, working toward the same goals, and not duplicating effort.

The structure of health-care organizations is changing rapidly. For example, many formerly independent organizations are considering joining together into accountable care organizations that provide a continuum of care, from primary care to inpatient care and long-term care for the people they serve. The goal is to provide the best quality care while keeping costs under control (Evans, 2013).

Processes

Organizations have formal processes for getting things done and informal ways to get around the formal processes (Perrow, 1969). The *formal* processes are the written policies and procedures present in all health-care organizations. The *informal* processes are not written and often not discussed. They exist in organizations as a kind of "shadow" organization that is harder to see but equally important to recognize and understand (Purser & Cabana, 1999).

The informal route is often much simpler and faster to use than the formal one. Because the

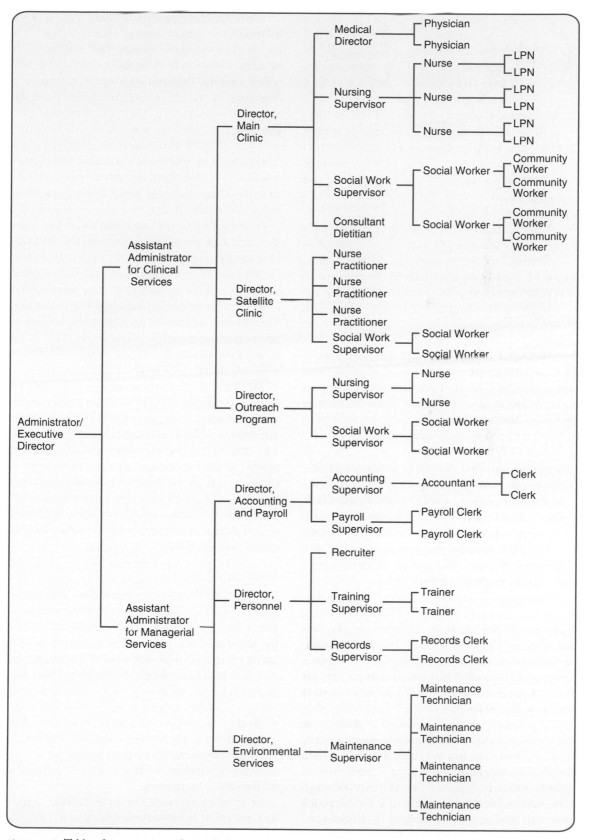

Figure 5.2 Table of organization of an ambulatory care center. *Adapted from DelBueno, D.J. (1987). An organizational checklist. Journal of Nursing Administration, 17(5), 30 33.*

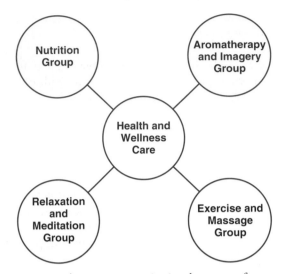

Figure 5.3 An organic organizational structure for a nontraditional wellness center. Based on Morgan, A. [1993]. *Imaginization: The art of creative management.* Newbury Park, Calif.: Sage.

informal ways of getting things done are seldom discussed (and certainly not a part of a new employee's orientation), it may take some time for you to figure out what they are and how to use them. Once you know they exist, they may be easier for you to identify. The following is an example:

> *Jocylene noticed that Harold seemed to get STAT x-rays done on his patients faster than she did. At lunch one day, Jocylene asked Harold why that happened. "That's easy," he said. "The people in x-ray feel unappreciated. I always tell them how helpful they are. Also, if you call and let them know that the patients are coming, they will get to them faster." Harold has just explained an informal process to Jocylene.*

Here is another example. Community Hospital recently installed a new EHR (electronic health record) system. Both the labs and the emergency department already had computerized record systems, but these old systems did not interface with the new hospital-wide system. Eventually, they would transition to the new system as well, but in the meantime they had to continue sharing information across departments. To do this, they created "workarounds," going back to paper reports that had to be sent to nursing units (Clancy, 2010). Although Community Hospital was officially paperless, the informal system had to develop a workaround during the transition to a hospital-wide EHR.

Sometimes, people are unwilling to discuss the informal processes. However, careful observation of the most experienced "system-wise" individuals in an organization will eventually reveal these processes. This will help you do things as efficiently as they do.

Power

There are times when one's attempts to influence others are overwhelmed by other forces or individuals. Where does this power come from? Who has it? Who does not?

In the earlier section on hierarchy, it was noted that although people at the top of the hierarchy have most of the *authority* in the organization, they do not have all of the *power*. In fact, the people at the bottom of the hierarchy also have some sources of power. This section explains how this can be true. First, power is defined, and then the sources of power available to people on the lower rungs of the ladder are considered.

Definition

Power is the ability to influence other people despite their resistance. Using power, one person or group can impose its will on another person or group (Haslam, 2001). The use of power can be positive, as when the nurse manager gives a staff member an extra day off in exchange for working an extra weekend, or negative, as when a nurse administrator transfers a "bothersome" staff nurse to another unit after that staff nurse pointed out a physician error (Talarico, 2004).

Sources

Isosaari (2011) calls organizations "systems of power" (p. 385). There are numerous sources of power. Many of them are readily available to nurses, but some of them are not. The following is a list derived primarily from the work of French, Raven, and Etzioni (Barraclough & Stewart, 1992; Isosaari, 2011):

- **Authority.** The power granted to an individual or a group to control resources and decision making by virtue of position within the organizational hierarchy.
- **Reward.** The promise of money, goods, services, recognition, or other benefits.
- **Control of Information.** The special knowledge an individual is believed to possess.

As Sir Francis Bacon said, "Knowledge is power" (Bacon, 1597, quoted in Fitton, 1997, p. 150).

- **Coercion.** The threat of pain or of some type of harm, which may be physical, economic, or psychological.

Power at Lower Levels of the Hierarchy

There is power at the bottom of the organizational ladder as well as at the top. Patients also have sources of power (Bradbury-Jones, Sambrook, & Irvine, 2007). Various groups of people in a health-care organization have different types of power available to them:

- *Managers* are able to reward people with salary increases, promotions, and recognition. They can also cause economic or psychological pain for the people who work for them, particularly through their authority to evaluate and fire people but also through the way they make assignments, grant days off, and so on.
- *Patients.* Considerable power over health-care decisions is associated with health-care professionals: their guidance is not often questioned by patients (Fredericks et al., 2012). The patient-centered care movement is directed to redistributing this power, involving patients and their families in decisions about their health care. For the most part, patients have not exerted the potential power that they possess. If patients refused to use the services of a particular organization, that organization would eventually cease to exist. Patients can reward health-care workers by praising them to their supervisors. They can also cause problems by complaining about them.
- *Assistants and technicians* may also appear to be relatively powerless because of their low positions in the hierarchy. Imagine, however, how the work of the organization (e.g., hospital, nursing home) would be impeded if all the nursing aides failed to appear one morning.
- *Registered nurses* have expert power and authority over licensed practical nurses, aides, and other personnel by virtue of their position in the hierarchy. They are critical to the operation of most health-care organizations and could cause considerable

trouble if they refused to work, another source of nurse power.

Fralic (2000) offered a good example of the power of information that nurses have always had: Florence Nightingale showed very graphically in the 1800s that far fewer wounded soldiers died when her nurses were present, and many more died when they were not. Think of the power of that information. Immediately, people were saying, "What would you like, Miss Nightingale? Would you like more money? Would you like a school of nursing? What else can we do for you?" She had solid data, she knew how to collect it, and she knew how to interpret and distribute it in terms of things that people valued (p. 340).

Empowering Nurses

This final section looks at several ways in which nurses, either individually or collectively, can maximize their power and increase their feelings of empowerment.

Power is the actual or potential ability to "recognize one's will even against the resistance of others," according to Max Weber (quoted in Mondros & Wilson, 1994, p. 5). *Empowerment* is a psychological state, a feeling of competence, control, and entitlement. Given these definitions, it is possible to be powerful and yet not feel empowered. *Power* refers to ability, and *empowerment* refers to feelings. Both are of importance to nursing leaders and managers.

Feeling empowered includes the following:

- **Self-determination.** Feeling free to decide how to do your work
- **Meaning.** Caring about your work, enjoying it, and taking it seriously
- **Competence.** Confidence in your ability to do your work well
- **Impact.** Feeling that people listen to your ideas, that you can make a difference (Spreitzer & Quinn, 2001)

The following contribute to nurse empowerment:

- **Decision making.** Control of nursing practice within an organization
- **Autonomy.** Ability to act on the basis of one's knowledge and experience (Manojlovich, 2007)

- **Manageable workload.** Reasonable work assignments
- **Reward and recognition.** Appreciation, both tangible (raises, bonuses) and intangible (praise) received for a job well done
- **Fairness.** Consistent, equitable treatment of all staff (Spence & Laschinger, 2005)

The opposite of empowerment is *disempowerment*. Inability to control one's own practice leads to frustration and sometimes failure. Work overload and lack of meaning, recognition, or reward produce emotional exhaustion and burnout (Spence, Laschinger, & Finegan, 2005). Nurses, like most people, want to have some power and to feel empowered. They want to be heard, to be recognized, to be valued, and to be respected. They do not want to feel unimportant or insignificant to society or to the organization in which they work.

Participation in Decision Making

The amount of power available to or exercised by a given group (e.g., nurses) *within* an organization can vary considerably from one organization to the next. Three sources of power are particularly important in health-care organizations:

- **Resources.** The money, materials, and human help needed to accomplish the work
- **Support.** Authority to take action without having to obtain permission
- **Information.** Patient care expertise and knowledge about the organization's goals and activities of other departments

In addition, nurses also need access to *opportunities:* opportunities to be involved in decision making, to be involved in vital functions of the organization, to grow professionally, and to move up the organizational ladder (Sabiston & Laschinger, 1995). Without these, employees cannot be empowered (Bradford & Cohen, 1998). Nurses who are part-time, temporary, or contract employees are less likely to feel empowered than full-time permanent employees, who generally feel more secure in their positions and connected to the organization (Kuokkanen & Katajisto, 2003). Managers and higher-level administrators can take actions to empower nursing staff by providing these opportunities.

Shared Governance

Nursing practice councils are an effective, although not simple, way to share decision making (Brody, Barnes, Ruble, & Sakowsk, 2012). Under shared governance, staff nurses may be included in the highest levels of decision making within the nursing department through representation on various councils that govern practice and management issues. These councils may set standards for patient safety, diversity, staffing, career ladders, evaluations, promotion, and the like. In many cases, a change in the organizational culture is necessary before shared governance can work (Currie & Loftus-Hills, 2002; Moore & Wells, 2010).

Genuine sharing of decision making is difficult to accomplish, partly because managers are reluctant to relinquish control or to trust their staff members to make wise decisions. Yet genuine empowerment of the nursing staff cannot occur without this sharing. Having some control over one's work and the ability to influence decisions are essential to empowerment (Manojlovich & Laschinger, 2002). For example, if staff members cannot control the budget for their unit, they cannot implement a decision to replace aides with registered nurses without approval from higher-level management. If they want increased autonomy in decision making about the care of individual patients, they cannot do so if opposition by another group, such as physicians, is given greater credence by the organization's administration.

Return to the example of the staff of the critical care department (Scenario 2). Why did the vice president for nursing tell the nurse manager that the plan would not be implemented?

Actually, the vice president for nursing thought the plan had some merit. He believed that the proposal to create a geriatric intensive care unit could save money, provide a higher quality of patient care, and result in increased nursing staff satisfaction. However, the critical care department was the centerpiece of the hospital's agreement with a nearby medical school. In this agreement, the medical school provided the services of highly skilled intensivists in return for the learning opportunities afforded their students. In its present form, the nurses' plan would not allow sufficient autonomy for the medical students, a situation that would not be acceptable to the medical school. The vice president knew that the board of trustees of the hospital believed their affiliation with the medical school brought a great deal of prestige to the organization and that they would not allow anything to interfere with this relationship.

"If shared governance were in place here, I think we could implement this or a similar model of care," he told the nurse manager.

"How would that work?" she asked.

"If we had shared governance, the nursing practice council would review the plan and, if they approved it, forward it to a similar medical practice council. Then committees from both councils would work together to figure out a way for this to benefit everyone. It wouldn't necessarily be easy to do, but it could be done if we had real collegiality between the professions. I have been working toward this model but haven't convinced the rest of the administration to put it into practice yet. Perhaps we could bring this up at the next nursing executive meeting. I think it is time I shared my ideas on this subject with the rest of the nursing staff."

In this case, the organizational goals and processes existing at the time the nurses developed their proposal did not support their idea. However, the vice president could see a way for it to be accomplished in the future. Implementation of genuine shared governance would make it possible for the critical care nurses to accomplish their goal.

Professional Organizations

Although the purposes of the American Nurses Association and other professional organizations are discussed in Chapter 14, these organizations are considered here specifically in terms of how they can empower nurses.

A collective voice, expressed through these organizations, can be stronger and is more likely to be heard than one individual voice. By joining together in professional organizations, nurses make their viewpoint known and their value recognized more widely. The power base of nursing professional organizations is derived from the number of members and their expertise in health matters.

Why there is power in numbers may need some explanation. Large numbers of active, informed members of an organization represent large numbers of potential voters to state and national legislators, most of whom wish to be remembered favorably in forthcoming elections. Large groups of people also have a "louder" voice: they can write

more letters, speak to more friends and family members, make more telephone calls, and generally attract more attention than small groups can.

Professional organizations can empower nurses in a number of ways:

- Collegiality, the opportunity to work with peers on issues of importance to the profession
- Commitment to improving the health and well-being of the people served by the profession
- Representation at the state or province and national level when issues of importance to nursing arise
- Enhancement of nurses' competence through publications and continuing education
- Recognition of achievement through certification programs, awards, and the media

Collective Bargaining

Like professional organizations, collective bargaining uses the power of numbers, in this case for the purpose of equalizing the power of employees and employer to improve working conditions, gain respect, increase job security, and have greater input into collective decisions (empowerment) and pay increases (Tappen, 2001). It can provide nurses with a stronger "voice," providing support and reducing fearfulness in speaking out about concerns (Seago et al., 2011). It may reduce staff turnover (Porter et al., 2010; Temple et al., 2011).

When people join for a common cause, they can exert more power than when they attempt to bring about change individually. Large numbers of people have the potential to cause more psychological or economic pain to an "opponent" (the employer in the case of collective bargaining) than an individual can. For example, the resignation of one nursing assistant or one nurse may cause a temporary problem, but it is usually resolved rather quickly by hiring another individual. If 50 or 100 aides or nurses call in "sick" or resign, however, the organization can be paralyzed and will have much more difficulty replacing these essential workers. Collective bargaining takes advantage of this power in numbers.

An effective collective bargaining contract can provide considerable protection to employees. However, the downside of collective bargaining (as with most uses of coercive power) is that it may encourage conflict rather than cooperation between employees and managers, an "us" against "them" environment (Haslam, 2001). Many nurses are also concerned about the effect that going out on strike might have on their patients' welfare and on their own economic security. Most administrators and managers prefer to operate within a union-free environment (Hannigan, 1998). Others are able to develop cooperative working relationships with their collective bargaining units, finding ways to work within the restrictions of a union contract and work together toward shared goals. For example, a Nursing Labor Management Partnership, part of a hospital-wide labor management partnership, was developed at Mt. Sinai Medical Center in New York (Porter, Kolcaba, McNulty, & Fitzpatrick, 2010). The mission of this partnership was for nurses and management to work together to achieve "unprecedented excellence" in patient care and create a positive work environment (p. 273). By respecting each other's differences and searching for common ground, nursing management and nursing union leaders worked together on shared goals such as reduction of nosocomial (due to hospitalization) pressure ulcers by 75% in 2 years. Another example of collaboration is from Shands Jacksonville Medical Center in Jacksonville, Florida. Nursing management wanted to institute a clinical ladder whereby nurses could achieve higher pay and higher clinical levels by completing certain requirements such as obtaining a higher degree, conducting a research study, or working on implementing an evidence-based change in practice. A traditional clinical ladder would conflict with the union's efforts to achieve pay equity, so the achievements were instead rewarded with bonuses for staff that did not affect their annual salaries (Lawson et al., 2011). It was a good way to achieve a win-win outcome for all involved.

Enhancing Expertise

Most health-care professionals, including nurses, are empowered to some extent by their professional knowledge and competence. You can take steps to enhance your competence, thereby increasing your sense of empowerment (Fig. 5.4):

- Participate in interdisciplinary team conferences and patient-centered conferences on your unit.
- Participate in continuing education offerings to enhance your expertise.

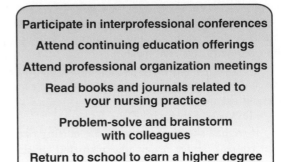

Figure 5.4 How to increase your expert power.

- Attend local, regional, and national conferences sponsored by relevant nursing and specialty organizations.
- Read journals and books in your specialty area.
- Participate in nursing research projects related to your clinical specialty area.
- Discuss with colleagues in nursing and other disciplines how to handle a difficult clinical situation.
- Observe the practice of experienced nurses.
- Return to school to earn a bachelor's degree and higher degrees in nursing.

You can probably think of more, but this list at least gives you some ideas. You can also share your knowledge and experience with other people. This means not only using your knowledge to improve your own practice but also communicating what you have learned to your colleagues in nursing and other professions. It also means letting your supervisors know that you have enhanced your professional competence. You can share your knowledge with your patients, empowering them as well. You may even reach the point at which you have learned more about a particular subject than most nurses have and want to write about it for publication.

Conclusion

Although most nurses are employed by health-care organizations, too few have taken the time to analyze the operation of their employing health-care organization and the effect it has on their practice. Understanding organizations and the power relationships within them will increase the effectiveness of your leadership.

Study Questions

1. Describe the organizational characteristics of a facility in which you currently have a clinical assignment. Include the following: the type of organization, its organizational culture, its structure, and its formal and informal goals and processes.

2. Define power, and describe how power affects the relationships between people of different disciplines (e.g., nursing, medicine, physical therapy, housekeeping, administration, finance, social work) in a health-care organization.

3. Discuss ways in which nurses can become more empowered. How can you use your leadership skills to do this?

Case Study to Promote Critical Reasoning

Tanya Washington will finish her associate's degree nursing program in 6 weeks. Her preferred clinical area is pediatric oncology, and she hopes to become a pediatric nurse practitioner one day. Tanya has received two job offers, both from urban hospitals with large pediatric units. Because several of her friends are already employed by these facilities, she asked them for their thoughts.

"Central Hospital is a good place to work," said one friend. "It is a dynamic, growing institution, always on the cutting edge of change. Any new idea that seems promising, Central is the first to try it. It's an exciting place to work."

"City Hospital is also a good place to work," said her other friend. "It is a strong, stable institution where traditions are valued. Any new idea must be carefully evaluated before it is adapted. It's been a pleasure to work there."

1. How would the organizational culture of each hospital affect a new graduate?

2. Which organizational culture do you think would be best for a new graduate, Central's or City's?

3. Would your answer differ if Tanya were an experienced nurse?

4. What do you need to know about Tanya before deciding which hospital would be best for her?

5. What else would you like to know about the two hospitals?

References

Aiken, L.H., Clarke, S.P., Sloane, D.M., Lake, C.T., et al. (2008). Effects of hospital care environments on patient mortality and nurse outcomes. *Journal of Nursing Administration, 38*(5), 223–229.

Armstrong, K.J., & Laschinger, H. (2006). Structural empowerment, magnet hospital characteristics, and patient safety culture. *Journal of Nursing Care Quality, 21*(2), 124–132.

Barraclough, R.A., & Stewart, R.A. (1992). Power and control: Social science perspectives. In Richmond, V.P., & McCroskey, J.C. (eds.). *Power in the classroom: Communication, control and concern.* Hillsdale, N.J.: Lawrence Erlbaum.

Berkow, S., Workman, J., Arson, S., Stewart, J., Virkotis, K., & Kahn, M. (2012). Strengthening frontline nurse investment in organizational goals. *Journal of Nursing Administration, 42*(3), 165–169.

Bradbury-Jones, C., Sambrook, S., & Irvine, F. (2007). Power and empowerment in nursing: A fourth theoretical approach. *Journal of Advanced Nursing, 62*(2), 258–266.

Bradford, D.L., & Cohen, A.R. (1998). *Power up: Transforming organizations through shared leadership.* New York: John Wiley & Sons.

Brody, A., Barnes, K., Ruble, C., & Sakowksi, J. (2012). Evidence-based practice councils: Potential path to staff nurse empowerment and leadership growth. *Journal of Nursing Administration, 42*(1), 28–33.

Cameron, K., & Quinn, R. (2006). *Diagnosing and changing organizational culture.* San Francisco: Jossey-Bass.

Clancey, T.R. (2010). Technology and complexity: Trouble brewing? *Journal of Nursing Administration, 40*(6), 247–249.

Connaughton, M.J., & Hassinger, J. (2007). Leadership character: Antidote to organizational fatigue. *Journal of Nursing Administration, 37*(10), 464–470.

Currie, L., & Loftus-Hills, A. (2002). The nursing view of clinical governance. *Nursing Standard, 16*(27), 40–44.

DelBueno, D.J. (1987). An organizational checklist. *Journal of Nursing Administration, 17*(5), 30–33.

Evans, M. (2013). Redesigning healthcare: Accountable care organization. *Modern Healthcare, 43*(12), 7.

Fitton, R.A. (1997). *Leadership: Quotations from the world's greatest motivators.* Boulder, Colo.: Westview Press.

Fralic, M.F. (2000). What is leadership? *Journal of Nursing Administration, 30*(7/8), 340–341.

Fredericks, S., Lapeim, J., Schwind, J., Beanlands, H., Romaniuk, D., & McCay, E. (2012). Discussion of patient-centered care in health care organizations. *Quality Management in Health Care, 21*(3), 127–134.

Frusti, D.K., Niesen, K.M., & Campion, J.K. (2003). Creating a culturally competent organization. *Journal of Nursing Administration, 33*(1), 33–38.

Hannigan, T.A. (1998). *Managing tomorrow's high-performance unions.* Westport, Conn.: Greenwood Publishing.

Haslam, S.A. (2001). *Psychology in organizations.* Thousand Oaks, Calif.: Sage.

Hinshaw, A.S. (2008). Navigating the perfect storm: Balancing a culture of safety with workforce. *Nursing Research, 57*(1S), S4–10.

Isosaari, U. (2011). Power in health care organizations: Contemplations from the first-line management perspective. *Journal of Health Organization and Management, 25*(4), 385–399.

Kuokkanen, L., & Katajisto, J. (2003). Promoting or impeding empowerment? *Journal of Nursing Administration, 33*(4), 209–215.

Laschinger, H.K.S., Wong, C., McMahon, L., & Kaufman, C. (1999). Leader behavior impact on staff nurse empowerment, job tension, and work effectiveness. *Journal of Nursing Administration, 29*(5), 28–39.

Lawson, L., Miles, K., Vallish, R., & Jenkins, S. (2011). Recognizing nursing professional growth and development in a collective bargaining environment. *Journal of Nursing Administration, 41*(5), 197–200.

Mackoff, B.L., & Triolo, P.K. (2008). Why do nurses, managers stay? Building a model of engagement: Part 2: Cultures of engagement. *Journal of Nursing Administration, 38*(4), 166–171.

Manojlovich, M. (2007). Power and empowerment in nursing: Looking backward to inform the future. *New Hampshire Nursing News, 12*(1), 14–16.

Manojlovich, M., & Laschinger, H.K. (2002). The relationship of empowerment and selected personality characteristics to nursing job satisfaction. *Journal of Nursing Administration, 32*(11), 586–595.

Mondros, J.B., & Wilson, S.M. (1994). *Organizing for power and empowerment.* New York: Columbia University Press.

Moore, S.C., & Wells, N.J. (2010). Staff nurses lead the way for improvement to shared governance structure. *Journal of Nursing Administration, 40*(11), 477–482.

Morgan, A. (1997). *Images of organization.* Thousand Oaks, Calif.: Sage.

Morgan, A. (1993). *Imaginization: The art of creative management.* Newbury Park, Calif.: Sage.

Nelson, W. (2013). The imperative of a moral compass-driven healthcare organization. *Frontiers of a Health Services Management, 30*(1), 39–45

Perera, F. & Peiro, M. (2012). Strategic planning in healthcare organizations. *Revista Española de Cardiología, 65*(8), 749–754.

Perrow, C. (1969). The analysis of goals in complex organizations. In Etzioni, A. (ed.). *Readings on modern organizations.* Englewood Cliffs, N.J.: Prentice-Hall.

Porter, C., Kolcaba, K., McNulty, S.R., & Fitzpatrick, J.J. (2010). A nursing labor management partnership model. *Journal of Nursing Administration, 40*(6), 272–276.

Purser, R.E., & Cabana, S. (1999). *The self-managing organization.* New York: Free Press (Simon & Schuster).

Redman, R.W. (2008). Symposium in tribute to a nursing leader: Ada Sue Hinshaw. *Nursing Research, 51*(15), S1–S3.

Roark, D.C. (2005). Managing the healthcare supply chain. *Nursing Management, 36*(2), 36–40.

Rosen, R.H. (1996). *Leading people: Transforming business from the inside out.* New York: Viking Penguin.

Sabiston, J.A., & Laschinger, H.K.S. (1995). Staff nurse work empowerment and perceived autonomy. *Journal of Nursing Administration, 28*(9), 42–49.

Schein, E.H. (2004). *Organizational culture and leadership.* New York: Jossey-Bass.

Scott-Findley, S., & Golden-Biddle, K. (2005). Understanding how organizational culture shapes research use. *Journal of Nursing Administration, 35*(7/8), 359–365.

Seago, J., Spetz, J., Ash, M., Herrera, C., & Keane, D. (2011). Hospital RN job satisfaction and nurse unions. *Journal of Nursing Administration, 41*(3), 109–114.

Spence, H.K., & Laschinger, J.F. (2005). Using empowerment to build trust and respect in the workplace: A strategy for addressing the nursing shortage. *Nursing Economics, 23*(1), 6–13.

Spreitzer, G.M., & Quinn, R.E. (2001). *A company of leaders.* San Francisco: Jossey-Bass.

Talarico, K.M. (2004, April 27). A look at power in nursing. *Vital Signs, 6–7,* 21.

Tappen, R.M. (2001). *Nursing leadership and management: Concepts and practice,* 4th ed. Philadelphia: F.A. Davis.

Temple, A., Dobbs, D., & Andel, R. (2011). Exploring correlates of turnover among nursing assistants in the hospital nursing home survey. *Journal of Nursing Administration, 41*(7/8), S34–S44.

Trinh, H.Q., & O'Connor, S.J. (2002). Helpful or harmful? The impact of strategic change on the performance of U.S. urban hospitals. *Health Services Research, 37*(1), 145–171.

Vogus, T.J., & Sutcliffe, K.M. (2007). The safety organizing scale: Development and validation of a behavioral measure of safety culture in hospital nursing units. *Medical Care, 45*(1), 46–54.

Weber, M. (1969). Bureaucratic organization. In A. Etzioni (ed.). *Readings on modern organizations.* Englewood Cliffs, N.J.: Prentice-Hall.

Weissman, J.S., Rothschild, J.M., Bendavid, E., Sprivulis, P., et al. (2007). Hospital workload and adverse events. *Medical Care, 45*(5), 448–455.

Yourstone, S.A., & Smith, H.L. (2002). Managing system errors and failures in health care organizations: Suggestions for practice and research. *Health Care Management Review, 27*(1), 50–61.

chapter 6

Communicating With Others and Working With the Interprofessional Team

Claude has been working in a busy oncology center for several years. The center uses an interprofessional team approach to client care. Claude manages a caseload of six to eight clients daily, and he believes that he provides safe, competent care and collaborates with other members of the interprofessional team. While Claude was on his way to deliver chemotherapy to a client recently diagnosed with osteosarcoma, the team nutritionist, Sonja, called to him, "Claude, come with me, please."

Claude responded, "Wait one minute. I need to hang the chemo on Mr. Juniper. I will come right after that. Where will you be?"

Sonja responded, "I need you now. There have been changes in Mrs. Alejandro's home care and medication regimen. I am trying to discuss how she needs to change her diet due to the medication changes. I can't seem to explain this to her. She keeps telling me she needs to eat 'cold foods' because she has

a 'hot stomach.' You seem to understand her better than I do." Claude stopped what he was doing and went to speak with Sonja and Mrs. Alejandro. While engaged in this conversation, the oncology nurse practitioner re-evaluated Mr. Juniper's lab values and physical condition. The advanced practice nurse (APRN) determined that Mr. Juniper should not receive his chemotherapy that day and should be sent to the hospital for further evaluation. The APRN wrote the order and went on to evaluate other patients without communicating the change to Claude. After Claude finished with Sonja, he returned to Mr. Juniper and proceeded to administer the chemotherapy. That night Mr. Juniper was admitted to the hospital with uncontrollable bleeding and sepsis.

Health-care professionals need to communicate clearly and effectively with each other. When they fail to do so, patient safety is at risk. In this case, the APRN failed to communicate a change in the patient's status. This resulted in a situation causing the patient's death.

Today's health-care system requires nurses to interact with more than physicians. Primary health-care providers include APRNs and physician assistants who work with physicians. Other disciplines involved in direct patient care include pharmacists, physical and occupational therapists, speech-language pathologists, and ancillary unlicensed personnel. Effective communication among all members of the health-care team is essential in the provision of safe patient care. Based on the changes in health care, the report from the Institute of Medicine (IOM), and the move toward an interprofessional model of providing health care, this chapter focuses on communication skills needed to work with members of the interprofessional team and providing information in a multicultural society.

Communication

People often assume that communication is simply giving information to another person. In fact, giving information is only a small part of communication. Communication models demonstrate that communication occurs on several levels and includes more than just giving information. Communication involves the spoken word as well as the nonverbal message, the emotional state of people involved, outside distractions, and the cultural background that affects their interpretation of the message. Superficial listening often results in misinterpretation of the message. An individual's attitude also influences what is heard and how the message is interpreted. Active listening is necessary to pick up all these levels of meaning in a communication.

Assertiveness in Communication

Nurses are integral members of the health-care team and often find themselves acting as "navigators" for patients as they guide them through the system. For this reason nurses need to develop assertive communication skills. Assertive behaviors allow people to stand up for themselves and their rights without violating the rights of others. Assertiveness is different from aggressiveness. People use aggressive behaviors to force their wishes or ideas on others. In assertive communication, an individual's position is stated clearly and firmly, using "I" statements. When working in an interprofessional environment, assertiveness assumes a greater importance as nurses need to act as patient advocates to ensure that patients receive safe, effective, and appropriate care. Using assertive communication helps in expressing your ideas and position; however, it does not necessarily guarantee that you will get what you want.

Interpersonal Communication

Communication is an integral part of our daily lives. Most daily communication qualifies as impersonal, such as interactions with salespeople or service personnel. Interpersonal communication is a process that gives people the opportunity to reflect, construct personal knowledge, and develop a sense of collective knowledge about others. Individuals use this form of communication to establish relationships to promote their personal and professional growth. This type of communication remains key to working effectively with others.

Interpersonal communication differs from general communication in that it includes several criteria. First, it is a selective process in that most general communication occurs on a superficial level. Interpersonal communication occurs on a more intimate level. It is a systemic process as it occurs within various systems and among the members within those systems (Wood, 2010). The work of the system influences how we communicate, where we communicate, and the meaning of the communication.

Interpersonal communication is also unique in that the individuals engaged in the communication are unique. Each person holds a specific role that influences the form and process of the communication, thus impacting the outcome. Finally, interpersonal communication is a dynamic and ongoing process. The communication changes based on the need and the existing situation.

Transactional models of communication differ from earlier linear models in that the transactional models label all individuals as communicators and not specifically as "senders" or "receivers." They highlight the dynamic process of interpersonal communication and the many roles individuals assume in these interactions. These models also allow for the fact that communication among and between individuals occurs simultaneously as the participants may be sending, receiving, and interpreting messages at the same time.

Transactional models acknowledge that noise, which interrupts communication, occurs in all interactions. Noise may assume many forms such as background conversations within the workplace or even spam or instant messages in the electronic milieu. Transactional models also include the concept of time, as communication among and between individuals changes over time and acknowledges that communication occurs within systems. These systems influence what people communicate and how they relay and process information.

Barriers to Communication Among Health-Care Providers and Health-Care Recipients

Successful interactions among health care providers and between those providers and their patients require effective communication. Many challenges exist that impede this communication. These include: (a) low health literacy; (b) cultural diversity; (d) cultural competence of health-care providers; and (d) lack of interprofessional communication education of providers (Schwartz, Lowe, & Sinclair, 2010).

Low Health Literacy

The IOM reports that approximately 90 million Americans lack the health literacy needed to meet their health-care needs (IOM, 2012). In the United States the estimated cost of low health literacy is between $106 and $236 billion (National Patient Safety Foundation, 2012). Individuals who lack the skills necessary to acquire and use health-care information are less likely to manage their chronic conditions and/or medication regimens effectively. For this reason they utilize health-care facilities more frequently and have higher mortality rates.

Cultural Diversity

Nurses work in environments rich in cultural diversity. This diversity exits among both professionals and patients. Culture affects communication in how the content is conveyed, emphasized, and understood. These factors affect how the communicators process and act on the information.

Cultural Competence

Cultural competence affects the way health-care providers interact with each other and with the populations they service. Cultural competence includes a set of similar behaviors, attitudes, and policies that, when joined together, enable individuals or groups to work effectively in cross-cultural situations (DHS, Office of Minority Health, 2013). To practice cultural competence, health-care professionals need to recognize and relate to how culture is reflected in each other and in the individuals with whom they interface.

Interprofessional Communication Education of Health-Care Providers

Challenges exist when communicating with professionals in other disciplines. Some difficulties in interprofessional communication are related to the use of concepts and terminology common to one specific discipline but not well understood by members of other professions. This interferes with another professional's understanding of the meaning or value of the situation.

Effective and safe health-care delivery requires nurses to be cognizant of these possible barriers to communication with patients and among members of the health-care team. When nurses and other members of the health-care team lack effective communication skills, patient safety is at risk. These barriers are outlined in Table 6-1.

Electronic Forms of Communication

Information Systems and E-Mail

Electronic Medical Records and Electronic Health Records

Communication through the use of computer technology is the norm today in nursing practice and health-care institutions. Electronic medical records (EMR) and documentation are used throughout health care. The Health Information Technology for Economic and Clinical Health (HITECH) Act mandated the use of the electronic health record (EHR) by the year 2015 (CMS, 2013). This organization developed Medicare and Medicaid incentive payment programs to help physicians and health-care institutions transition from traditional

table 6-1	
Barriers to Effective Communication in Health Care	
Low health literacy	Lack of the skills needed to access and use health information
Cultural diversity	Impedes the ability to access, understand, and utilize services and information.
Cultural competency of health-care providers	Lack of the ability of health-care providers to identify and consider cultural practices
Communication skills of health-care providers	Health-care providers lack the training needed for communicating with each other (interprofessional communication)

Source: Adapted from Schwartz, Lowe, & Sinclair (2010). Communication in health care: Consideration and strategies for successful consumer and team dialogue. Hypothesis, 8(1), 1–8.

record-keeping to EHR. According to the Department of Health and Human Services (DHHS), "EHR adoption has tripled since 2010, increasing to 44 percent in 2012 and computerized physician order entry has more than doubled (increased 168 percent) since 2008" (CMS, 2013).

Although the terms *electronic medical record* (EMR) and *electronic health record* (EHR) are used interchangeably, they differ in the types of information they contain. EMRs are the computerized clinical records produced in the health-care institution and health-care provider offices. They are considered legal documents regarding patient care within these settings. The EHR includes summaries of the EMR. EMRs are digital versions of the paper charts in the health-care provider's office. They contain the medical and treatment history of the patients within that specific health-care provider's practice. Some advantages of the EMR over paper charts include the ability of the health-care provider to:

■ Track data over time
■ Identify which patients need preventive screenings or checkups
■ Monitor patients status regarding health maintenance and prevention, such as blood pressure readings or vaccinations
■ Evaluate and improve overall quality of care within the specific practice

A disadvantage of the EMR is that it does not easily move *out* of the specific practice. Often the patient record needs to be printed and delivered by mail to specialists and other members of the care team.

EHR documents are shared among varying institutions/individuals such as insurance companies, the government, and the patients themselves

(CMS, 2013). EHRs focus on the total health of a patient extending beyond the data collected in the health-care provider's office. They provide a more inclusive view of a patient's care and are designed to share information with other health-care providers, such as laboratories and specialists, so they contain information from *all the clinicians involved in the patient's care.*

The use of electronic patient records allows health-care providers to retrieve and distribute patient information precisely and quickly. Decisions regarding patient care can be made more efficiently with less waiting time. Errors are reduced, patient safety is increased, and quality is improved. Information systems in many organizations also provide opportunities to access current, high-quality clinical and research data to support evidence-based practice (Gartee & Beal, 2012).

Because security safeguards are in place, EHRs also assist in maintaining patient confidentiality when compared to traditional paper systems. Health-care providers and institutions need to enforce processes to protect patient information through the use of passwords, limited accessibility, and compliance with laws, regulations, and acceptable standards. If a nurse attempts to obtain information on a patient not under his or her care, the institution may consider this a breach of security and patient confidentiality. Many institutions have strict policies in place that may result in a nurse losing his or her position if an electronic record is accessed when it is not necessary for the nurse's job. It is important to remember to always log off when using a computerized system. This helps to prevent security breaches.

The goal of computerized record-keeping is to provide safe, quality care to patients. It allows for tracking of quality controls. The use of BAR scanning prior to administering medications or obtain-

Potential Benefits of Computer-Based Patient Information Systems

- Increased hours for direct patient care
- Patient data accessible at bedside
- Improved accuracy and legibility of data
- Immediate availability of all data to all members of the team
- Increased safety related to positive patient identification, improved standardization, and improved quality
- Decreased medical errors
- Increased staff satisfaction

Adapted from Arnold, J., & Pearson, G. (eds.). (1992). Computer applications in nursing education and practice. New York: National League for Nursing.

ing blood samples for laboratory testing maintains quality and assists in ensuring patient safety.

Additional benefits of computerized systems for health-care applications are listed in Box 6-1.

E-Mail

E-mail has become a communication standard. Organizations use e-mail to communicate both within (intranet) and outside (Internet) of their systems. The same communication principles that apply to traditional letter writing pertain to e-mail. Using e-mail competently and effectively requires good writing skills. Remember, when communicating by e-mail, you are not only making an impression but also leaving a written record (Shea, 2000).

The rules for using e-mail in the workplace are somewhat different than for using e-mail among friends. Much of the humor and wit found in personal e-mail is not appropriate for the work setting. Emoticons are cute but not necessarily appropriate in the work setting.

Professional e-mail may remain informal. However, the message must be clear, concise, and courteous. Avoid common text abbreviations such as "LOL" or "BZ." Think about what you need to say before you write it. Then write it, read it, and reread it. Once you are satisfied that the message is appropriate, clear, and concise, send it.

Many executives read personal e-mail sent to them, which means that it is often possible to contact them directly. Many systems make it easy to send e-mail to everyone at the health-care institution. For this reason, it is important to keep e-mail professional. Remember the "chain of command": always go through the proper channels.

The fact that you have the capability to send e-mail instantly to large groups of people does not necessarily make sending it a good idea. Be careful if you have access to an all-company mailing list. It is easy to unintentionally send e-mail throughout the system. Consider the following example:

A respiratory therapist and a department administrator at a large health-care institution were engaged in a relationship. They started sending each other personal notes through the company e-mail system. One day, one of them accidentally sent one of these notes to all the employees at the health-care institution. Both employees were terminated. The moral of this story is simple: do not send anything by e-mail that you would not want published on the front page of a national newspaper or broadcasted on your favorite radio station.

Although voice tone cannot be "heard" in e-mail, the use of certain words and writing styles indicates emotion. A rude tone in an e-mail message may provoke extreme reactions. Follow the "rules of netiquette" (Shea, 2000) when communicating through e-mail. Some of these rules are listed in Box 6-2.

Text Messaging

Text messaging has evolved as a non-voice cell phone function among individuals. What started as a simple informal method of communication has evolved far beyond its initial intent. The average number of texts sent and received daily per cell phone user is growing rapidly. Texting as a brief, informal method of electronic communication between friends, close acquaintances, or automated systems has become the rule more than the exception.

Rules of Netiquette

1. If you were face-to-face, would you say this?
2. Follow the same rules of behavior online that you follow when dealing with individuals personally.
3. Send information only to those individuals who need it.
4. Avoid flaming; that is, sending remarks intended to cause a negative reaction.
5. Do not write in all capital letters; this suggests anger.
6. Respect other people's privacy.
7. Do not abuse the power of your position.
8. Proofread your e-mail before sending it.

Adapted from Shea, V. (2000). Netiquette. San Rafael, CA: Albion.

Presently, there are not any texting "rules." This permits mobile phone users to express themselves however they see fit. "Texters" frequently use short-hand abbreviations during such exchanges to replace longer, more commonly used phrases. Although texting has evolved as a widely accepted, even preferred, form of "talking," messages may be misinterpreted with the absence of voiced emotion and body language.

Business consultants predict that texting will evolve as an accepted form of electronic communication for certain occasions that require only simple questions and answers. When texting colleagues or departments, follow the same guidelines as you would for e-mail (Ruggieri, 2012). Confidential information should never be sent in a text message.

Reporting Patient Information

In today's health-care system, delivery methods involve multiple encounters and patient hand-offs among numerous health-care practitioners who have various levels of education and occupational training. Patient information needs to be communicated effectively and efficiently to ensure that critical information is relayed to each professional responsible for care delivery (O'Daniel and Rosenstein, 2008). If health care professionals fail to communicate effectively, patient safety is at risk for several reasons: (a) critical information may not be given, (b) information may be misinterpreted, (c) verbal or telephone orders may not be clear, and (d) changes in status may be overlooked. Medical errors easily occur given any one of these situations.

Hand-Off Communications

The transmission of crucial information and the accountability for care of the patient from one health-care provider to another is a fundamental component of communication in health care. Nurses traditionally give one another a "report." The hand-off report, often referred to as the change of shift report, has become the accepted method of communicating patient care needs from one nurse to another. However, with multiple providers involved in patient care, other professionals in addition to nurses are included in the hand-off report.

In the report, pertinent information related to events that occurred is given to the individuals responsible for providing continuity of care (Box 6-3). Although historically the report has been given face to face, there are newer ways to share information. Many health-care institutions use audiotape and computer printouts as mechanisms for sharing information. These mechanisms allow the nurses and other providers from the previous shift to complete their tasks and those assuming care to make inquiries for clarification as necessary.

In 2009, the Joint Commission incorporated "managing hand-off communications" in its national patient safety goals (TJC, 2013). The report should be organized, concise, and complete, with relevant details. Not every unit uses the same system for giving a hand-off report. The system is easily modified according to the pattern of nursing care delivery and the types of patients serviced. For example, many intensive care units, because of their small size and the more acute needs of their patients, use walking rounds as a means for giving the report.

---

box 6-3

Information for Change-of-Shift Report (Hand-Off)

- Identify the patient, including the room and bed numbers.
- Include the patient diagnosis.
- Account for the presence of the patient on the unit. If the patient has left the unit for a diagnostic test, surgery, or just to wander, it is important for the oncoming staff members to know the patient is off the unit.
- Provide the treatment plan that specifies the goals of treatment. Note the goals and the critical pathway steps either achieved or in progress. Personalized approaches can be developed during this time and patient readiness for those approaches evaluated. It is helpful to mention the patient's primary care physician. Include new orders and medications and treatments currently prescribed.
- Document patient responses to current treatments. Is the treatment plan working? Present evidence for or against this. Include pertinent laboratory values as well as any negative reactions to medications or treatments. Note any comments the patient has made regarding the hospitalization or treatment plan that the oncoming staff members need to address.
- Omit personal opinions and value judgments about patients as well as personal/confidential information not pertinent to providing patient care. If you are using computerized information systems, make sure you know how to present the material accurately and concisely.

This system allows nurses and others involved in patient care to discuss the current patient status and to set goals for care for the next several hours. Together, the nurses gather objective data as one nurse ends a shift and another begins. This way, there is no confusion as to the patient's status at shift change. This same system is often used in emergency departments and labor and delivery units. Larger patient care units may find the "walking report" time-consuming and an inefficient use of resources.

It is helpful to take notes or create a worksheet while listening to the report. Many institutions now provide a computerized action plan to assist with gathering accurate and concise information during the hand-off report. A worksheet helps organize the work for the day (Fig. 6.1). As specific tasks are mentioned, the nurse assuming responsibility makes a note of the activity in the appropriate time slot. Patient status, medications, and treatments should be documented. Any priority interventions should also be identified at this time. Many institutions are now using electronic tablets to assist nurses and other health-care providers to organize and track activities.

Any changes from the previous day are noted, particularly when the nurse is familiar with the patient. Recording changes counteracts the tendency to remember what was done the day before and repeat it, often without checking for new orders. During the day, the worksheet acts as a reminder of the tasks that have been completed and of those that still need to be done.

Reporting skills improve with practice. When presenting information in a hand-off report, certain details must be included. Begin the report by identifying the patient, room number, age, gender, and health-care provider. Also include the admitting as well as current diagnoses. Address the expected treatment plan and the patient's responses to the treatment. For example, if the patient has had multiple antibiotics and a reaction occurred, this information must be relayed to the next nurse. Avoid making value judgments and offering personal opinions about the patient (Fig. 6.2).

Communicating With the Health-Care Provider

The function of professional nurses in relation to their patients' health-care providers is to communicate changes in the patient's condition, share other pertinent information, discuss modifications of the treatment plan, and clarify orders. This can be stressful for a new graduate who still has some role insecurity. Using good communication skills and having the necessary information at hand are helpful when discussing patient needs.

Before calling a health-care provider, make sure that all the information needed is available. The provider may want more clarification about the situation. If calling to report a drop in a patient's blood pressure, be sure to have the list of the patient's medications, the last time the patient received the medications, laboratory results, vital signs, and blood pressure trends. Also be prepared to provide a general assessment of the patient's present status.

There are times when a nurse calls a physician or health-care provider and the health-care provider does not return the call. It is important to document all health-care provider contacts in the patient's record. Many units keep calling logs. In the log, enter the health-care provider's name, the date, the time, the reason for the call, and the time the health-care provider returned the call. If the provider does not return the call in a reasonable amount of time, or patient safety is in jeopardy, the nurse should follow chain of command to make sure patient safety is maintained.

ISBARR

In response to the number of patients who die from or confront a preventable adverse event during hospitalization, health-care institutions have been challenged to improve patient safety standards. This challenge forced health-care institutions to look at the causes of most sentinel events within their environments. Originally known as SBAR (Situation, Background, Assessment, and Recommendation), the communication technique has recently been updated to ISBARR or ISBAR. ISBARR is an acronym for *I*ntroduction, *S*ituation, *B*ackground, *A*ssessment, *R*ecommendation, and *R*ead-back (Enlow, Shanks, Guhde, & Perkins, 2010; Haig, Sutton, & Whittingdon, 2006). Whether referred to as SBAR or ISBARR, the technique provides a framework for communicating critical patient information in a systemized and organized fashion. The ISBARR method focuses on the immediate situation so that decisions regarding patient care may be made quickly and safely.

Name _____ Room # _____ Allergies _____

0700	0800	0900	1000	1100	1200	1300	1400	1500	1600	1700	1800

Name _____ Room # _____ Allergies _____

0700	0800	0900	1000	1100	1200	1300	1400	1500	1600	1700	1800

Name _____ Room # _____ Allergies _____

0700	0800	0900	1000	1100	1200	1300	1400	1500	1600	1700	1800

Figure 6.1 Organization and time management schedule for patient care.

Although originally established by the U.S. Navy as SBAR to accurately communicate critical information, the technique was adapted by Kaiser-Permanente as an "escalation tool" to be implemented when a rapid change in patient status occurs or is imminent. Both the Joint Commission and the Institute for Health Care Improvement have mandated that health-care institutions employ a standardized reporting/hand-off system and promote the use of the SBAR technique (Haig,

Room # _____ Patient Name _____ Diagnoses _____

Diet _____ Activity _____

1900	0100
2000	0200
2100	0300
2200	0400
2300	0500
2400	0600

Figure 6.2 Patient information report.

Sutton, & Whittingdon; www.rwjf.org, 2013; IHI, 2006; TJC, 2009). The use of the ISBARR format helps to standardize a communication system to effectively transmit needed information to provide safe and effective patient care. Table 6-2 defines the steps of the ISBARR communication model.

The implementation of ISBARR as a communication technique has demonstrated success in reducing adverse events and improving patient safety. It also allows nurses, health-care providers, and members of the interprofessional team to communicate in a collegial and professional manner.

Health-Care Provider Orders

Professional nurses are responsible for accepting, transcribing, and implementing health-care provider orders. It is important to remember that nurses may only receive orders from physicians, dentists, podiatrists, and advanced practice registered nurses (APRNs) who are licensed and credentialed in the state in which they are working.

table 6-2

ISBARR (Introduction, Situation, Background, Assessment, Recommendation, Read-Back)

Elements	Description	Example
Introduction	Identification of yourself, your role, and location	Hello, my name is ●●●. I am the nurse at (location) for your patient <name>.
Situation	Brief description of the existing situation	Critical laboratory value that needs to be addressed (critical blood gas value, International Normalized Ratio [INR], etc.)
Background	Medical, nursing, or family information that is significant to the care and/or patient condition	Patient admitted with a pulmonary embolus and on heparin therapy, receiving oxygen at 4 L via nasal cannula; what steps have been taken
Assessment	Recent assessment data that indicate the most current clinical state of the patient	Vital signs, results of laboratory values, lung sounds, mental status, pulse oximetry results, electrocardiogram results
Recommendation	Information for future interventions and/or activities	Monitor patient Change heparin dose Repeat INR Repeat computed tomography or ventilation- perfusion scan
Read-Back	Repeat or re-state any new orders or recommendations for clarity	Repeat the recommendations back to the HCP, or member of the interprofessional health-care team Repeat the INR and change the heparin dose to 1,500 units; repeat the VQ scan and call with the results.

Orders written by medical students need to be countersigned by a physician or APRN before implementation.

The three main types of orders are written, telephone, and faxed. Some health-care institutions are looking into the possibility of receiving health-care provider orders through e-mail. These orders include the provider's name, date, and time and provide an electronic record of the order.

Written orders are dated and placed on the appropriate institutional form. The health-care provider gives *telephone orders* directly to the nurse by telephone. Faxed orders come directly from the health-care provider office and need to be initialed by the provider. Telephone orders, e-mail orders, and faxed orders also need to be signed when the health-care provider comes to the nursing unit. It is important to verify the institution's policy on telephone, e-mail, and faxed orders.

Many health-care institutions are moving to maintaining the EMR and away from verbal orders as the health-care provider is present and can enter the order on the appropriate form in the patient's record. A telephone order needs to be written on the appropriate institutional form, the time and date noted, and the form signed as a telephone order by the nurse.

When receiving a telephone order, repeat it back to the physician for confirmation. If the health-care provider is speaking too rapidly, ask him or her to speak more slowly. Then repeat the information for confirmation. If a faxed document is unclear, call the health-care provider for clarification. Most institutions require the health-care provider to cosign the order within 24 hours.

Professionalism and a courteous attitude by all parties are necessary to maintain collegial relationships with physicians and other health-care professionals. One nurse explained their importance as follows:

RN satisfaction simply is not about money. A major factor is how well nurses feel supported in their work. Do people listen to us—our managers, upper management, human resources? Being able to communicate with each other—to be able to speak directly with your peers, physicians, or managers in a way that is nonconfrontational—is really important to having good working relationships and to providing good care. You need to have mutual respect. (Quoted by Trossman, 2005, p. 1.)

This statement finds support in the IOM report (2010) and research conducted by the American Nurses Credentialing Center (ANCC), which holds responsibility for MAGNET designation (ANCC, 2012).

Teams

Teams and teamwork are everyday terms in today's organizations. Teams bring together the variety of skills, perspectives, and talents that create an effective work environment. Nursing is a "team sport." In other words, nurses bring a specific set of skills and talents and need to work together with other professionals to achieve a common goal. The goal in this case is quality patient care. Health-care providers understand that safe quality patient care thrives in an environment that promotes interprofessional teamwork and collaboration. Not all teams are interprofessional teams, and it is important to understand that a team does not necessarily infer collaboration.

In 2004, the IOM revealed that issues surrounding nursing competency contributed in part to ensuring patient safety. Some of the issues revolved around the lack of communication among nurses and other members of the health-care team, including medicine, pharmacy, and other supportive services. The Quality and Safety Education for Nurses (QSEN) addressed these concerns and looked at collaboration and teamwork as a way of decreasing medical errors and promoting quality care.

QSEN (2011) defined *teamwork* as the ability to perform "effectively within nursing and interprofessional teams, fostering open communication, mutual respect, and shared decision-making to achieve quality patient care" (http://qsen.org/competencies/pre-licensure-ksas/#teamwork_collaboration). Kalisch and Lee (2011) conducted a study that looked at staffing, teamwork, and collaboration. The study supported the fact that teamwork contributes to safe quality care; however, health-care institutions need to provide adequate staffing to ensure collaboration and teamwork. Health-care institutions that choose to apply for MAGNET status must demonstrate how they provide adequate staffing that promotes teamwork and interprofessional collaboration.

Learning to Be a Team Player

When asking for assistance, nothing is more frustrating to hear than "Oh, he's not my patient" or "I have my own mess to deal with, I certainly can't help you." A team player states, "I have not seen that patient yet today, but let me help get that information for you," or ""How can I be of assistance?"

Every team member brings value to the team through personal strengths and specific skill sets. To develop a strong team, members must treat each other with dignity and respect. They also must understand the role and scope of practice of each discipline. It is important for each member to identify personal strengths, limitations, and competencies in order to function as a contributing member of the team.

Team players consistently treat other members with courtesy and consideration. They demonstrate commitment, understand the team's goals, and support other team members appropriately. They care about the work and purpose of the team and they contribute to its success. Team players with commitment look beyond their own workload and provide support and assistance when and where needed (Nelson & Economy, 2010). The goal in the health-care setting is safe, quality patient care.

Building a Working Team

Building a strong team takes time and talent. Assuming that all the team members possess the skills sets that are needed, how do you create an efficient team? Brounstein (2002) identified 10 qualities of an effective team player (Box 6-4). These qualities provide the foundation for a strong professional team.

To build an effective team, first identify the team players and focus on the strengths and weaknesses of each. While building on the strengths, devise a plan to assist team members in improving their weaknesses. Second, make sure that the team understands the goal and is committed to achieving that outcome. In health care the primary goal is safe, quality patient care. Third, act as a role model and exhibit the expected behaviors. Fourth, reward the team for accomplishments and achievements, discuss setbacks, and together create an improvement plan.

---

box 6-4

Ten Qualities of an Effective Team Player

1. Demonstrates dependability
2. Communicates constructively
3. Engages in active listening
4. Actively participates
5. Shares information openly and willingly
6. Supports and offers assistance
7. Displays flexibility
8. Exhibits loyalty to the team
9. Acts as a problem solver
10. Treats others in a courteous and considerate manner

Adapted from Brounstein, M. (2002). Managing teams for dummies. NY: John Wiley & Sons.

Interprofessional Collaboration and the Interprofessional Team

Although building an interprofessional team seems practical, it requires a commitment and collaboration among members of all the disciplines (O'Daniel & Rosenstein, 2008). The IOM (2010), the National League for Nursing (NLN) (2012), the American Association of Colleges of Nursing (AACN) (2011), and the American Organization of Nurse Executives (AONE) (2012) issued statements supporting collaboration among all members of the health-care team with the purpose of providing safe, effective care and achieving positive patient outcomes. Research demonstrates that patient care provided by integrated teams composed of health-care professionals who understand each other's functions and goals results in better clinical outcomes and greater patient satisfaction (Hale, 2011). As simple as this concept seems, it takes an integrated and dedicated approach to form a collaborative interprofessional team.

Interprofessional Collaboration

The World Health Organization (WHO) (2010) defines *interprofessional collaboration* as occurring when "multiple health workers from different professional backgrounds work together with patients, families, caregivers, and communities to deliver the highest quality care." Collaboration differs from cooperation. Cooperation means working with someone in the sense of enabling: making them more able to do something (typically by providing information or resources they wouldn't otherwise have). Collaborating (from Latin *laborare,* to work) requires working alongside someone to achieve something (Martin, Ummenhofer, Manser, & Spirig, 2010).

The fundamental difference between collaboration and cooperation is the level of formality in the relationships between agencies and/or stakeholders. For many years members of other health-care disciplines cooperated with each other. Nurses and physicians cooperated with each other in patient care delivery. However, inequalities existed between the disciplines regarding shared expertise and power (Robert Woods Johnson Foundation, 2013).

A true collaborative effort comprises the following key components: sharing, partnership, interdependency, and power (O'Brien, 2013). Collaboration assumes that members share responsibility, values, and resources. To engage in partnership, members need to be honest and open with each other, demonstrate mutual trust and respect, and value each other's contributions and perspectives. Members of an interprofessional team are dependent on each other and work with each other to achieve a common goal. Finally, power is shared among the members. The health professionals recognize their own individual scope of practice and skill set, while demonstrating an appreciation for the other members' capabilities and contributions. They also share in the accountability for the delivery of patient care. This shared effort among health-care professionals helps to coordinate care and promote patient safety.

Interprofessional Communication

Breakdowns in verbal and written communication among health-care providers present a major concern in the health-care delivery system. The Joint Commission (www.tjc.org) attributes a high percentage of sentinel events to poor communication among health-care providers (2009, 2013). Communication is considered to be a core competency to promote interprofessional collaborative practice. Using a common language among the professions assists in understanding and overcoming barriers to interprofessional communication.

The SBAR method was discussed earlier in the chapter. A team-related method of communication, Team STEPPS, developed by the Department of Defense (DoD) and the Agency for Healthcare Research and Quality (AHRQ), is another method. The purpose of this teamwork system is to improve collaboration and communication related to patient safety (AHRQ, 2013). This method includes four skills: leadership, situation monitoring, mutual support, and communication. The program goals focus on (a) creating highly effective medical teams that optimize the use of information, people, and resources to achieve the best clinical outcomes for patients; (b) increasing team awareness and clarifying team roles and responsibilities; (c) resolving conflicts and improving information sharing; and (d) eliminating barriers to quality and safety. The program is composed of training modules available to health-care institutions.

With the goal of collaboration among health-care professionals, to promote continuity of care and facilitate communication, many health-care institutions have created a position known as the "nurse navigator." The function of the navigator is to coordinate patient care by guiding patients through the diagnostic process, educating and supporting them, integrating care with other members of the interprofessional team, and assisting them in making informed decisions (Brown, Cantril, McMullen, Barkly, Dietz, Murphy, & Fabrey, 2012).

Nurses remain an integral part of the interprofessional health-care team. Nurses usually have the most contact with the patients and their families. They often find themselves in the particularly advantageous position to observe the patient's responses to treatments and report these back to the interprofessional team. For example:

> *Mr. Richards, a 68-year-old man, was in a motor vehicle accident and sustained a traumatic brain injury. He had right-sided weakness and dysphagia. The health-care provider requested evaluations and treatment plans from speech pathology, physical therapy, and social services. The speech pathologist conducted a swallow study and determined that Mr. Richards should receive pureed foods for the next 2 days. The RN assigned an LPN to feed Mr. Richards a pureed lunch. The LPN reported that although Mr. Richards had done well the previous day, he had difficulty swallowing even pureed foods today. The RN immediately notified the speech pathologist, and a new treatment plan was developed.*

Building an Interprofessional Team

Effective interprofessional teams include several characteristics and focus on the needs of the patient or client, not the individual contributions of the team members. Each member understands the characteristics of collaboration and demonstrates a willingness to share, recognize the others' expertise, and participate in open communication. Members of a team share information through verbal and written communication in an interprofessional team conference. The characteristics of an effective interprofessional health-care team are listed in Box 6-5.

Interprofessional teams communicate by engaging in conferences. The conference begins with the presenter stating the patient's name, age, and diagnoses. Each team member then explains the goal of his or her discipline, the interventions, and the intended outcome. Effectiveness of treatment, development of new interventions, and the setting

box 6-5
Characteristics of Effective Interprofessional Health-care Teams
1. Members provide care to a common group of patients/clients.
2. Members develop common goals for patient/client outcomes and work together to achieve the goals.
3. Members have roles and functions and understand their roles and the roles of others.
4. The team develops a mechanism for sharing information.
5. The team creates a system to supervise the implementation of plans, evaluate outcomes, and make adjustments based on the results.

of new goals are discussed. All members contribute and participate, demonstrating mutual respect and valuing the expertise of the others. A method to oversee the implementation of the plan is devised in order to assess outcomes, and make adjustments as needed. The nurse (or nurse navigator) is often the individual who assumes the responsibility for this oversight. The key to a successful interprofessional conference is presenting information in a clear, concise manner and ensuring input from all disciplines and levels of care providers, from nursing assistive personnel (NAP) to health-care providers.

Conclusion

The responsibility for delivering and coordinating patient care is an important part of the role of the professional nurse. To accomplish this, nurses need good communication skills. Being assertive without being aggressive and interacting with others in a professional manner enhance the relationships that nurses develop with colleagues, health-care providers, and other members of the interprofessional team.

A major focus of the national safety goals is improved communication among health-care professionals and the development of interprofessional health-care teams. In an effort to improve patient safety, health-care institutions have implemented communication protocols referred to as the SBAR method or Team STEPPS. SBAR sets a specific procedure that reminds nurses how to relay information quickly and effectively to the patient's health-care provider, which ultimately leads to improved patient outcomes. Team STEPPS, developed by the DoD, assists health-care institutions in promoting patient safety through communication and coordination of patient care.

Collaboration and teamwork encourage interprofessional collegial relationships that promote safe quality patient care. Key nursing organizations, the IOM, QSEN, and MAGNET criteria address the need for collaboration and teamwork. Nurses act as the key players in ensuring interprofessional communication and collaboration in patient care delivery.

Finally, health-care institutions need to be committed to creating an environment that promotes communication and team collaboration. This needs to come from the top down and the bottom up to create an organizational culture that promotes patient safety. Nurses are in a unique position to act as change agents within their organizations by practicing safe, effective patient care, promoting collegial communications, and committing themselves to interprofessional collaboration.

Study Questions

1. This is your first position as an RN, and you are working with an LPN who has been on the unit for 20 years. On your first day she says to you, "The only difference between you and me is the size of the paycheck." Demonstrate how you would respond to this statement, using assertive communication techniques.

2. A health-care provider orders "Potassium Chloride 20 milliequivalents IV over 20 minutes." You realize that this is a dangerous order. How would you approach the health-care provider?

3. A patient is admitted to the same-day surgical center for a breast biopsy. Her significant other, who has just had an altercation with an admissions secretary about their insurance, accompanies her. The patient is met by a nurse navigator who notes that the mammogram and blood work are not in the electronic medical record. The patient's significant other says, "What is wrong with you people? Can't you ever get anything straight? If you can't get the insurance right, and you can't get the diagnostic tests right, how can we expect you to get the surgery right?" How should the nurse navigator assist the patient and her significant other?

4. Your nurse manager asks you to develop an interprofessional team on the unit. This team is to serve as a model for other nursing units. How would you start the process? What qualities would you look for in the team members?

Case Study to Promote Critical Reasoning

Corel Jones is a new nursing assistive personnel (NAP) who has been assigned to your acute rehabilitation unit. Corel is a hard worker; he comes in early and often stays late to finish his work. However, Corel is gruff with the patients, especially with the male patients. If a patient is reluctant to get out of bed, Corel often challenges him, saying, "Hey, let's go. Don't be such a wimp. Move your big butt." Today, you overheard Corel telling a female patient who said she did not feel well, "You're just a phony. You like being waited on, but that's not why you're here." The woman started to cry.

1. You are the newest staff nurse on this unit. How would you handle this situation? What would happen if you ignored it?

2. If you decided to pursue the issue, with whom should you speak? What would you say?

3. What do you think is the reason Corel speaks to patients this way?

References

Agency for Healthcare Research and Quality (AHRQ). (2013). *Team STEPPS*. Retrieved September 25, 2013, from http://teamstepps.ahrq.gov

American Association of Colleges of Nursing (AACN). (2011). Core competencies for interprofessional collaboration. Retrieved September 23, 2013, from www.aacn.nche.edu/leading-initiatives/IPECReport.pdf

American Nurses Credentialing Center (ANCC). (2012). MAGNET designated hospitals demonstrate lower mortality rates. Retrieved from www.medscape.com/viewarticle/773611

American Organization of Nurse Executives (AONE). (2012). AONE guiding principles: AACN-AONE task force on academic-practice partnerships. American Organization of Nurse Executives.

Bello, J., Quinn, P., & Horrell, L. (2011). Maintaining Patient Safety Through Innovation: An Electronic SBAR Communication Tool. *Computers Informatics and Nursing, 29*(9), 481–483.

Brounstein, M. (2002). *Managing teams for dummies.* NY: John Wiley & Sons.

Brown, C.G., Cantril, C., McMullen, L., Barkely, D.L., Dietz, M., Murphy, C.M., & Fabrey, L.J. (2012). Oncology nurse navigator role delineation study: An oncology nursing society report. *Clinical Journal of Oncology Nursing, 16*(6), 581–585.

Centers for Medicare and Medicaid Services (CMS), (2013). Research, statistics data and systems. Retrieved from www.cms.gov/Research-Statistics-Data-and-Systems/Statistics-Trends-and-Reports/MedicareMedicaidStatSupp/2010.html

Centers for Medicare and Medicaid Services (CMS). (2013). Meaningful use. Retrieved from www.cms.gov/apps/media/press/release.asp?Counter=4554&intNumPerPage=10&checkDate=&checkKey=&srchType=1&numDays=3500&sr.

Centers for Medicare and Medicaid Services (CMS). (2013). EHR Incentive programs. Retrieved from www.cms.gov/ cmsincentiveprograms

Department of Health and Human Services Office of Minority Health. (2013). Retrieved from http://minorityhealth.hhs.gov/templates/browse.aspx?lvl=2&lvlID=11

Enlow, M., Shanks, L., Guhde, J., & Perkins, M. (2010). Incorporating interprofessional communication Skills (ISBARR) into an undergraduate nursing curriculum. *Nurse Educator, 35*(4), 176–180.

Gabor, D. (1994). *Speaking your mind in 101 difficult situations.* New York: Stonesong Press (Simon & Schuster).

Gartee, R., & Beal, S. (2012). *Electronic health records and nursing.* Boston, MA: Pearson.

Haig, K.M., Sutton, S., & Whittingdon, J. (2006). SBAR: A shared mental model for improving communication between clinicians. *Journal on Quality and Patient Safety, 32*(3), 167–175.

Hale, J. F. (2011). The value and imperative for health professions engaging in interprofessional learning. Retrieved September 28, 2013, from www.umassmed.edu/uploadedFiles/fmch/Community_Health/IPE%20%20Update%20for%20Clerkship%20Booklet_hale2011.docx

Institute for Healthcare Improvement. (2006). Using SBAR to improve communication between caregivers. Retrieved November 30, 2008, from www.ihi.org/IHI/Programs/AudioAndWebPrograms/WebACTIONUsingSBARtoImproveCommunication.htm?TabId=7

Institute of Medicine (IOM), (2010). The future of nursing: leading change, advancing health. Committee on the Robert Wood Johnson Foundation Initiative on the Future of Nursing at the Institute of Medicine; Institute of Medicine. www.nap.edu/catalog/12956.html.

Institute of Medicine (IOM). (2012). Public health literacy. Retrieved September 26, 2013, from www.iom.edu/~/media/Files/Activity%20Files/PublicHealth/HealthLiteracy/HealthLiteracyFactSheets_Feb6_2012_Parker_JacobsonFinal1.pdf

Kalisch, B.J., & Lee, K.H. (2011). Nurse staffing levels and teamwork: A cross-sectional study of seven patient care units in acute care hospitals. *Journal of Nursing Scholarship, 43*(1), 82–88.

Martin, J.S., Ummenhofer, W., Manser, T., & Spirig, R. (2010). Interprofessional collaboration among nurses and physicians: Making a difference in patient outcome. *Swiss Medical Weekly.* May 4, 2010, 1–12. Retrieved September 26, 2013, from www.snw.ch

National Patient Safety Foundation. (2012). Health literacy: Statistics at a glance. Retrieved September 26, 2013, from www.npsf.org/wpcontent/uploads/2011/12/AskMe3_Stats_English.pdf

Nelson, B., & Economy, P. (2010). *Managing for dummies (3rd ed.).* New York: John Wiley & Sons.

O'Brien, J. (2013). Interprofessional collaboration. *AMN Healthcare Education.* Retrieved September 26, 2013, from www.rn.com

O'Daniel, M., & Rosenstein, A. H. (2008). Professional communication and team collaboration. In Hughes, R.G., *Patient Safety and Quality: An Evidence-Based Handbook for Nurses.* Retrieved September 26, 2013, from www.ncbi.nlm.nih.gov/books/NBK2651

O'Malley, P.A. (2008). Profile of a professional. *Nursing Management, 39*(6), 24–27.

Robert Woods Johnson Foundation. (2013). How to foster interprofessional collaboration between physicians and nurses? Robert Woods Johnson Foundation. January 9, 2013. Retrieved September 25, 2013, from www.sjcg.net/departments/education/faq/aspx

Ruggieri, C. (2012). Is texting appropriate in business communication? Washington University School of Business. Retrieved February 28, 2013, from managerialcommunication.wordpress.com

Schwartz, F., Lowe, M., & Sinclair, L. (2010). Communication in health care: Consideration and strategies for successful consumer and team dialogue. *Hypothesis, 8*(1), 1–8.

Shea, V. (2000). *Netiquette.* San Rafael, CA: Albion.

The Joint Commission (TJC). (2013). Manual for Joint Commission national quality measures (v2013A1). Retrieved February 28, 2013, from https://manual.jointcommission.org/releases/TJC2013A/

Trossman, S. (2005). Who you work with matters. *American Nurse, 37*:4, 1, 8. American Nurses Association.

Wood, J.T. (2010). The interpersonal imperative. In *Interpersonal Communication: Everyday encounters* (6th ed.). Boston, MA: Cengage Learning.

World Health Organization (WHO). (2010). Framework for Action on Interprofessional Education & Collaborative Practice. Retrieved September 26, 2013, from http://whqlibdoc.who.int/hq/2010/WHO_HRH_HPN_10.3_eng.pdf

chapter 7

Delegation and Prioritization of Client Care

Ora, a new graduate, just completed her orientation. She works from 7 p.m. to 7 a.m. on a busy, monitored neuroscience unit. The client census is 48, making this a full unit. Although there is an associate nurse manager for the shift, Ora acts as the charge nurse. Her responsibilities include receiving and confirming orders, contacting physicians with any information or requests, accessing laboratory reports from the computer, reviewing them and giving them to the appropriate staff members, checking any new medication orders and placing them in the appropriate medication administration records, relieving the monitor technician for dinner and breaks, and assigning staff to dinner and breaks. When Ora arrives to work, she discovers that one registered nurse (RN) called in sick. Her staff tonight consists of two RNs and three nursing assistive personnel (NAP). To complicate matters, the

institution just rolled out a new computerized acuity-based staffing model last week, and she needs to enter the complexity level of care for each client. She panics and wants to refuse to take report. After a discussion with the charge nurse from the previous shift, she realizes that refusing to take report is not an option. She sits down to evaluate the acuity of the clients and the capabilities of her staff.

Introduction to Delegation

Delegation is not a new concept. In her *Notes on Nursing,* Florence Nightingale (1859) clearly stated: "Don't imagine that if you, who are in charge, don't look to all these things yourself, those under you will be more careful than you are . . . ." She continued by directing, "But then again to look to all these things yourself does not mean to do them yourself. If you do it, it is by so much the better certainly than if it were not done at all. But can you not insure that it is done when not done by yourself? Can you insure that it is not undone when your back is turned? This is what being in charge means. And a very important meaning it is, too. The former only implies that just what you can do with your own hands is done. The latter that what ought to be done is always done. Head in charge must see to house hygiene, not do it herself" (p. 17).

Today, nurses find that there is more nursing needed than nurses available to deliver the care. Changes in demographics, improved life expectancy, and newer, more complex therapies continue to generate an increased demand for nursing care. Changes in the health-care law compound this need, requiring nurses to learn how to work effectively with other members of the health-care delivery team, particularly nursing assistive personnel. Knowing how and when to delegate are critical skills for nurses entering the profession today and in the future.

Definition of Delegation

In 2005, the American Nurses Association (ANA) and the National Council of State Boards of Nursing (NCSBN) approved papers regarding delegation in nursing practice (NCSBN, 2006). Previously the ANA (1996) defined delegation as the reassigning of responsibility for the performance of a job from one person to another. The NCSBN describes delegation as the transferring of authority. Both organizations agree that this means the registered nurse (RN) has the ability to request another person to do something that this individual may not usually be permitted to do. However, registered nurses maintain accountability for supervising those to whom tasks are delegated (ANA, 2005). Nightingale referred to this delegation responsibility when she implied that the "head in charge" does not necessarily carry out the task but still sees that it is completed.

Assignments and Delegation

Making or giving an assignment is not the same as delegation. In an assignment, power is not transferred (the directive to do something not necessarily described as part of the job, does not occur). Both the NCSBN and the ANA define an assignment as the allocation of duties that each staff member is responsible for during a specific work period (2006). Assignments relate to situations where an RN directs another individual to do something that the person is already authorized to do. For example, the RN assigns the NAP the responsibility of taking vital signs on three patients. The NAP is already authorized to take vital signs. However, if the RN directed the NAP to check the amount of drainage on a fresh postoperative abdominal dressing, this would be considered delegation because the RN retains responsibility for this action. Matching the skill set of the appropriately educated health-care personnel with the needs of the client and family defines the difference between delegation and assignment (Weydt, 2010).

The individual state nurse practice acts define the legal boundaries for professional nursing practice (www.ncsbn.org). Individual nursing organizations also set standards of practice for their specialties that fall within the guidelines of the nurse practice acts. Nurses need to understand the guidelines and provisions of their state's nurse practice acts regarding delegation of patient care (Cipriano, 2010). However, according to the ANA, specific overlying principles remain firm regarding delegation. These include the following:

- The nursing profession delineates the scope of nursing practice.
- The nursing profession identifies and supervises the necessary education, training, and use of ancillary roles concerned with the delivery of direct client care.
- The RN assumes responsibility and accountability for the provision of nursing care and expertise.
- The RN directs care and determines the appropriate utilization of any ancillary personnel involved in providing direct client care.
- The RN accepts assistance from ancillary nursing personnel in delivering nursing care for the client (ANA, 2005, p. 6).

Nurse-related principles are also designated by the ANA. These are important when considering what tasks may be delegated and to whom. These principles are:

- The RN has the duty to be accountable for personal actions related to the nursing process.

- The RN considers the knowledge and skills of any ancillary personnel to whom aspects of care are delegated.
- The decision to delegate or assign is based on the RN's judgment regarding the following: the condition of the patient; the competence of the members of the nursing team; and the amount of supervision that will be required of the RN if a task is delegated.
- The RN uses critical thinking and professional judgment when following the Five Rights of Delegation delineated by the National Council of State Boards of Nursing (NCSBN) (Box 7-1).
- The RN recognizes that a relational aspect exists between delegation and communication. Communication needs to be culturally appropriate, and the individual receiving the communication should be treated with respect.
- Chief nursing officers are responsible for creating systems to assess, monitor, verify, and communicate continuous competence requirements in areas related to delegation.
- RNs monitor organizational policies, procedures, and job descriptions to ensure they are in compliance with the nurse practice act, consulting with the state board of nursing as needed (ANA, 2005, p. 6).

Delegation may be direct or indirect. *Direct delegation* is usually "verbal direction by the RN delegator regarding an activity or task in a specific nursing care situation" (ANA, 1996, p. 15). In this case, the RN decides which staff member is capable of performing the specific task or activity. *Indirect delegation* is "an approved listing of activities or tasks that have been established in policies and procedures of the health care institution or facility" (ANA, 1996, p. 15).

Permitted tasks vary from institution to institution. For example, a certified nursing assistant (CNA) performs specific activities designated by the job description approved by the particular health-care institution. Although the institution

box 7-1

The Five Rights of Delegation

1. Right task
2. Right circumstances
3. Right person
4. Right direction/communication
5. Right supervision/evaluation

delineates tasks and activities, this does not mean that the RN cannot decide to assign other personnel in specific situations. Take the following example:

Ms. Ross was admitted to the neurological unit from the neuroscience intensive care unit. She suffered a right hemisphere intracerebral bleed 2 weeks ago and has a left hemiplegia. She has difficulty with swallowing and receives tube feedings through a percutaneous endoscopic gastrostomy (PEG) tube; however, she has been advanced to a pureed diet. She needs assistance with personal care, toileting, and feeding. A physical therapist comes twice a day to get her up for gait training; otherwise, the primary health-care provider wants Ms. Ross in a chair as much as possible.

Assessing this situation, the RN might consider assigning a licensed practical nurse (LPN) to this client. The swallowing problems place the client at risk for aspiration, which means that feeding may present a problem. Based on education and skill level, the LPN is capable of managing the PEG tube feeding. While assisting with bathing, the LPN can perform range-of-motion exercises to all the client's extremities and assess her skin for breakdown. The LPN also knows the appropriate way to assist the client in transferring from the bed to the chair (Zimmerman and Schultz, 2013).

Supervision

The term *supervisor* implies that an individual holds authority over others (National Labor Relations Act [NLRA], 1935). While nurses supervise others on a daily basis, they do not necessarily hold "authority" over those they supervise. Therefore, it is important to differentiate between supervision and delegation (Matthews, 2010). Supervision is more direct and requires directly overseeing the work or performance of others. Supervision includes checking with individuals throughout the day to see what activities they completed and what they may still need to finish. When one RN works with another, then supervision is not needed. This is a collaborative relationship and includes consulting and giving advice when needed.

The following gives an example of supervision:

A NAP has been assigned to take all the vital signs on the unit and give the morning baths to eight patients. Three hours into the morning, the NAP is far behind in the assignment. At this point, it is important that the RN discover the reason the NAP has not been able to complete the assignment. Perhaps one of the clients required more care than expected, or the NAP needed to complete an errand off the unit. Reevaluation of the assignment may be necessary.

Individuals who supervise others also delegate tasks and activities. Chief nursing officers often delegate tasks to associate directors. This may include record reviews, unit reports, or client acuities. Certain administrative tasks, such as staff scheduling, may be delegated to another staff member, such as an associate manager. The delegator remains accountable for ensuring the activities are completed.

Supervision sometimes entails more direct evaluation of performance, such as performance evaluations and discussions regarding individual interactions with clients and other staff members.

Regardless of where you work, you cannot assume that only those in the higher levels of the organization delegate work to other people. You, too, will be responsible at times for delegating some of your work to other nurses, to technical personnel, or to other members of the interprofessional team. Decisions associated with this responsibility often cause some difficulty for new nurses. Knowing each person's capabilities and job description can help you decide which personnel can assist with a task.

The Nursing Process and Delegation

Before deciding who should care for a particular client, the nurse needs to assess each client's care requirements, set client-specific goals, and match the skills of the person assigned with the tasks that need to be accomplished *(assessment).* Thinking this through before delegating helps prevent problems later *(plan).* Next, the nurse assigns the tasks to the appropriate person *(implementation).* The nurse must then oversee the care and determine whether client care needs have been met *(evaluation)* (Zimmerman and Schultz, 2013). It is also important for the nurse to allow time for feedback during the day. This enables all personnel to see what has been accomplished and what still needs to be done.

Often, the nurse must first coordinate care for groups of clients before being able to delegate tasks to other personnel. The nurse also needs to consider his or her own responsibilities. This includes communicating clearly, assisting other staff members with setting priorities, clarifying instructions, and reassessing the situation.

The Need for Delegation

The 1990s brought rapid change to the health-care environment. These changes, including shorter hospital stays, increased patient acuity, and the intensification of the nursing shortage, have continued into the 21st century, requiring institutions to hire other personnel to assist nurses with client care (McHugh, Kelly, Smith, Wu, Vanak, & Aiken, 2013).

Based on the studies by McHugh et al. (2013) and the IOM (2001), it seems that registered nurses need to provide all care needs to ensure safety and quality in this complex and demanding health-care environment. While a lofty idea, this system of health-care delivery would be economically prohibitive. For this reason, health-care institutions often use nursing assistive personnel (NAP) to perform certain patient care tasks.

As the nursing shortage becomes more critical, there is a greater need for institutions to recruit the services of NAPs (ANA, 2002). A survey conducted by the American Hospital Association (AHA) revealed that 97% of hospitals currently employ some type of NAP (Spetz, Donaldson, Aydin, & Brown, 2008). Because a high percentage of institutions employ these personnel, many nurses believe they know how to work with and safely delegate tasks to them. This is not the case. Therefore, many nursing organizations, such as the American Association of Critical Care Nurses (AACN) (2010), the Society of Gastroenterology Nurses (SGNA) (2009), and the Association for Women's Health, Obstetrics and Neonatal Nurses (AWHONN) (2010), have developed definitions for NAP and criteria regarding their responsibilities. The ANA defines NAP as follows:

Unlicensed assistive personnel/Nursing assistive personnel are individuals who are trained to function in an assistive role to the registered nurse in the provision of patient/client care activities as delegated by and under the supervision of the registered professional nurse. Although some of these people may be certified (e.g., certified nursing assistant [CNA]), it is important to remember that certification differs from licensure. When a task is delegated to an unlicensed person, the professional nurse remains personally responsible for the outcomes of these activities (ANA, 2005).

As work on the unlicensed assistive personnel/nursing assistive personnel (UAP/NAP) issue is ongoing, the ANA updated its position statements in 2012 to define direct and indirect patient care activities that may be performed by UAP/NAP. Included in these updates are specific definitions regarding UAP/NAP and technicians and acceptable tasks (www.nursingworld.org).

Use of the RN to provide all the care a client needs may not be the most efficient or cost-effective use of professional time. More hospitals are moving away from hiring LPNs and utilizing all RN staffing with UAP/NAP. In these facilities, the nursing focus is directed at diagnosing client care needs and carrying out complex interventions.

The ANA cautions against delegating nursing activities that include the foundation of the nursing process and that require specialized knowledge, judgment, or skill (ANA, 1996, 2002, 2005). Non-nursing functions, such as performing clerical or receptionist duties, taking trips or doing errands off the unit, cleaning floors, making beds, collecting trays, and ordering supplies, should not be carried out by the highest paid and most educated member of the team. These tasks are easily delegated to other personnel.

Safe Delegation

In 1990 the NCSBN adopted a definition of *delegation,* stating that delegation is "transferring to a competent individual the authority to perform a selected nursing task in a selected situation" (p. 1). In its publication *Issues* (1995), the NCSBN again presented this definition. Likewise, the ANA Code for Nurses (1985) stated, "The nurse exercises informed judgment and uses individual competence and qualifications as criteria in seeking consultation, accepting responsibilities, and delegating nursing activities to others" (p. 1). In 2005, the ANA defined *delegation* as "the transfer of responsibility for the performance of an activity from one individual to another while retaining accountability

---

box 7-2

Seven Components of the Delegation Decision-Making Grid

1. Level of client acuity
2. Level of unlicensed assistive personnel capability
3. Level of licensed nurse capability
4. Possibility for injury
5. Number of times the skill has been performed by the unlicensed assistive personnel
6. Level of decision making needed for the activity
7. Client's ability for self-care

Adapted from the National Council of State Boards of Nursing. Delegation Decision-Making Grid. National State Boards of Nursing, Inc., 1997 (ncsbn.org).

---

for the outcome" (p. 4). To delegate tasks safely, nurses must delegate appropriately and supervise adequately.

In 1997 the NCSBN developed a Delegation Decision-Making Grid (www.ncsbn.org). This grid is a tool to help nurses delegate appropriately. It provides a scoring instrument for seven categories that the nurse should consider when making delegation decisions. The categories for the grid are listed in Box 7-2.

Scoring the components helps the nurse evaluate the situations, the client needs, and the healthcare personnel available to meet the needs. A low score on the grid indicates that the activity may be safely delegated to personnel other than the RN, and a high score indicates that delegation may not be advisable. Figure 7.1 shows the Delegation Decision-Making Grid. The grid is also available on the NCSBN Web site at ncsbn.com.

Nurses who delegate tasks to UAP/NAP should evaluate the activities being considered for delegation (Keeney, Hasson, McKenna, & Gillen, 2005). The American Association of Critical Care Nurses (AACN) (1990; 2010) recommended considering five factors, which are listed in Box 7-3, in making a decision to delegate.

---

box 7-3

Five Factors for Determining If Client Care Activity Should Be Delegated

1. Potential for harm to the patient
2. Complexity of the nursing activity
3. Extent of problem solving and innovation required
4. Predictability of outcome
5. Extent of interaction

Adapted from American Association of Critical Care Nurses (AACN). (1990, 2010). Delegation of Nursing and Non-Nursing Activities in Critical Care: A Framework for Decision-Making. Irvine, CA: AACN.

Elements for Review		Client A	Client B	Client C	Client D
Activity/task	**Describe activity/task:**				
Level of Client Stability	**Score the client's level of stability:** 0. Client condition is chronic/stable/predictable 1. Client condition has minimal potential for change 2. Client condition has moderate potential for change 3. Client condition is unstable/acute/strong potential for change				
Level of NAP Competence	**Score the NAP competence in completing delegated nursing care activities in the defined client population:** 0. NAP - expert in activities to be delegated, in defined population 1. NAP - experienced in activities to be delegated, in defined population 2. NAP - experienced in activities, but not in defined population 3. NAP - novice in performing activities and in defined population				
Level of Licensed Nurse Competence	**Score the licensed nurse's competence in relation to both knowledge of providing nursing care to a defined population and competence in implementation of the delegation process:** 0. Expert in the knowledge of nursing needs/activities of defined client population and expert in the delegation process 1. Either expert in knowledge of needs/activities of defined client population and competent in delegation or experienced in the needs/activities of defined client population and expert in the delegation process 2. Experienced in the knowledge of needs/activities of defined client population and competent in the delegation process 3. Either experienced in the knowledge of needs/activities of defined client population or competent in the delegation process 4. Novice in knowledge of defined population and novice in delegation				
Potential for Harm	**Score the potential level of risk the nursing care activity has for the client (risk is probability of suffering harm):** 0. None 1. Low 2. Medium 3. High				
Frequency	**Score based on how often the NAP has performed the specific nursing care activity:** 0. Performed at least daily 1. Performed at least weekly 2. Performed at least monthly 3. Performed less than monthly 4. Never performed				
Level of Decision Making	**Score the decision making needed, related to the specific nursing care activity, client (both cognitive and physical status), and client situation:** 0. Does not require decision making 1. Minimal level of decision making 2. Moderate level of decision making 3. High level of decision making				
Ability for Self-Care	**Score the client's level of assistance needed for self-care activities:** 0. No assistance 1. Limited assistance 2. Extensive assistance 3. Total care or constant attendance				
	Total Score				

Figure 7.1 Delegation decision-making grid.

It is the responsibility of the RN to be well acquainted with the state's nurse practice act and regulations issued by the state board of nursing regarding UAP/NAP (ANA, 2005). State laws and regulations supersede any publications or opinions set forth by professional organizations. As stated earlier, the NCSBN provides criteria to assist nurses with delegation.

LPNs are trained to perform specific tasks, such as basic medication administration, dressing changes, and personal hygiene tasks. In some states, the LPN, with additional training, may start and monitor intravenous (IV) infusions and administer certain medications.

Criteria for Delegation

The purpose of delegation is not to assign tasks to others that you do not want to do yourself. When you delegate to others effectively, the result is you have more time to perform the tasks that only a professional nurse is permitted to do.

In delegating, the nurse must consider both the *ability* of the person to whom the task is delegated and the *fairness* of the task to the individual and the team (Whitehead, Weiss, & Tappen, 2010). In other words, both the *task aspects* of delegation (Is this a complex task? Is it a professional responsibility? Can this person do it safely?) and the *interpersonal aspects* (Does the person have time to do this? Is the work evenly distributed?) must be considered.

The ANA (2005) has specified tasks that RNs may not delegate because they are specific to the discipline of professional nursing. These activities include initial nursing and follow-up assessments if nursing judgment is indicated (Zimmerman & Schultz, 2013):

- Decisions and judgments about client outcomes
- Determination and approval of a client plan of care
- Interventions that require professional nursing knowledge, decisions, or skills
- Decisions and judgments necessary for the evaluation of client care

Task-Related Concerns

The primary task-related concern in delegating work is whether the person assigned to do the task has the ability to complete it. Team priorities and efficiency are also important considerations.

Abilities

To make appropriate assignments, the nurse needs to know the knowledge and skill level, legal definitions, role expectations, and job description for each member of the team. It is equally important to be aware of the different skill levels of caregivers within each discipline because ability differs with each level of education. Additionally, individuals within each level of skill possess their own strengths and weaknesses. Prior assessment of the strengths of each member of the team will assist in providing safe and efficient care to clients. Figure 7.2 outlines the skills of various health-care personnel.

People should not be assigned a task that they do not have the skills or knowledge to perform, regardless of their professional level. People are

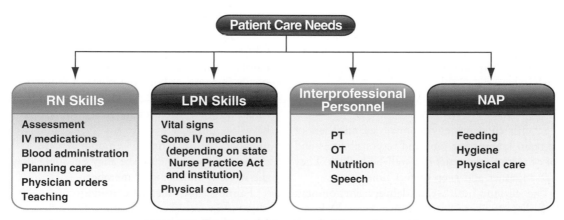

Figure 7.2 Diagram of delegation decision-making grid.

often reluctant to admit they cannot do something. Instead of seeking help or saying they are not comfortable with a task, they may avoid doing it, delay starting it, do only part of it, or even bluff their way through it, a risky choice in health care.

Regardless of the length of time individuals have been in a position, employees need orientation when assigned a new task. Those who seek assistance and advice are showing concern for the team and the welfare of their clients. Requests for assistance or additional explanations should not be ignored, and the person should be praised, not criticized, for seeking guidance (Whitehead, Weiss, & Tappen, 2010).

Priorities

The work of a busy unit rarely ends up going as expected. Dealing with sick people, their families, physicians, and other team members all at the same time is a difficult task. Setting priorities for the day should be based on client needs, team needs, and organizational and community demands. The values of each may be very different, even opposed. These differences should be discussed with team members so that decisions can be made based on team priorities.

One way to determine patient priorities is to base decisions on Maslow's hierarchy of needs. Maslow's hierarchy is frequently used in nursing to provide a framework for prioritizing care to meet client needs. The basic physiological needs come first because they are necessary for survival. For example, oxygen and medication administration, IV fluids, and enteral feedings are included in this group.

Identifying priorities and deciding the needs to be met first help in organizing care and in deciding which other team members can meet client needs. For example, nursing assistants can meet many hygiene needs, allowing licensed personnel to administer medications and enteral feedings in a timely manner.

Efficiency

In an efficient work environment, all members of the team know their jobs and responsibilities and work together like gears in a well-built clock. They mesh together and keep perfect time.

The current health-care delivery environment demands efficient, cost-effective care. Delegating appropriately can increase efficiency and save money. Likewise, incorrect delegation can decrease efficiency and cost money. When delegating tasks to individuals who cannot perform the job, the RN must often go back to perform the task.

Although institutions often need to "float" staff to other units, maintaining continuity, if at all possible, is important. Keeping the same staff members on the unit all the time, for example, allows them to develop familiarity with the physical setting and routines of the unit as well as the types of clients the unit services. Time is lost when staff members are reassigned frequently to different units. Although physical layouts may be the same, client needs, unit routines, use of space, and availability of supplies are often different. Time spent to orient reassigned staff members takes time away from delivery of client care. However, when staff members are reassigned, it is important for them to indicate their skill level and comfort in the new setting. It is just as important for the staff members who are familiar with the setting to identify the strengths of the reassigned person and build on them.

Appropriateness

Appropriateness is another task-related concern. Nothing can be more counterproductive than, for example, floating a coronary care nurse to labor and delivery. More time will be spent teaching the necessary skills than providing safe mother-baby care. Assigning an educated, licensed staff member to perform non-nursing functions to protect safety is also poor use of personnel.

Relationship-Oriented Concerns

Relationship-oriented concerns include fairness, learning opportunities, health concerns, compatibility, and staff preferences.

Fairness

Fairness requires the workload to be distributed evenly in terms of both the physical requirements and the emotional investment in providing health care. The nurse who is caring for a dying client may have less physical work to do than another team member, but in terms of emotional care to the client and family, he or she may be doing double the work of another staff member.

Fairness also means considering equally all requests for special consideration. The quickest way to alienate members of a team is to be unfair. It is important to discuss with team members any decisions that have been made that may appear unfair to any one of them. Allow the team members to participate in making decisions regarding assignments. Their participation will decrease resentment and increase cooperation. In some health-care institutions, team members make such decisions as a group.

Learning Opportunities

Including assignments that stimulate motivation, learning, and assisting team members to learn new tasks and take on new challenges is part of the role of the RN.

Health

Some aspects of caregiving jobs are more stressful than others. Rotating team members through the more difficult jobs may decrease stress and allow empathy to increase among the members. Special health needs, such as family emergencies or special physical problems of team members, also need to be addressed. If some team members have difficulty accepting the needs of others, the situation should be discussed with the team, bearing in mind the employee's right to privacy when discussing sensitive issues.

Compatibility

No matter how hard you may strive to get your team to work together, it just may not happen. Some people work together better than others. Helping people develop better working relationships is part of team building. Creating opportunities for people to share and learn from each other increases the overall effectiveness of the team.

As the leader, you may be forced to intervene in team member disputes. Many individuals find it difficult to work with others they do not like personally. It sometimes becomes necessary to explain that liking another person is a plus but not a necessity in the work setting and that personal problems have no place in the work environment. For example:

Laura had been a labor and delivery room supervisor in a large metropolitan hospital for 5 years before she moved to another city. Because a position similar to the one she left was not available, she became a staff nurse at a small local hospital. The hospital had just opened its new birthing center. The first day on

the job went well. The other staff members seemed cordial. As the weeks went by, however, Laura began to have problems getting other staff to help her. No one would offer to relieve her for meals or a break. She noticed that certain groups of staff members always went to lunch together but that she was never invited to join them. She attempted to speak to some of the more approachable coworkers, but she did not get much information. Disturbed by the situation, Laura went to the nurse manager. The nurse manager listened quietly while Laura related her experiences. She then asked Laura to think about the last staff meeting. Laura realized that she had alienated the staff during the meeting because she had said repeatedly that in "her hospital" things were done in a particular way. Laura also realized that, instead of asking for help, she was in the habit of demanding it. Laura and the nurse manager discussed the difficulties of her changing positions, moving to a new place, and trying to develop both professional and social ties. Together, they came up with several solutions to Laura's problem.

Staff Preferences

Considering the preferences of individual team members is important but should not supersede other criteria for delegating responsibly. Allowing team members to always select what they want to do may cause the less assertive members' needs to be unmet.

It is important to explain the rationale for decisions made regarding delegation so that all team members may understand the needs of the unit or organization. Box 7-4 outlines basic rights for

---

box 7-4

Basic Entitlements of Nurses in the Workplace

Professionals in the workplace are entitled to:
- Respect from other members of the interprofessional health-care team
- A work assignment that matches skills and education and does not exceed that of other members with the same education and skills set
- Wages commensurate with the job
- Autonomy in setting work priorities
- Ability to speak out for self and others
- A healthy work environment
- Accountability for his/her own behaviors
- Act in the best interest of the client
- Be human

Adapted from ANA Resolutions: Workplace Abuse (2006).

professional health-care team members. Although written originally for women, the concepts are applicable to all professional health-care providers.

Barriers to Delegation

Many nurses, particularly new ones, have difficulty delegating. The reasons for this include experience issues, licensure issues, legal issues, and quality-of-care issues.

Experience Issues

Many nurses working today graduated during the 1980s, when primary care was the major delivery system. These nurses lacked the education and skill needed for delegation. Nurses educated in the 1970s and before worked in settings with LPNs and nursing assistants, where they routinely delegated tasks. However, client acuity was lower and the care less complex. More expert nurses have considerable delegation experience and can be a resource for younger nurses.

The added responsibility of delegation creates some discomfort for nurses. Many believe they are unprepared to assume this responsibility, especially in deciding the competency of another person. To decrease this discomfort, nurses need to participate in establishing guidelines for NAP within their institution. The ANA Position Statements on Nursing Assistive Personnel/Unlicensed Assistive Personnel address this. Table 7-1 lists the direct and indirect client care activities that may be performed by NAP.

Licensure Issues

Although the current health-care environment requires nurses to delegate, many nurses voice concerns about the personal risk regarding their licensure if they delegate inappropriately. The courts have usually ruled that nurses are not liable for the negligence of other individuals, provided that the nurse delegated appropriately. Delegation is within the scope of nursing practice. The art and skill of delegation are acquired with practice.

Legal Issues and Delegation

State nurse practice acts establish the legal boundaries for nursing practice. Professional nursing organizations define practice standards, and the policies of the health-care institution create job descriptions and establish policies that guide appropriate delegation decisions for the organization.

Inherent in today's health-care environment is the safety of the client. The quality of client care and the delivery of safe and effective care are central to the concept of delegation. RNs are held accountable when delegating care activities to others. This means that they have an obligation to intervene whenever they deem the care provided is unsafe or unethical. It is also important to realize that a delegated task may not be "sub-delegated." In other words, if the RN delegated a task to the LPN, the LPN cannot then delegate the task to the NAP, even if the LPN has decided that it is within the abilities of that particular NAP. There may be legal implications if a client is injured as a result of inappropriate delegation. Consider the following case:

In Hicks v. New York State Department of Health, a nurse was found guilty of patient neglect because of her failure to appropriately train and supervise the UAP working under her. In this particular situation, a security guard discovered an elderly nursing home client in a totally dark room undressed and covered with urine and fecal material. The client

table 7-1	
Direct and Indirect Client Care Activities	
Direct Client Care Activities	**Indirect Client Care Activities**
Assisting with feeding and drinking	Providing a clean environment
Assisting with ambulation	Providing a safe environment
Assisting with grooming	Providing companion care
Assisting with toileting	Providing transportation for noncritical clients
Assisting with dressing	Assisting with stocking nursing units
Assisting with socializing	Providing messenger and delivery services

Source: Adapted from American Nurses Association. (2002). Position statement on utilization of unlicensed assistive personnel/nursing assistive personnel. Washington, DC: American Nurses Association.

was partially in his bed and partially restrained in an overturned wheelchair. The court found the nurse guilty on the following: the nurse failed to assess whether the UAP had delivered proper care to the client, and this subsequently led to the inadequate delivery of care (1991).

Quality-of-Care Issues

Nurses have expressed concern over the quality of patient care when tasks and activities are delegated to others. Activities typically delegated include turning, ambulating, personal care, and blood glucose monitoring. When these care activities are missed, either delayed or omitted, the probability of untoward and costly outcomes increases (Kalish, Landstrom, & Hinshaw, 2009). Failure to carry out these delegated activities appropriately also affects patient safety (IOM, 2001). Remember Nightingale's words earlier in the chapter, "Don't imagine that if you, who are in charge, don't look to all these things yourself, those under you will be more careful than you are." She added that you do not need to do everything yourself to see that it is done correctly. When you delegate, you control the delegation. You decide to whom you will delegate the task.

Assigning Work to Others

Assigning work can be difficult for several reasons:

1. Some nurses think they must do everything themselves.
2. Some nurses distrust subordinates to do things correctly.
3. Some nurses think that if they delegate all the technical tasks, they will not reinforce their own learning.
4. Some nurses are more comfortable with the technical aspects of patient care than with the more complex issues of patient teaching and discharge planning.

Families and clients do not always see professional activities. Rather, they see direct patient care (Keeney, Hasson, McKenna, & Gillen, 2005). Nurses believe that when they do not participate directly in client care, they do not accomplish anything for the client. The professional aspects of nursing, such as planning care, teaching, and discharge planning, help to promote positive outcomes for clients and their families. When working with

LPNs, knowing their scope of practice helps in making delegation decisions.

Prioritization

Nurses need to know how to effectively prioritize care for their patients. Prioritizing requires making a decision regarding the importance of choosing a specific action or activity from several options. Sometimes nurses base these choices on personal values; other times nurses make decisions based on imperatives (Lake, Moss, & Duke, 2009). *Prioritization* is defined as "deciding which needs or problems require immediate action and which ones could be delayed until a later time because they are not urgent" (Silvestri, 2008, p. 68). While it is important to know what to do first, it is just as imperative to understand the result of delaying an action. If postponing the activity may result in an unfavorable outcome, then this activity assumes a level of priority.

Nurses focus care based on the intended outcome of the care or intervention. Alfaro-Lefevre (2011) provides three levels of priority setting:

- Use the ABCs plus V (airway, breathing, circulation, and vital signs). These are the most critical.
- Address mental status, pain, untreated medical issues, and abnormal laboratory results.
- Consider long-term health (chronic) problems, health education, and coping.

Nurses need to evaluate and assess the situation or need for completion of each task. Certain skills such as assessment, planning, and evaluating nursing care always remain within the purview of the registered nurse. Understanding the process for evaluating and setting patient care priorities is essential when coordinating assignments and delegating care to others.

Coordinating Assignments

One of the most difficult tasks for new nurses to master is coordinating daily activities. Often, you have clients for whom you provide direct care while at the same time you must supervise the work of others, such as non-nurse caregivers (NAP), LPNs, or licensed vocational nurses (LVNs). Although critical (or clinical) pathways, concept maps, and computer information sheets are available to help identify patient needs, these items do not provide a mechanism for coordinating the delivery of care. Developing a personalized worksheet helps prioritize tasks to perform for each patient. Using the worksheets assists the nurse to identify tasks that require the knowledge and skill of an RN and those that can be carried out by NAP.

On the worksheet, tasks are prioritized on the basis of patient need, not nursing convenience. For example, an order states that a patient receives continuous tube feedings. Although it may be convenient for the nurse to fill the feeding container with enough supplement to last 6 hours, it is not the standard practice and may be unsafe for the patient. Instead, the nurse should plan to check the tube feeding every 2 hours.

As for Ora at the beginning of the chapter, a worksheet will help her determine how to delegate. First, she needs to decide which patients require the skill sets of a registered nurse. These include receiving and transcribing orders; contacting physicians with information or requests; accessing laboratory reports from the computer, reviewing them, deciding on an action, and giving them to the appropriate staff members; and checking any new medication orders and placing them in the medication administration records. Another RN may be able to relieve the monitor technician for dinner and breaks, and a second RN may be able to assign staff to dinner and breaks. Next, Ora needs to look at individual patient requirements on the unit and prioritize them. She is now ready to effectively delegate to her staff.

Some activities must be done at a certain time, and their timing may be out of the nurse's control. Examples include medication administration and patients who need special preparation for a scheduled procedure. The following are some tips for organizing work on personalized worksheets to help establish client priorities (Whitehead, Weiss, & Tappen, 2010):

▪ Plan your time around activities that need to occur at a specific time.
▪ Do high-priority activities first.
▪ Determine which activities are best done in a cluster.
▪ Remember that you are responsible for activities delegated to others.
▪ Consider your peak energy time when scheduling optional activities.

This list acts as a guideline for coordinating client care. The nurse needs to use critical thinking skills in the decision-making process. Remember that this is one of the ANA nurse-related principles of delegation (ANA, 2005). For example, activities that are usually clustered include bathing, changing linen, and parts of the physical assessment. Some patients may not be able to tolerate too much activity at one time. Take special situations into consideration when coordinating patient care and deciding who should carry out some of the activities. Remember, however, that even when you delegate, you remain accountable.

Figure 7.3 is an example of a personalized worksheet.

Models of Care Delivery

Functional nursing, team nursing, total client care, and primary nursing are models of care delivery that developed in an attempt to balance the needs of the client with the availability and skills of nurses. Regardless of the method of assignment or care delivery system, the majority of nursing care is delivered within a group practice model where coordination and continuity of care depend on sharing common practice values and establishing communication (Anthony & Vidal, 2010). Nurses need to develop strong delegation and communication skills to successfully follow through with any given model of care delivery.

Functional Nursing

Functional nursing or task nursing evolved during the mid-1940s due to the loss of RNs who left home to serve in the armed forces during the Second World War. Prior to the war, RNs comprised the majority of hospital staffing. Because of the lack of nurses to provide care at home, hospitals used more LPNs or LVNs and NAP to care for clients.

When implementing functional nursing, the focus is on the task and not necessarily holistic client care. The needs of the clients are categorized by task, and then the tasks are assigned to the "best person for the job." This method takes into consideration the skill set and licensure scope of practice of each caregiver. For example, the RN would perform and document all assessments and administer all IV medications; the LPN or LVN would administer treatments and perform dressing changes. NAP would be responsible for meeting hygiene needs of clients, obtaining and recording vital signs, and assisting in feeding clients. This method is efficient and effective; however, when implemented, continuity in client care is lost. Many times, reevaluation of client status and follow-up does not occur, and a breakdown in communication among staff occurs.

Team Nursing

Team nursing grew out of functional nursing; nursing units often resort to this model when appropriate staffing is unavailable. A group of nursing personnel or a team provides care for a cluster of clients. The manner in which clients are

---

Nurse/Team_____DNR 8607/Code 99

Patient Room # _____ Name _____ Age_____

Allergies_____

Diagnosis_____

Diet _____Fluids: PO _____IV_____ Type _____

Restrictions: BR _____ BRP _____OOB/Chair_____ Ambulate with assist_____

Activity _____

Assessment_____

Treatments

1. _____

2. _____

3. _____

4. _____

5. _____

Monitor

1. Vital signs: Temp_____Pulse_____AHR_____BP_____Parameters _____

2. Cardiac Monitor: Rhythm_____ Rate _____

3. Neurologic Status _____

4. CMS: _____ Traction: _____

Figure 7.3 Personalized patient worksheet.

divided varies and depends on several issues: the layout of the unit, the types of clients on the unit, and the number of clients on the unit. The organization of the team is based on the number of available staff and the skill mix within the group.

An RN assumes the role of the team leader. The team may consist of another RN, an LPN, and NAP. The team leader directs and supervises the team, which provides client care. The team knows the condition and needs of all the clients on the team.

The team leader acts as a liaison between the clients and the health-care provider/physician. Responsibilities include formulating a client plan of care, transcribing and communicating orders and treatment changes to team members, and solving problems of clients and/or team members. The nurse manager confers with the team leaders, supervises the client care teams and, in some institutions, conducts rounds with the health-care providers.

For this method to be effective, the team leader needs strong delegation and communication skills. Communication among team members and the nurse manager avoids duplication of efforts and decreases competition for control of assignments that may not be equal based on client acuity and the skills sets of team members.

Total Patient Care

During the 1920s total patient care was the original model of nursing care delivery. Much nursing was in the form of private duty nursing. In this model, nurses cared for patients in homes and in hospitals. Hospital schools of nursing provided students who staffed the nursing units and delivered care under the watchful eyes of nursing supervisors and directors. In this model, one RN assumes the responsibility of caring for one client. This includes acting as a direct liaison among the patient, family, health-care provider, and other members of the health-care team. Today, this model is seen in high-acuity areas such as critical care units; postanesthesia recovery units; and labor, delivery, and recovery (LDR) units. This model requires RNs to engage in non-nursing tasks that might be assumed by NAP.

Primary Nursing

In the 1960s, nursing care delivery models started to move away from team nursing and placed the RN in the role of giving direct patient care. The central principle of this model distributes nursing decision making to the nurses who care for the client. As the primary nurse, the RN devises, implements, and maintains responsibility for the nursing care of the patient during the time the patient remains on the nursing unit. The primary nurse, along with associate nurses, gives direct care to the client.

In its ideal form, primary nursing requires an all-RN staff. Although this model provides continuity of care and nursing accountability, staffing is difficult and expensive, especially in today's health-care environment. Some view it as ineffective as other personnel could carry out many tasks that consume the time of the registered nurse.

Conclusion

The concept of delegation is not new. In today's health-care environment and the need for cost containment, using full RN staffing is unrealistic. Knowing the principles of delegation remains an essential skill for registered nurses. Personal organizational skills and the ability to prioritize patient care are prerequisites to delegation. Before the nurse can delegate tasks to others, he or she needs to identify individual patient needs. Using worksheets, the ABC plus V method, and Maslow's hierarchy helps the nurse understand these individual patient needs, set priorities, and identify which tasks can be delegated to others. Using the Delegation Decision-Making Grid helps the nurse delegate safely and appropriately.

Nurses need to be aware of the capabilities of each staff member, the tasks that may be delegated, and the tasks that the RN needs to perform. When delegating, the RN uses critical thinking and professional judgment in making decisions. Professional judgment is directed by state nurse practice acts, evidence-based practice, and approved national nursing standards. Institutions develop their own job descriptions for NAP and other health-care professionals, but institutional policies must remain compliant with state nurse practice acts. Although the nurse delegates the task or activity, he or she remains accountable for the delegated decision.

Understanding the concept of delegation helps the new nurse organize and prioritize client care. Knowing the staff and their capabilities simplifies delegation. Utilizing staff members' capabilities creates a pleasant and productive working environment for everyone involved.

Study Questions

1. What are the responsibilities of the professional nurse when delegating tasks to an LPN/LVN or NAP?

2. What factors need to be considered when delegating tasks?

3. What is the difference between delegation and assignment?

4. What are the nurse manager's legal responsibilities in supervising nursing assistive personnel?

5. Review the scenario on p. 111. If you were the nurse manager, how would you have handled Laura's situation?

6. Bring the patient diagnosis census from your assigned clinical unit to class. Using the Delegation Decision-Making Grid, decide which patients you would assign to the personnel on the unit. Give reasons for your decision.

7. What type of nursing delivery model is implemented on your assigned clinical unit? Give examples of the roles of the personnel engaged in client care to support your answer.

Case Study to Promote Critical Reasoning

Julio works at a large teaching hospital in a major metropolitan area. This institution services the entire geographical region, including indigent clients, and, because of its reputation, administers care to international clients and individuals who reside in other states. Like all health-care institutions, this one has been attempting to cut costs by using more NAP. Nurses are often floated to other units. Lately, the number of indigent and foreign clients on Julio's unit has increased. The acuity of these clients has been quite high, requiring a great deal of time from the nursing staff.

Julio arrived at work at 6:30 a.m., his usual time. He looked at the census board and discovered that the unit was filled, and Bed Control was calling all night to have clients discharged or transferred to make room for several clients who had been in the emergency department since the previous evening. He also discovered that the other RN assigned to his team called in sick. His team consists of himself, two NAP, and an LPN who is shared by two teams. He has eight patients on his team:

- Two need to be readied for surgery, including preoperative and postoperative teaching, one of whom is a 35-year-old woman scheduled for a modified radical mastectomy for the treatment of breast cancer.

- Three are second-day postoperative clients, two of whom require extensive dressing changes, are receiving IV antibiotics, and need to be ambulated.

- One postoperative client who is required to remain on total bedrest, has a nasogastric tube to suction as well as a chest tube, is on total parenteral nutrition and lipids, needs a central venous catheter line dressing change, has an IV, is taking multiple IV medications, and has a Foley catheter.

- One client who is ready for discharge and needs discharge instruction.

- One client who needs to be transferred to a subacute unit, and a report must be given to the RN of that unit.

Once the latter client is transferred and the other one is discharged, the emergency department will be sending two clients to the unit for admission.

1. How should Julio organize his day? Set up an hourly schedule.

2. Make a priority list based on the ABC plus V method.

3. What type of client management approach should Julio consider in assigning staff appropriately?

4. If you were Julio, which clients and/or tasks would you assign to your staff? List all of them, and explain your rationale.

5. Using the Delegation Decision-Making Grid, make staff and client assignments.

References

Alfaro-Lefevre, R. (2011). Critical thinking, clinical reasoning, and clinical judgment: A practical approach (5th ed.). St. Louis, MO. Mosby: Elsevier.

American Association of Critical Care Nurses (AACN). (1990). *Delegation of nursing and non-nursing activities in critical care: A framework for decision making.* Irvine, CA: AACN.

American Association of Critical Care Nurses (AACN). (2010). *Delegation handbook.* Irvine, CA: AACN.

American Nurses Association (ANA). (1985). *Code for nurses.* Washington, DC: ANA.

American Nurses Association (ANA). (1996). *Registered professional nurses and unlicensed assistive personnel.* Washington, DC: ANA.

American Nurses Association (ANA). (2002). *Position statements on registered nurse utilization of unlicensed assistive personnel.* Washington, DC: ANA.

American Nurses Association (ANA). (2005). *Principles for delegation.* Washington, DC: ANA.

American Nurses Association (ANA). (2012). ANA's principles for delegation: For registered nurses to unlicensed assistive personnel (UAP). Bethesda, MD: ANA.

Anthony, M.K., & Vidal, K. (2010). Mindful communication: A novel approach to improving delegation and increasing patient safety. *The Online Journal of Issues in Nursing, 15*(2), 1–3. Retrieved September 22, 2013, from www.nursingworld.org/MainMenuCategories/ANAMarketplace/ANAPeriodicals/OJIN/JournalTopics/Delegation-Dilemmas

Association for Women's Health, Obstetrics and Neonatal Nurses (AWHONN). (2010). *Guidelines for professional nurse staffing on perinatal units.* Washington, DC: AWHONN.

Cipriano, R.F. (2010). Overview and summary: Delegation dilemmas: Standards and skills for practice. *The Online Journal of Issues in Nursing, 15*(2), 1–3. Retrieved September 22, 2013, from www.nursingworld.org/MainMenuCategories/ANAMarketplace/ANAPeriodicals/OJIN/JournalTopics/Delegation-Dilemmas.

Hicks v. New York State Department of Health. (1991). 570 N.Y.S. 2d 395 (A.D. 3 Dept).

Institute of Medicine. (2001). *Crossing the quality chasm: A new health system for the 21st century.* Washington, DC: National Academy Press.

Kalisch, B.J., Landstrom, G.L., & Hinshaw, A.S. (2009). Missed nursing care: A concept analysis. *Journal of advanced nursing, 65*(7), 1509–1517.

Keeney, S., Hasson, F., McKenna, H., & Gillen, P. (2005). Health care assistants: The view of managers of health care agencies on training and employment. *Journal of Nursing Management, 13*(1), 83–92.

Keeney, S., Hasson, F., & McKenna, H. (2005). Nurses', midwives', and patients' perceptions of trained health care assistants. *Journal of Advanced Nursing, 50*(4), 345–355.

Lake, S., Moss, C., & Duke, J. (2009). Nursing prioritization of the patient need for care: A tacit knowledge embedded in the clinical decision-making literature. *International Journal of Nursing Practice, 15*(5), 376–388.

Matthews, J. (2010). When does delegating make you a supervisor? *The Online Journal of Issues in Nursing, 15*(2). Retrieved September 22, 2013, from www.nursingworld.org/MainMenuCategories/ANAMarketplace/ANAPeriodicals/OJIN/JournalTopics/Delegation-Dilemmas

McHugh, M.D., Kelly, L.A., Smith, H.L., Wu, E.S., Vanak, J.M., & Aiken, L.H. (2013). Lower mortality in magnet hospitals. *Medical Care, 51*(5), 382–388.

National Council of State Boards of Nursing. (1990). *Concept paper on delegation.* Chicago: NCSBN.

National Council of State Boards of Nursing. (1995). Delegation: Concepts and decision-making process. *Issues* (December), 1–2.

National Council of State Boards of Nursing. (1997). *Delegation decision-making grid.* Chicago: NCSBN. Retrieved on from https://www.ncsbn.org/delegation _grid_NEW.pdf

National Council of State Boards of Nursing. (2006). Joint Statement on delegation. Retrieved September 20, 2013, from https://www.ncsbn.org/Delegation_joint _statement_ NCSBN

National Council of State Boards of Nursing. (2007). The five rights of delegation. Retrieved from www.ncsbn. org/Joint_statement.pdf

National Labor Relations Act (NLRA). (1935). Retrieved September 22, 2013, from www.dol.gov/olms/regs/compliance/EmployeeRightsPoster11x17_Final .pdf

Nightingale, F. (1859). *Notes on nursing: What it is and what it is not.* London: Harrison and Sons. (Reprint 1992. Philadelphia: JB Lippincott.)

Silvestri, L. (2008). *Saunders comprehensive review for the NCLEX-RN examination* (4th ed.). St. Louis, MO: Saunders.

Society of Gastroenterology Nurses and Associates, Inc. (2009). Position statement: Role delineation of nursing assistive personnel in gastroenterology.

Spetz, J., Donaldson, N., Aydin, C., & Brown D.S. (2008). How many nurses per patient? Measurements of nurse staffing in health services research. *Health Services Research, 43*(5), 1674–1692.

Weydt, A. (2010). Developing delegation skills. *The Online Journal of Issues in Nursing, 15*(2). Retrieved September 22, 2013, from www.nursingworld.org/MainMenuCategories/ANAMarketplace/ANAPeriodicals/OJIN/JournalTopics/Delegation-Dilemmas

Whitehead, D.K., Weiss, S.A., & Tappen, R. (2010). *Essentials of leadership and management.* (5th ed.). Philadelphia: F.A. Davis.

Zimmerman, P.G., & Schultz, M.J. (2013). Delegating to unlicensed assistive personnel. Gannet Education Publishing.

Dealing With Problems and Conflicts

The pressures and demands of the workplace often generate conflicts among people that can seriously interfere with their ability to work together. If the various polls and surveys of nurses are correct, the amount of hostility and unresolved conflict experienced by nurses at work seems to be increasing (Lazoritz & Carlson, 2008; Siu, Laschinger, & Finegan, 2008). Conflicts with doctors, supervisors, managers, and colleagues can be very stressful (Laschinger et al., 2013; Vivar, 2006). Consider Case 1, which is the first of three that will be used to illustrate how to deal with problems and conflicts.

Conflict

There are no conflict-free work groups (Van de Vliert & Janssen, 2001). Small or large, conflicts are a daily occurrence in the life of nurses (McElhaney, 1996), and they can interfere with getting work done, as shown in Case 1.

Serious conflicts can be very stressful. Stress symptoms—such as difficulty concentrating, anxiety, sleep disorders, and withdrawal—and other inter-personal relationship problems can occur. Bitterness, anger, and, in rare occurrences, violence can erupt in the workplace if conflicts are not resolved.

Conflict also has a positive side, however. In the process of learning how to manage conflict constructively, people can develop more open, cooperative ways of working together (Tjosvold & Tjosvold, 1995). They can begin to see each other as people with similar needs, concerns, and dreams instead of as competitors or blocks in the way of progress. Being involved in successful conflict resolution can be an empowering experience (Horton-Deutsch & Wellman, 2002).

The goal in dealing with conflict is to create an environment in which conflicts are dealt with in as cooperative and constructive a manner as possible, rather than in a competitive and destructive manner.

Many Sources of Conflict

Why do conflicts occur? The workplace itself can be a generator of conflict. Some conflicts are focused on issues related to the work being done;

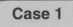

Case 1

Team A and Team B

Team A has stopped talking to Team B. If several members of Team A are out sick, no one on Team B will help Team A with their work. Likewise, Team A members will not take telephone messages for anyone on Team B. Instead, they ask the person to call back later. When members of the two teams pass each other in the hall, they either glare at each other or turn away to avoid eye contact. Arguments erupt when members of the two teams need the same computer terminal or another piece of equipment at the same time.

When a Team A nurse reached for a glucometer at the same moment as a Team B nurse did, the second nurse said, "You've been using that all morning."

"I've got a lot of patients to monitor," was the response.

"Oh, you think you're the only one with work to do?"

"We take good care of our patients."

"Are you saying we don't?"

The nurses fell silent when the nurse manager entered the room.

"Is something the matter?" she asked. Both nurses shook their heads and left quickly.

"I'm not sure what's going on here," the nurse manager thought to herself, "but something's wrong, and I need to find out what it is right away."

We will return to this case later as we discuss workplace problems and conflicts, their sources, and how to resolve them.

---

these are *task-related conflicts*. Others are primarily related to personal and social issues; these are *relationship conflicts* (Jordan & Troth, 2004).

Power Plays and Competition between Groups

Differences in status and authority within the health-care team may generate conflicts. Physicians often feel that they have authority over other members of the team, sometimes causing them to disregard input from other team members (Sun, 2011) or refuse to engage in conflict resolution. The most common problem is disrespect or incivility, but sarcasm, finger-pointing, throwing things, and use of inappropriate language also occur (Lazoritz & Carlson, 2008). In one study of new graduate nurses, 12% reported daily workplace incivility from coworkers, 4.87% reported incivility from supervisors, and 7% reported daily incivility from physicians (Laschinger et al., 2013). The amount of incivility from fellow nurses is especially significant since they are an important source of guidance and support for new graduates.

Bullying involves behavior intended to exert power over another person. It is more than being overly demanding. Workplace bullies often single out one individual as a target, adding a degree of personal malice to their behavior. The effect on the targeted individual can be devastating and the cost to the organization is huge. A 2007 Gallup poll of over a million workers found that having an overbearing boss was the most common reason given for leaving a job (Wescott, 2012).

In some settings, nurses feel powerless, trapped by the demands of tasks they must complete and frustrated that they cannot provide quality care (Ramos, 2006). Union-management conflicts occur in some workplaces. Disagreements over professional "territory" can occur in any setting. Nurse practitioners and physicians may disagree over the scope of nurse practitioner practice, for example. Gender-based issues, including equal pay for women and sexual harassment, and diversity issues such as speaking languages other than English or feelings of being accepted by others may also occur (Howard & Wellins, 2009; Osterberg & Lorentsson, 2010).

Increased Workload

Emphasis on cost reduction has resulted in *work intensification*, a situation in which employees are required to do more in less time (Willis, Taffoli,

Henderson, & Walter, 2008). Common responses are skipping breaks, doing paperwork over lunch, and working overtime without pay. This leaves many health-care workers believing that their employers are taking advantage of them and causes even more conflict if they believe others are not working as hard as they are.

Multiple Role Demands

Inappropriate task assignments (e.g., asking nurses to clean patient rooms as well as nurse their patients) are often the result of cost-control efforts. Such assignments can lead to disagreements about who does what task and who is responsible for the outcome.

Threats to Safety and Security

When cost saving is emphasized and staff members face layoffs, people's economic security is threatened. This can be a source of considerable stress and tension.

Scarce Resources

Limited resources almost inevitably lead to competition to get one's fair share (or more), often resulting in conflict between individuals and between departments (Isosaari, 2011). Inadequate money for pay raises, equipment, supplies, or additional help can increase competition between or among individuals and departments as they scramble to grab their share of what little is available.

Cultural Differences

Language differences may make communication challenging. Some cultures emphasize the importance of the individual while others emphasize the importance of the group (Osterberg & Lorentsson, 2010). Different beliefs about how hard a person should work, what constitutes productivity, and even what it means to arrive at work "on time" can lead to conflicts if they are not reconciled.

Ethical Conflicts

Moral distress occurs when a nurse encounters a situation that violates his or her personal or professional ethics, especially when others ignore it or pretend it is not a concern (Lachman, Murray, Iseminger, & Ganske, 2012). Examples of such conflicts are recording care that was not given or failing to fully explain a procedure before obtaining patient consent.

Invasion of Personal Space

Crowded conditions and the constant interactions that occur at a busy nurses' station can increase interpersonal tension and lead to battles over scarce work space (McElhaney, 1996).

When Conflict Occurs

Conflict can occur at any level and involve any number of people. On the individual level, conflict can occur between two people on a team, in different departments, or between a staff member and a patient or family member. On the group level, conflict can occur between two teams (as in Case 1), two departments, or two different professional groups (e.g., between nurses and social workers over who is responsible for advance care planning). Conflict can also occur between two organizations (e.g., when two home health agencies compete for a contract with a large hospital). The focus in this chapter is primarily on the first two levels: among individuals and groups of people within a health-care organization.

Health care–oriented workplaces have been especially resistant to effective conflict management in the past, but several forces are reducing this resistance. The Institute of Medicine report *To Err is Human* (IOM, 1999) exposed serious threats to patient safety due to preventable errors and made it clear that problems need to be resolved, not buried. The Joint Commission added several standards that focus on better communication and problem resolution (Feldman et al., 2011). Nurses also find themselves in patient care situations where an ethical response might cause some conflict about which they cannot remain silent if this puts a patient at risk. Developing competency in dealing with conflict is an important leadership skill (Kritek, 2011). Box 8-1 lists situations in which conflict resolution is needed.

Resolving Problems and Conflicts

Win, Lose, or Draw?

Some people think about problems and conflicts that occur at work in the same way they think about a basketball game or tennis match: someone has to win and someone has to lose. There are some problems with this sports comparison. First, the aim of conflict resolution is to work together more effectively, not to win. Second, if people really do lose they are likely to feel bad about it. As a result, they may spend their time gearing up to win the next round rather than concentrating on their work.

A win-win result in which both sides gain some benefit is the best resolution (Haslan, 2001). Sometimes people cannot reach agreement (consensus) but can recognize and accept their differences and get on with their work (McDonald, 2008).

Other Conflict Resolution Myths

Many people think of what can be "won" as a fixed amount: "I get half, and you get half." This is the *fixed pie* myth of conflict resolution (Thompson & Fox, 2001). Another erroneous assumption is called the *devaluation reaction:* "If the other side is getting what they want, then it has to be bad for us." These erroneous beliefs can be serious barriers to achievement of a mutually beneficial conflict resolution.

When disagreements first arise, *problem solving* may be sufficient. If the situation has already developed into a full-blown conflict, however, *negotiation,* either informal or formal, of a settlement may be necessary.

Problem Resolution

The use of the problem-solving process in patient care should be familiar. The same approach can be used when staff problems occur. The goal is to find a solution that satisfies everyone involved. The process illustrated in Figure 8.1 includes identifying the issue, generating solutions, evaluating the suggested solutions, choosing what appears to be the best solution, implementing that solution, evaluating the extent to which the problem has been resolved, and, finally, concluding either that the problem has been resolved or that it will be

necessary to repeat the process to find a better solution.

Identify the Problem or Issue

First, ask participants in the conflict what they want (Sportsman, 2005). If the issue is not highly charged, they may be able to give a direct answer. Other times, however, some discussion and exploration of the issues will be necessary before the real problem emerges. "It would be nice," wrote Browne and Keeley, "if what other people were really saying was always obvious, if all their essential thoughts were clearly labeled for us . . . and if all knowledgeable people agreed about answers to important questions" (Browne & Keeley, 1994, p. 5). Of course, this is not what usually happens. People are often vague about what their real concern is; sometimes they are genuinely uncertain about what the real problem is. Strong emotions may further cloud the issue. All this needs to be sorted out so that the problem is clearly identified and a solution can be sought.

Generate Possible Solutions

Here, creativity is especially important. Try to discourage people from using old solutions for new problems. It is natural for people to try a solution that has already worked well, but previously successful solutions may not work in the future.

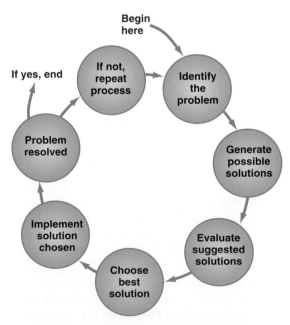

Figure 8.1 The process of resolving a problem.

When an innovative solution is needed, suggest that the group take some time to *brainstorm*. Ask everyone to write down (or call out as you write on a board, screen, or flip chart) as many solutions as they can come up with (Rees, 2005). Then give everyone a chance to consider each suggestion on its own merits.

Review Suggested Solutions and Choose the Best Solution

An open-minded evaluation of each suggestion is needed, but accomplishing this is not always easy. Some groups get "stuck in a rut," unable to "think outside the box." Other times, groups find it difficult to separate the suggestion from its source. On an interdisciplinary team, for example, the status of the person who made the suggestion may influence whether the suggestion is judged to be useful. Yet the best suggestions often come from those closest to the problem (McChrystal, 2012). This may be the care assistants who spend the most time with their patients. Whose solution is most likely to be the best one, the physician's or the unlicensed assistant's? A suggestion should be judged on its merits, not its source. Which of the suggested solutions is most likely to work? A combination of suggestions is often the best solution.

Implement the Solution Chosen

The true test of any suggested solution is how well it actually works. Once a solution has been imple-

mented, it is important to give it time to work. Impatience sometimes leads to premature abandonment of a good solution.

Evaluate: Is the Problem Resolved?

Not every problem is resolved successfully on the first attempt. If the problem has not been resolved, then the process needs to be resumed with even greater attention to what the real problem is and how it can be resolved successfully.

Consider the following situation in which problem-solving was helpful (Case 2)

The nurse manager asked Ms. Deloitte to meet with her to discuss the problem. The following is a summary of their problem-solving:

- **The Issue.** Ms. Deloitte wanted to take her vacation from the end of December through early January. Making the assumption that she was going to be permitted to go, she had purchased nonrefundable tickets. The policy forbids vacations from December 20 to January 5. The former nurse manager had not enforced this policy with Ms. Deloitte, but the new nurse manager thought it fair to enforce the policy with everyone, including Ms. Deloitte.
- **Possible Solutions**
  1. Ms. Deloitte resigns.
  2. Ms. Deloitte is fired.
  3. Allow Ms. Deloitte to take her vacation as planned.

Case 2

The Vacation

Francine Deloitte has been a unit secretary for 10 years. She is prompt, efficient, accurate, courteous, flexible, and productive—everything a nurse manager could ask for in a unit secretary. When nursing staff members are very busy, she distributes afternoon snacks or sits with a family for a few minutes until a nurse is available. There is only one issue on which Ms. Deloitte is insistent and stubborn: taking her 2-week vacation over the Christmas and New Year holidays. This is forbidden by hospital policy, but every nurse manager has allowed her to do this because it is the only special request she ever makes and because it is the only time she visits her family during the year.

A recent reorganization of the administrative structure had eliminated several layers of nursing managers and supervisors. Each remaining nurse manager was given responsibility for two or three units. The new nurse manager for Ms. Deloitte's unit refused to grant her request for vacation time at the end of December. "I can't show favoritism," she explained. "No one else is allowed to take vacation time at the end of December." Assuming that she could have the time off as usual, Francine had already purchased a nonrefundable ticket for her visit home. When her request was denied, she threatened to quit. On hearing this, one of the nurses on Francine's unit confronted the new nurse manager saying, "You can't do this. We are going to lose the best unit secretary we've ever had if you do."

4. Allow everyone to take vacations between December 20 and January 5 as requested.
5. Allow no one to take a vacation between December 20 and January 5.

■ **Evaluate Suggested Solutions.** Ms. Deloitte preferred solutions 3 and 4. The new nurse manager preferred 5. Neither wanted 1 or 2. They could agree only that none of the solutions satisfied both of them, so they decided to try again.

■ **Second List of Possible Solutions**
1. Reimburse Ms. Deloitte for the cost of the tickets.
2. Allow Ms. Deloitte to take one last vacation between December 20 and January 5.
3. Allow Ms. Deloitte to take her vacation during Thanksgiving instead.
4. Allow Ms. Deloitte to begin her vacation on December 26 so that she would work on Christmas Day but not on New Year's Day.
5. Allow Ms. Deloitte to begin her vacation earlier in December so that she could return in time to work on New Year's Day.

■ **Choose the Best Solution.** As they discussed the alternatives, Ms. Deloitte said she could change the day of her flight without a penalty. The nurse manager said she would allow solution 5 on the second list if Ms. Deloitte understood that she could not take vacation time between December 20 and January 5 in the future. Ms. Deloitte agreed to this.

■ **Implement the Solution.** Ms. Deloitte returned on December 30 and worked both New Year's Eve and New Year's Day.

■ **Evaluate the Solution.** The rest of the staff members had been watching the situation very closely. Most believed that the solution had been fair to them as well as to Ms. Deloitte. Ms. Deloitte thought she had been treated fairly. The nurse manager believed both parties had found a solution that was fair to Ms. Deloitte but still reinforced the manager's determination to enforce the vacation policy.

■ **Resolved, or Resume Problem Solving?** Ms. Deloitte, staff members, and the nurse manager all thought the problem had been solved satisfactorily.

Negotiating an Agreement Informally

When a disagreement has become too big, too complex, or too heated for problem resolution to be successful, a more elaborate process may be required to resolve it. On evaluating Case 1, the nurse manager decided that the tensions between Team A and Team B had become so great that negotiation would be necessary.

The process of negotiation is a complex one that requires much careful thought beforehand and considerable skill in its implementation. Box 8-2 is an outline of the most essential aspects of negotiation. Case 1 is used to illustrate how it can be done.

Scope the Situation

For a strategy to be successful, it is important that the entire situation be understood thoroughly. Walker and Harris (1995) suggested asking three questions:

1. *What am I trying to achieve?* The nurse manager in Case 1 is very concerned about the tensions between Team A and Team B. She wants the members of these two teams to be able to work together in a cooperative manner, which they are not doing at the present time.
2. *What is the environment in which I am operating?* The members of Teams A and B were openly hostile to each other. The overall climate of the organization, however, was benign. The nurse manager knew that teamwork was encouraged and that her actions to resolve the conflict would be supported by administration.
3. *What problems am I likely to encounter?* The nurse manager knew that she had allowed the problem to go on too long. Even physicians, social workers, and visitors to the unit were getting caught up in the conflict. Team members were actively encouraging other staff to take sides, making clear that "if you're not with us, you're against us." This made people

---

box 8-2

The Informal Negotiation Process

- Scope the situation. Ask yourself:
  What am I trying to achieve?
  What is the environment in which I am operating?
  What problems am I likely to encounter?
  What does the other side want?
- Set the stage.
- Conduct the negotiation.
- Set the ground rules.
- Clarify the problem.
- Make your opening move.
- Continue with offers and counteroffers.
- Agree on the resolution of the conflict.

from other departments very uncomfortable because they had to work with both teams. The nurse manager knew that resolution of the conflict would be a relief to many people.

It is important to ask one additional question in preparation for negotiations.

4. *What does the other side want?* In this situation, the nurse manager was not certain what either team really wanted. She realized that she needed this information before she could begin to negotiate.

Set the Stage

When a conflict such as the one between Teams A and B has gone on for some time, the opposing sides are often unwilling to meet to discuss the problem. This avoidance prevents an exchange of information between the two groups (Sun, 2011). If this occurs, it may be necessary to confront them with direct statements designed to open communications between the two sides, challenging them to seek resolution of the situation. At the same time, it is important to avoid any suggestion of blame because this provokes defensiveness.

To confront Teams A and B with their behavior toward one another, the nurse manager called them together at the end of the day shift. "I am very concerned about what I have been observing," she told them. "It appears to me that instead of working together, our two teams are working against each other." She continued with some examples of what she had observed, taking care not to mention names or blame anyone for the problem. She was also prepared to take responsibility for having allowed the situation to deteriorate before taking this much-needed action.

Conduct the Negotiation

As indicated earlier, conducting a negotiation requires a great deal of skill.

1. **Manage the emotions.** When people are very emotional, they have trouble thinking clearly. Acknowledging these emotions is essential to negotiating effectively (Fiumano, 2005). When faced with a highly charged situation, do not respond with added emotion. Take time out if you need to get your own feelings under control. Then find out why emotions are high (watch both verbal and nonverbal cues

carefully) and refocus the discussion on the issues. Allow disagreements to be expressed. Those who are willing to voice their differences play an important role in helping the group move toward resolution of the problem. The leader's role is to encourage group members to listen to and consider these differences, the first step in moving toward resolution of the conflict (Sarkar, 2009). Without effective leadership to prevent disagreements, emotional outbursts, and personal attacks, a mishandled negotiation can worsen a situation. With effective leadership, the conflict may be resolved (Box 8-3).

2. **Set ground rules.** Members of Teams A and B began throwing accusations at each other as soon as the nurse manager made her statement. The nurse manager stopped this quickly and said, "First, we need to set some ground rules for this discussion. Everyone will get a chance to speak but not all at once. Please speak for yourself, not for others. And please do not make personal remarks or criticize your coworkers. We are here to resolve this problem, not to make it worse." She had to remind the group of these ground rules several times during the meeting.

3. **Clarification of the problem.** The nurse manager wrote a list of problems raised by team members on a chalkboard. As the list grew longer, she asked the group, "What do you see here? What is the real problem?" The group remained silent. Finally, someone said,

---

box 8-3

Tips for Leading the Discussion

- Create a climate of comfort.
- Let others know the purpose is to resolve a problem or conflict.
- Freely admit your own contribution to the problem.
- Begin with the presentation of facts.
- Recognize your own emotional response to the situation.
- Set ground rules.
- Do not make personal remarks.
- Avoid placing blame.
- Allow each person an opportunity to speak.
- Do speak for yourself but not for others.
- Focus on solutions.
- Keep an open mind.

Adapted from Patterson, K., Grenny, J., McMillan, R., & Surtzler, A. (18 March 2003). Crucial conversations: Making a difference between being healed and being seriously hurt. Vital Signs, 13(5), 14–15.

"We don't have enough people, equipment, or supplies to get the work done." The rest of the group nodded in agreement.

4. **Opening move.** Once the problem is clarified, it is time to obtain everyone's agreement to seek a way to resolve the conflict. In a more formal negotiation, you may make a statement about what you wish to achieve. This first statement sets the stage for the rest of the negotiation (Suddath, 2012). For example, if you are negotiating a salary increase, you might begin by saying, "I am requesting a 10% increase for the following reasons: . . ." Of course, your employer will probably make a counteroffer, such as, "The best I can do is 3%." These are the opening moves of a negotiation.

5. **Continue the negotiations.** The discussion should continue in an open, nonhostile manner. Each side's concerns may be further explained and elaborated. Additional offers and counteroffers are common. As the discussion continues, it is helpful to emphasize areas of agreement as well as disagreement so that both parties are encouraged to continue the negotiations (Tappen, 2001).

Agree on a Resolution of the Conflict

After much testing for agreement, elaborating each side's positions and concerns, and making offers and counteroffers, the people involved should finally reach an agreement.

The nurse manager of Teams A and B led them through a discussion of their concerns related to working with severely limited resources. The teams soon realized that they had a common concern and that they might be able to help each other rather than compete with each other. The nurse manager agreed to become more proactive in seeking resources for the unit. "We can simultaneously seek new resources and develop creative ways to use the resources we already have," she told the teams. Relationships between members of Team A and Team B improved remarkably after this meeting. They learned that they could accomplish more by working together than they had ever achieved separately.

Formal Negotiation: Collective Bargaining

There are many varieties of formal negotiations, from real estate transactions to international peace treaty negotiations. A formal negotiation process of special interest to nurses is collective bargaining, which is highly formalized because it is governed by laws and contracts called *collective bargaining agreements*.

Collective bargaining involves a formal procedure governed by labor laws, such as the National Labor Relations Act in the United States. Nonprofit health-care organizations were added to the organizations covered by these laws in 1974. Once a union or professional organization has been designated as the official bargaining agent for a group of nurses, a contract defining such important matters as salary increases, benefits, time off, unfair treatment, safety issues, and promotion of professional practice is drawn up. This contract governs employee-management relations within the organization.

A collective bargaining contract is a legal document that governs the relationship between management and staff, who are represented by the union (for nurses, it may be the nurses' association or another health-care workers' union). The contract may cover some or all of the following:

■ **Economic issues:** Salaries, shift differentials, length of the workday, overtime, holidays, sick leave, breaks, health insurance, pensions, severance pay

■ **Management issues:** Promotions, layoffs, transfers, reprimands, grievance procedures, hiring and firing procedures

■ **Practice issues:** Adequate staffing, standards of care, code of ethics, safe working environment, other quality-of-care issues, staff development opportunities

Better patient-nurse staffing ratios, more reasonable workloads, opportunities for professional development, and better relationships with management are among the most important issues for practicing nurses (Budd, Warino, & Patton, 2004).

Case 3 is an example of how collective bargaining agreements can influence the outcome of a conflict between management and staff in a health-care organization.

The Pros and Cons of Collective Bargaining

Some nurses believe it is unprofessional to belong to a union. Others point out that physicians and teachers are union members and that the protections offered by a union outweigh the downside. There is no easy answer to this question.

Case 3

Collective Bargaining

The chief executive officer (CEO) of a large home health agency in a southwestern resort area called a general staff meeting. She reported that the agency had grown rapidly and was now the largest in the area. "Much of our success is due to the professionalism and commitment of our staff members," she said. "With growth come some problems, however. The most serious problem is the fluctuation in patient census. Our census peaks in the winter months when seasonal residents are here and troughs in the summer. In the past, when we were a small agency, we all took our vacations during the slow season. This made it possible to continue to pay everyone his or her full salary all year. However, given pressures to reduce costs and the large number of staff members we now have, we cannot continue to do this. We are very concerned about maintaining the high quality of patient care currently provided, but we have calculated that we need to reduce staff by 30 percent over the summer in order to survive financially."

The CEO then invited comments from the staff members. The majority of the nurses said they wanted and needed to work full-time all year. Most supported families and had to have a steady income all year. "My rent does not go down in the summer," said one. "Neither does my mortgage payment or the grocery bill," said another. A small number said that they would be happy to work part-time in the summer if they could be guaranteed full-time employment from October through May. "We have friends who would love this work schedule," they added.

"That's not fair," protested the nurses who needed to work full-time all year. "You can't replace us with part-time staff." The discussion grew louder and the participants more agitated. The meeting ended without a solution to the problem. Although the CEO promised to consider all points of view before making a decision, the nurses left the meeting feeling very confused and concerned about the security of their future income. Some grumbled that they probably should begin looking for new positions "before the ax falls."

The next day the CEO received a telephone call from the nurses' union representative. "If what I heard about the meeting yesterday is correct," said the representative, "your plan is in violation of our collective bargaining contract." The CEO reviewed the contract and found that the representative was correct. A new solution to the financial problems caused by the seasonal fluctuations in patient census would have to be found.

Probably the greatest advantages of collective bargaining are protection of the right to fair treatment and the availability of a written grievance procedure that specifies both the employee's and the employer's rights and responsibilities if an issue arises that cannot be settled informally (Forman & Merrick, 2003). Another advantage is salary: nurses working under a collective bargaining agreement can earn as much as 28% more than those who do not (Pittman, 2007).

The greatest disadvantage of using collective bargaining as a way to deal with conflict is that it clearly separates management from staff, often creating an adversarial relationship. Any nurses who make staffing decisions may be classified as supervisors and, therefore, may be ineligible to join the union, separating them from the rest of their colleagues (Martin, 2001). The result is that management and staff are treated as opposing parties rather than as people who are trying to work together to provide essential services to their patients. The collective bargaining contract also adds another layer of rules and regulations between staff members and their supervisors. Because management of such employee-related rules and regulations can take almost a quarter of a manager's time (Drucker, 2002), this can become a drain on a nurse manager's time and energy.

Conclusion

Conflict is inevitable within any large, diverse group of people who are trying to work together over an extended period. However, conflict does not have to be destructive, nor does it have to be an entirely negative experience. If it is handled skillfully, conflict can stimulate people to learn more about each other and how to work together in more effective ways. Resolving a conflict, when done well, can lead to improved working relationships, more creative methods of operation, and higher productivity.

Study Questions

1. Debate the question of whether conflict is constructive or destructive. How can good leadership affect the outcome of a conflict?

2. Give an example of how each of the seven sources of conflict listed in this chapter can lead to a serious problem. Then discuss ways to prevent the occurrence of conflict from each of the seven sources.

3. What is the difference between problem resolution and negotiation? Under what circumstances would you use one or the other?

4. Identify a conflict (actual or potential) in your clinical area, and explain how either problem resolution or negotiation could be used to resolve it.

5. In what ways does collective bargaining increase conflict? How does it help resolve conflicts?

Case Study to Promote Critical Reasoning

A not-for-profit hospice center in a small community received a generous gift from the grateful family of a patient who had died recently. The family asked only that the money be "put to the best use possible."

Everyone in this small facility had an opinion about the "best" use for the money. The administrator wanted to renovate the old, rundown headquarters. The financial officer wanted to put the money in the bank "for a rainy day." The chaplain wanted to add a small chapel to the building. The nurses wanted to create a food bank to help the poorest of their clients. The social workers wanted to buy a van to transport clients to health-care provider offices. The staff agreed that all the ideas had merit, that all of the needs identified were important ones. Unfortunately, there was enough money to meet only one of them.

The more the staff members discussed how to use this gift, the more insistent each group became that their idea was best. At their last meeting, it was evident that some were becoming frustrated and that others were becoming angry. It was rumored that a shouting match between the administrator and the financial officer had occurred.

1. In your analysis of this situation, identify the sources of the conflict that are developing in this facility.

2. What kind of leadership actions are needed to prevent the escalation of this conflict?

3. If the conflict does escalate, how could it be resolved?

4. Which idea do you think has the most merit? Why did you select the one you did?

5. Try role-playing a negotiation among the administrator, the financial officer, the chaplain, a representative of the nursing staff, and a representative of the social work staff. Can you suggest a creative solution?

References

Browne, M.N., & Keeley, S.M. (1994). *Asking the right questions: A guide to critical thinking.* Englewood Cliffs, NJ: Prentice-Hall.

Budd, K., Warino, L., & Patton, M. (2004). Traditional and non-traditional collective bargaining: Strategies to improve the patient care environment. *The Online Journal of Nursing.* Retrieved on December 4, 2013, from www.nursingworld.org/MainMenuCategories/ANAMarketplace/ANAPeriodicals/OJIN/TableofContents/Volume92004/No1Jan04/CollectiveBargainingStrategies.aspx

Drucker, P.F. (2002). They're not employees, they're people. *Harvard Business Review, 80*(2), 70–77, 128.

Feldman, H.R., & Greenberg, M.J. (Eds.). (2011). *Nursing leadership: A concise encyclopedia.* New York, NY: Springer Publishing Company.

Fiumano, J. (2005). Navigate through conflict, not around it. *Nursing Management, 36*(8), 14, 18.

Forman, H., & Merrick, F. (2003). Grievances and complaints: Valuable tools for management and for staff. *Journal of Nursing Administration, 33*(3), 136–138.

Haslan, S.A. (2001). *Psychology in organizations.* Thousand Oaks, CA: Sage.

Horton-Deutsch, S.L., & Wellman, D.S. (2002). Christman's principles for effective management. *Journal of Nursing Administration, 32,* 596–601.

Howard, A., & Wellins, R. (2009). *Holding women back: Troubling discoveries—and best practices for helping female leaders succeed.* A special report from Development Dimensions International's Global Leadership Forecast.

Institute of Medicine. (1999). *To err is human: Building a safer health care system.* Washington, DC: National Academies Press.

Isosaari, V. (2011). Power in health care organizations. *Journal of Health Organization and Management, 25*(4), 385–399.

Jordan, P., & Troth, A.C. (2004). Managing emotions during team problem solving: Emotional intelligence and conflict resolution. *Human Performance, 17*(2), 195–218.

Kritek, P.B. (2011). Conflict management in *nursing leadership: A concise encyclopedia (2nd ed.).* New York: Springer Publishing Company.

Lachman, V.D., Murray, J.S., Iseminger, K., & Ganske, K.M. (2012). Doing the right thing: Pathways to moral courage. *American Nurse Today, 7*(5), 24–29.

Laschinger, H., Wong, C., Regan, S., Young-Ritchie, C., & Bushell, P. (2013). Workplace incivility and new gradate nurses' mental health. The protective role of incivility. *The Journal of Nursing Administration, 43*(7/8), 415–421.

Lazoritz, S., & Carlson, P.J. (2008). Descriptive physician behavior. *American Nurse Today, 3*(3), 20–22.

Martin, R.H. (June 2001). Ruling may limit ability to unionize. *Advance for Nurses, 9.*

McChrystal, S. (2012). (Quoted by R. Safian). Secrets of the flux leader. *Fast Company, 170,* 105.

McDonald, D. (2008). Revisiting a theory of negotiation: The utility of Markiewicz (2005) proposed six principles. *Evaluation and Program Planning, 31*(3), 259–265.

McElhaney, R. (1996). Conflict management in nursing administration. *Nursing Management, 27*(3), 49–50.

Osterberg, C., & Lorentsson, T. (2010). Organizational conflict and socialization processes in healthcare. (Thesis). University of Gothenburg, Göteborg, Sweden.

Patterson, K., Grenny, J., McMillan, R., & Surtzler, A. (18 March 2003). Crucial conversations: Making a difference between being healed and being seriously hurt. *Vital Signs, 13*(5), 14–15.

Pittman, J. (2007). Registered nurse job satisfaction and collective bargaining unit membership status. *Journal of Nursing Administration, 37*(10), 471–476.

Ramos, M.C. (2006). Eliminate destructive behaviors through example and evidence. *Nursing Management, 37*(9), 34–41.

Rees, F. (2005). *25 Activities for developing team leaders.* San Francisco: Pfeiffer.

Sarkar, S. (2009). The dance of dissent: Managing conflict in healthcare organizations. *Psychoanalytic Psychotherapy. 23*(2), 121–135.

Siu, H., Laschinger, H.R.S., & Finegan, J. (2008). Nursing professional practice environments: Setting the stage for constructive conflict resolution and work effectiveness. *Journal of Nursing Administration, 38*(5), 250–257.

Sportsman, S. (2005). Build a framework for conflict assessment. *Nursing Management, 36*(4), 32–40.

Suddath, C. (2012). The art of haggling: When fighting for a new salary, it's all about the first number on the table. *Bloomberg Businessweek,* November 26–December 2012. Retrieved December 4, 2013, from http://www.businessweek.com/articles/2012-11-21/the-art-of-haggling

Sun, K. (2011). Inter-unit conflict, conflict resolution methods, and post-merger, organizational integration in healthcare organizations. (Dissertation.) University of Minnesota, Minneapolis.

Tappen, R.M. (2001) *Nursing leadership and management: Concept and practice.* Philadelphia: F.A. Davis.

Thompson, L., & Fox, C.R. (2001). Negotiation within and between groups in organizations: Levels of analysis. In Turner, M.E. (ed.), *Groups at Work,* 221–266. Mahwah, NJ: Laurence Erlbaum.

Tjosvold, D., & Tjosvold, M.M. (1995). *Psychology for leaders: Using motivation, conflict, and power to manage more effectively.* New York: John Wiley & Sons.

Van de Vliert, E., & Janssen, O. (2001). Description, explanation, and prescription of intragroup conflict behaviors. *Groups at work: Theory and research,* 267–297.

Vivar, C.G. (2006). Putting conflict management into practice: A nursing case study. *Journal of Nursing Management, 14,* 201–206.

Walker, M.A., & Harris, G.L. (1995). *Negotiations: Six steps to success.* Upper Saddle River, NJ: Prentice-Hall.

Wescott, D. (2012). Field guide to office bullies. *Bloomberg Businessweek.* Retrieved from http://images.businessweek.com/slideshows/2012-11-21/field-guide-to-office-bullies

Willis, E., Taffoli, L., Henderson, J., & Walter, B. (2008). Enterprise bargaining: A case study in the de-intensification of nursing work in Australia. *Nursing Inquiry, 15*(2), 148–157.

chapter 9

People and the Process of Change

When asked the theme of a nursing management conference, a top nursing executive answered, "Change, change, and more change." Whether it is called innovation, turbulence, or change, change is constant in the workplace today. Mismanaging change is common. In fact, as many as three out of four major change efforts fail (Cameron & Quinn, 2006; Hempel, 2005; Shirey, 2012), often because of resistant staff or a resistant organizational culture. This chapter discusses how people respond to change, how you can lead change, and how you can help people cope with change when it becomes difficult.

Change

A Natural Phenomenon

"Being scared by change doesn't help" (Carter quoted by Safian, 2012, p. 97). Change is a part of everyone's lives. People have new experiences, meet new people, and learn something new. People grow up, leave home, graduate from college, begin a

career, and perhaps start a family. Some of these changes are milestones, ones for which people have prepared and have anticipated for some time. Many are exciting, leading to new opportunities and challenges. Some are entirely unexpected, sometimes welcome and sometimes not. When change occurs too rapidly or demands too much, it can make people uncomfortable, even anxious or stressed.

Macro and Micro Change

The "ever-whirling wheel of change" (Dent, 1995, p. 287) in health care seems to spin faster every year. Medicare and Medicaid cuts, large numbers of people who are uninsured or underinsured, restructuring, downsizing, and staff shortages are major concerns. Increasingly diverse patient populations, rapid advances in technology, and new research findings necessitate frequent changes in nursing practice (Boyer, 2013; Cornell et al., 2010; Rodts, 2011). When first introduced, managed care had a tremendous impact on the provision of health care, and the recent Patient Protection and Affordable

Care Act may revolutionize health-care delivery yet again (Leonard, 2012; Webb & Marshall, 2010). Such changes sweep through the health-care system, affecting patients and caregivers alike. They are the *macro-level* (large-scale) changes that affect virtually every health-care facility.

A change may be local (confined to one nursing care unit, for example) or organization-wide. The change may be small, affecting just one care practice or one aspect of system operation, or sweeping, revolutionizing the structure and operation of the entire organization. Finally, the change may be implemented gradually or happen swiftly (Chreim, & Williams, 2012).

A series of small-scale changes to improve care on a pediatric care unit are described by MacDavitt (2011). They used a two-phase approach, designing the change in Phase I and implementing it in Phase II. One of the changes was initiation of bedside rounding including family members if they were available. Most of the pediatricians were enthusiastic supporters. However, the pulmonologists were more resistant, agreeing to test it first with only one patient, increasing the number by one each day. This had to begin all over again the next week when there was a new attending pulmonologist. The team persisted, patiently working through each new rotation of attending pulmonologists. Families were enthusiastic about the bedside rounds and complained if they didn't happen. This was critical to successful implementation of bedside rounds including families for all patients on this unit.

Change anywhere in a system creates ripples across the system (Parker & Gadbois, 2000). Every change that occurs at the system (organization or macro) level filters down to the *micro level*, to nursing units, teams, and individuals. Nurses, colleagues in other disciplines, and patients are participants in these changes. The micro level of change is the primary focus of this chapter.

New graduates may find themselves given responsibility for helping to bring about change. The following change-related activities are examples of the kinds of changes in which they might be asked to participate:

- Introducing a new technical procedure
- Implementing evidence-based practice guidelines
- Providing new policies for staff evaluation and promotion
- Participating in quality improvement and patient safety initiatives
- Preparing for surveys and safety inspections

Change and the Comfort Zone

The basic stages of the change process originally described by Kurt Lewin in 1951 are *unfreezing, change*, and *refreezing* (Lewin, 1951; Schein, 2004).

- *Unfreezing* involves actions that create readiness to change.
- *Change* is the implementation phase, the actions needed to put the change into effect.
- *Refreezing* is the restabilizing phase during which the change that was made becomes a regular part of everyday functions.

Imagine a work situation that is basically stable. People are generally accustomed to each other, have a routine for doing their work, know what to expect, and know how to deal with whatever problems come up. They are operating within their "comfort zone" (Farrell & Broude, 1987; Lapp, 2002). A change of any magnitude is likely to move people out of this comfort zone into discomfort. This move out of the comfort zone is called *unfreezing* (Fig. 9.1). For example:

Many health-care institutions offer nurses the choice of weekday or weekend work. Given these choices,

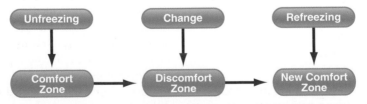

Figure 9.1 The change process. *Based on Farrell, K., & Broude, C. (1987]]. Winning the Change Game: How to Implement Information Systems With Fewer Headaches and Bigger Paybacks. Los Angeles: Breakthrough Enterprises; and Lewin, K. (1951). Field Theory in Social Science: Selected Theoretical Papers. New York: Harper & Row.*

nurses with school-age children are likely to find their comfort zone on weekday shifts. Imagine the discomfort they would experience if they were transferred to weekends. Such a change would rapidly unfreeze their usual routine and move them into the discomfort zone. They might have to find a new babysitter or begin a search for a new child-care center that is open on weekends. An alternative would be to establish a child-care center where they work. Yet another alternative would be to find a position that offers more suitable working hours.

Whatever alternative they chose, the nurses were being challenged to find a solution that enabled them to move into a new comfort zone. To accomplish this, they would have to find a consistent, dependable source of child care suited to their new schedule and to the needs of their children and then refreeze their situation. If they did not find a satisfactory alternative, they could remain in an unsettled state, in a discomfort zone, caught in a conflict between their personal and professional responsibilities.

As this example illustrates, what seems to be a small change can greatly disturb the people involved in it. The next section considers the many reasons why change can be unsettling and why change provokes resistance.

Resistance to Change

People resist change for a variety of reasons that vary from person to person and situation to situation. You might find that one patient-care technician is delighted with an increase in responsibility, whereas another is upset about it. Some people are eager to make changes; others prefer the status quo (Hansten & Washburn, 1999). Managers may find that one change in routine provokes a storm of protest and that another is hardly noticed. Why does this happen? We will first consider why people may be ready for change and why they may resist change.

Receptivity to Change
Preference for Certainty
An interesting research study on nurses' preferred information processing styles suggests that nurse managers were more receptive to change than were their staff members (Kalisch, 2007). Nurse manag-

ers were found to be innovative and decisive, whereas staff nurses preferred "proven" approaches and were resistant to change. Nursing assistants, unit secretaries, and licensed practical nurses were also unreceptive to change, adding layers of people who formed a "solid wall of resistance" to change. Kalisch suggests that helping teams recognize their preference for certainty (as opposed to change) will increase their receptivity to necessary changes in the workplace.

Speaking to People's Feelings
Although both thinking and feeling responses to change are important, Kotter (1999) says that the heart of responses to change lies in the emotions surrounding it. He suggests that a *compelling story* will increase receptivity to a change more than a carefully crafted analysis of the need for change. It is more likely to create that sense of urgency needed to stimulate change (Braungardt & Fought, 2008; Shirey, 2011). How is this done? The following are some examples of appeals to feelings

- Instead of presenting statistics about the number of people who are re-admitted due to poor discharge preparation, providing a story may be more persuasive. For example, you can tell the staff about a patient who collapsed at home the evening after discharge because he had not been able to control his diabetes post-surgery. Trying to break his fall, he fractured both wrists and needed surgical repair. With broken wrists, he is now unable to return home or take care of himself.
- Even better, videotape an interview with this man, letting him tell his story and describe the repercussions of poor preparation for discharge.
- Drama may also be achieved through visual display. A culture plate of pathogens grown from swabs of ventilator equipment and patient room furniture is more attention-getting than an infection control report. A display of disposables with price tags attached for just one patient is more memorable than an accounting sheet listing the costs.

The purpose of these activities is to present a compelling image that will affect people emotionally, increasing their receptivity to change and moving them into a state of readiness to change (Kotter, 1999).

Sources of Resistance

Resistance to change comes from three major sources: technical concerns, relation to personal needs, and threats to a person's position and power (Araujo Group).

Technical Concerns

The change itself may have *design flaws*. Resistance may be based on concerns about whether the proposed change is a good idea.

The Professional Practice Committee of a small hospital suggested replacing a commercial mouthwash with a mixture of hydrogen peroxide and water in order to save money. A staff nurse objected to this proposed change, saying that she had read a research study several years ago that found peroxide solutions to be an irritant to the oral mucosa (Tombes & Gallucci, 1993). A later review of the research noted that this depended on the concentration used (Hossainian, Slot, Afennich, & Van der Weijden, 2011). Fortunately, the chairperson of the committee recognized that this objection was based on technical concerns and requested a thorough study of the evidence before instituting the change. "It's important to investigate the evidence supporting a proposed change thoroughly before recommending it," she said.

A change may provoke resistance for *practical* reasons. For example, if the bar codes on patients' armbands are difficult to scan, nurses may develop a way to work around this safety feature by taping a duplicate armband to the bed or to a clipboard, defeating the electronically monitored medication system (Englebright & Franklin, 2005).

Personal Needs

Change often creates anxiety, much of it related to what people fear they might lose (Berman-Rubera, 2008; Johnston, 2008). Human beings have a hierarchy of needs, from the basic physiological needs to the higher-order needs for belonging, self-esteem, and self-actualization (Fig. 9.2). Maslow (1970) observed that the more basic needs (those lower on the hierarchy) must be at least partially met before a person is motivated to seek fulfillment of the higher-order needs.

Change may make it more difficult for a person to meet any or all of his or her needs. It may threaten safety and security needs. For example, if

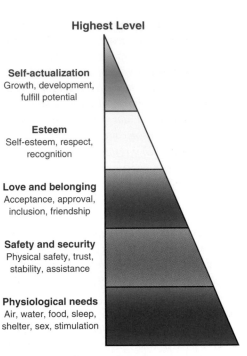

Highest Level

Self-actualization
Growth, development, fulfill potential

Esteem
Self-esteem, respect, recognition

Love and belonging
Acceptance, approval, inclusion, friendship

Safety and security
Physical safety, trust, stability, assistance

Physiological needs
Air, water, food, sleep, shelter, sex, stimulation

Lowest Level

Figure 9.2 Maslow's hierarchy of needs. *Based on Maslow, A.H. (1970). Motivation and Personality. New York: Harper & Row.*

a massive downsizing occurs and a person's job is eliminated, needs ranging from having enough money to pay for food and shelter to opportunities to fulfill one's career potential are likely to be threatened.

In other cases, the threat is subtler and may be harder to anticipate. For example, an institution-wide reevaluation of the effectiveness of the advanced practice role would be a great concern to a staff nurse who is working toward accomplishing a lifelong dream of becoming an advanced practice nurse in oncology. Staff reorganization that moves some staff members to different units could challenge the belonging needs of those who have close friends on the unit but few friends outside of work.

Position and Power

Once gained within an organization, status, power, and influence are hard to relinquish. This applies to people anywhere in the organization, not just those at the top. For example:

A clerk in the surgical suite had been preparing the operating room schedule for many years. Although his supervisor was expected to review the schedule before it was posted, she rarely did so because the clerk was skillful in balancing the needs of various parties, including some very demanding surgeons. When the supervisor was transferred to another facility, her replacement decided that she had to review the schedules before they were posted because they were ultimately her responsibility. The clerk became defensive. He tried to avoid the new supervisor and posted the schedules without her approval. This surprised her. She knew the clerk did this well and did not think that her review of them would be threatening.

Why did this happen? The supervisor had not realized the importance of this task to the clerk. The opportunity to tell others when and where they could perform surgery gave the clerk a feeling of power and importance. The supervisor's insistence on reviewing his work reduced the importance of his position. What seemed to the new supervisor to be a very small change in routine had provoked surprisingly strong resistance because it threatened the clerk's sense of importance and power.

Recognizing Resistance

Resistance may be *active* or *passive* (Heller, 1998). It is easy to recognize resistance to a change when it is expressed directly. When a person says to you, "That's not a very good idea," "I'll quit if you schedule me for the night shift," or "There's no way I'm going to do that," there is no doubt you are encountering resistance. Active resistance can take the form of outright refusal to comply, writing memos that destroy the idea, quoting existing rules that make the change difficult to implement, or encouraging others to resist.

When resistance is less direct, however, it can be difficult to recognize unless you know what to look for. Passive approaches usually involve avoidance: canceling appointments to discuss implementation of the change, being "too busy" to make the change, refusing to commit to changing, agreeing to it but doing nothing to change, and simply ignoring the entire process as much as possible (Table 9-1). Once resistance has been recognized, action can be taken to lower or even eliminate it.

Lowering Resistance

A great deal can be done to lower people's resistance to change. Strategies fall into four categories: sharing information, disconfirming currently held

table 9-1	
Resistance to Change	
Active	**Passive**
Attacking the idea	Avoiding discussion
Refusing to change	Ignoring the change
Arguing against the change	Refusing to commit to the change
Organizing resistance of other people	Agreeing but not acting

beliefs, providing psychological safety, and dictating (forcing) change (Tappen, 2001).

Sharing Information

Much resistance is simply the result of misunderstanding a proposed change. Sharing information about the proposed change can be done on a one-to-one basis, in group meetings, or through written materials distributed to everyone involved via print or electronic means.

Disconfirming Currently Held Beliefs

Disconfirming current beliefs is a primary force for change (Schein, 2004). Providing evidence that what people are currently doing is inadequate, incorrect, inefficient, or unsafe can increase people's willingness to change. For example, Lindberg and Clancy (2010) note a widespread belief in the inevitability of health-care associated infections, that they are unfortunate but unavoidable. To implement a successful campaign to reduce infection rates, this myth would have to be dispelled. The dramatic presentations described in the section on receptivity help to disconfirm current beliefs and practices. The following is a less dramatic example but still persuasive:

Jolene was a little nervous when her turn came to present information to the Clinical Practice Committee on a new enteral feeding procedure. Committee members were very demanding: they wanted clear, evidence-based information presented in a concise manner. Opinions and generalities were not acceptable. Jolene had prepared thoroughly and had practiced her presentation at home until she could speak without referring to her notes. The presentation went well. Committee members commented on how thorough she was and on the quality of the information presented. To her disappointment, however, no action was taken on her proposal.

Returning to her unit, she shared her disappointment with the nurse manager. Together, they used the unfreezing-change-refreezing process as a guide to review the presentation. The nurse manager agreed that Jolene had thoroughly reviewed the information on enteral feeding. The problem, she explained, was that Jolene had not attended to the need to unfreeze the situation. Jolene realized that she had not put any emphasis on the high risk of contamination and resulting gastrointestinal disturbances of the procedure currently in use. She had left members of the committee still comfortable with current practice because she had not emphasized the risk involved in failing to change it.

At the next meeting, Jolene presented additional information on the risks associated with the current enteral feeding procedures. This disconfirming evidence was persuasive. The committee accepted her proposal to adopt the new, lower-risk procedure.

Without the addition of the disconfirming evidence, it is likely that Jolene's proposed change would never have been implemented. The *inertia* (tendency to remain in the same state rather than to move toward change) exhibited by the Clinical Practice Committee is not unusual (Pearcey & Draper, 1996).

Providing Psychological Safety

As indicated earlier, a proposed change can threaten people's basic needs. Resistance can be lowered by reducing that threat, leaving people feeling more comfortable with the change. Each situation poses different kinds of threats and, therefore, requires different actions to reduce the levels of threat; the following is a list of useful strategies to increase psychological safety:

- Express approval of people's interest in providing the best care possible.
- Recognize the competence and skill of the people involved.
- Provide assurance (if possible) that no one will lose his or her position because of the change.
- Suggest ways in which the change can provide new opportunities and challenges (new ways to increase self-esteem and self-actualization).
- Involve as many people as possible in the design or plan to implement change.

- Provide opportunities for people to express their feelings and ask questions about the proposed change.
- Allow time for practice and learning of any new procedures before a change is implemented.

Dictating Change

This is an entirely different approach to change. People in authority in an organization can simply require people to make a change in what they are doing or can reassign people to new positions (Porter-O'Grady, 1996). This may not work well if there are ways for people to resist, however, such as in the following situations:

- When passive resistance can undermine the change
- When high motivational levels are necessary to make the change successful
- When people can refuse to obey the order without negative consequences

The following is an example of an unsuccessful attempt to dictate change:

A new, insecure nurse manager believed that her staff members were taking advantage of her inexperience by taking more than the two 15-minute coffee breaks allowed during an 8-hour shift. She decided that staff members would have to sign in and out for their coffee breaks and their 30-minute meal break. Staff members were outraged by this new policy. Most had been taking fewer than 15 minutes for coffee breaks or 30 minutes for lunch because of the heavy care demands of the unit. They refused to sign the coffee break sheet. When asked why they had not signed it, they replied, "I forgot," "I couldn't find it," or "I was called away before I had a chance." This organized passive resistance was sufficient to overcome the nurse manager's authority. The nurse manager decided that the coffee break sheet had been a mistake, removed it from the bulletin board, and never mentioned it again.

For people in authority, dictating a change often seems to be the easiest way to institute change: just tell people what to do, and do not listen to any arguments. There is risk in this approach, however. Even when staff members do not resist authority-based change, overuse of dictates can lead to a passive, dependent, unmotivated, and unempowered staff. Providing high-quality patient care requires staff members who are active, motivated, and highly committed to their work.

Leading Change

Now that you understand how change can affect people and have learned some ways to lower their resistance to change, consider what is involved in taking a leadership role in successful implementation of change.

The entire process of bringing about change can be divided into four phases: designing the change, deciding how to implement the change, carrying out the actual implementation, and following through to ensure the change has been integrated into the regular operation of the facility (Fig. 9.3).

Designing the Change

This is the starting point. The first step in bringing about change is to craft the change carefully. Not every change is for the better; some fail because they are poorly conceived in the first place.

Ask yourself the following questions:

- What are we trying to accomplish?
- Is the change necessary?
- Is the change technically correct?
- Will it work?
- Is this change a better way to do things?

Encourage people to talk about the changes planned, to express their doubts, and to provide their input (Fullan, 2001). Those who do are usually enthusiastic supporters later in the process.

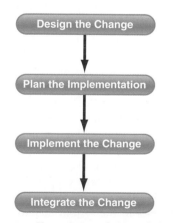

Figure 9.3 Four phases of planned change.

Planning

All the information presented previously about sources of resistance and ways to overcome that resistance should be taken into consideration when deciding how to implement a change.

For large-scale change, it is often helpful to appoint a champion, even a co-champion, to lead the innovation, helping staff prepare for the change and monitoring progress (Staren, Braun, & Denny, 2010).

The environment in which the change will take place is another factor to consider when assessing resistance to change. This includes the amount of change occurring at the same time and past history of change in the organization. Is there goodwill toward change because it has gone well in the past? Or have other changes gone badly? Bad experiences with previous changes can generate ill will and resistance to additional change (Maurer, 2008). There may be external pressure to change because of the competitive nature of the health-care market. In other situations, government regulations either may make it difficult to bring about a desired change or may force a change.

Almost everything you have learned about effective leadership is useful in planning the implementation of change: communicating the vision, motivating people, involving people in decisions that affect them, dealing with conflict, eliciting cooperation, providing coordination, and fostering teamwork. Consider all of these when formulating a plan to implement a change. Remember that people have to be moved out of their comfort zone to get them ready to change.

Implementing the Change

You are finally ready to embark on a journey of change and innovation that has been carefully planned. Consider the following factors:

- **Magnitude:** Is it a major change that affects almost everything people do, or is it a minor one?
- **Complexity:** Is this a difficult change to make? Does it require much new knowledge and skill? How much time will it take to acquire them?
- **Pace:** How urgent is this change? Can it be done gradually, or must it be implemented immediately?
- **Stress:** Is this the only change that is taking place, or is it just one of many? How stressful

are these changes? How can you help people keep their stress at tolerable levels?

A simple change, such as introducing a new type of thermometer, may be planned, implemented, and integrated easily into everyone's work routine. A complex change, such as introducing a new medication administration system, may require testing the new system, evaluating what works and what does not, and adapting the system before it works well in your facility.

Some discomfort is likely to occur with almost any change, and it is important to keep it within tolerable limits. You can exert some pressure to make people pay attention to the change process, but not so much pressure that they are overstressed. In other words, you want to raise the heat enough to get them moving but not so much that they boil over (Heifetz & Linsky, 2002).

Integrating the Change

This is the refreezing phase of change. After the change has been made, make sure that everyone has moved into a new comfort zone. Ask yourself:

- Is the change well integrated into everyday operations and routines?
- Is it working well?
- Are people comfortable with it?
- Is it well accepted? Is there any residual resistance that could still undermine it?

It may take some time before a change is fully integrated into everyday routines. As Kotter noted, change "sticks" when, instead of being the new way to do something, it has become "the way we always do things around here" (1999, p. 18).

Personal Change

The focus of this chapter is on leading others through the process of change. However, if you are leading change, you "have to be willing to change yourself" (Olivier quoted by Suddath, 2012, p. 85). Choosing to change may be an important part of your development as a leader.

Hart and Waisman (2005) used the story of the caterpillar and the butterfly to illustrate personal change:

Caterpillars cannot fly. They have to crawl or climb to find their food. Butterflies, on the other hand, can soar above an obstacle. They also have a different perspective on their world because they can fly. It is not easy to change from a caterpillar to a butterfly. Indeed, the transition (metamorphosis) may be quite uncomfortable and involves some risk. Are you ready to become a butterfly?

The process of personal change is similar to the process described throughout this chapter: first recognize the need for change, then learn how to do things differently, and then become comfortable with the "new you" (Guthrie & King, 2004). A more detailed step-by-step process is given in Table 9-2. You might, for example, decide that you need to stop interrupting people when they speak with you. Or you might want to change your leadership style from laissez-faire to participative.

Is a small change easier to accomplish than a radical change? Perhaps not. Deutschman (2005a) reports research that suggests radical change might be easier to accomplish because the benefits are evident much more quickly.

An extreme example: on the individual level, many people could avoid a second coronary bypass or angioplasty by changing their lifestyle, yet 90% do not do so. Deutschman compares the typical advice (exercise, stop smoking, eat healthier meals) with Ornish's radical vegetarian diet (only 10% of calories from fat). After 3 years, 77% of the patients who went through this extreme change had continued these lifestyle changes. Why? Ornish suggests several reasons: (1) after several weeks, people felt a change—they could walk or have sex without pain; (2) information alone is not enough—the emotional aspect is dealt with in support groups and through meditation, relaxation, yoga, and aerobic exercise; and (3) the motivation to pursue this change is redefined—instead of focusing on fear of death, which many find too frightening, Ornish focuses on the joy of living, feeling better, and being active without pain.

A large-scale, revolutionary change from fragmented, provider-centered care to fully integrated patient-centered primary care is described by Chreim and colleagues (2012). A family practice with eight physicians saw 9,000 patients a year. Some of the care they provided (well baby care, for example) overlapped with (duplicated) the public health nurses' care. To integrate care would require radical changes in the system including electronic sharing of patient records, paying physicians per patient per year (called capitation) instead of per

table 9-2

Which Stage of Change Are You In?

While studying how smokers quit the habit, Dr. James Prochaska, a psychologist at the University of Rhode Island, developed a widely influential model of the "stages of change." What stage are you in? See if any of the following statements sound familiar.

Typical Statement	Stage	Risks
"As far as I'm concerned, I don't have any problems that need changing."	1 Precontemplation	You are in denial. You probably feel coerced by other people who are trying to make you change. But they are not going to shame you into it—their meddling will backfire.
"I guess I have faults, but there's nothing that I really need to change."	("Never")	
"I've been thinking that I wanted to change something about myself."	2 Contemplation	Feeling righteous because of your good intentions, you could stay in this stage for years. But you might respond to the emotional persuasion of a compelling leader.
"I wish I had more ideas on how to solve my problems."	("Someday")	
"I have decided to make changes in the next 2 weeks."	3 Preparation	This "rehearsal" can become your reality. Some 85% of people who need to change their behavior for health reasons never reach this stage or progress beyond it.
"I am committed to join a fitness club by the end of the month."	("Soon")	
"Anyone can talk about changing. I'm actually doing something about it."	4 Action	It is an emotional struggle. It is important to change quickly enough to feel the short-term benefits that give a psychic lift and make it easier to stick with the change.
"I am doing okay, but I wish I was more consistent."	("Now")	
"I may need a boost right now to help me maintain the changes I've already made."	5 Maintenance	Relapse. Even though you have created a new mental pathway, the old pathway is still there in your brain, and when you are under a lot of stress, you might fall back on it.
"This has become part of my day, and I feel it when I don't follow through."	("Forever")	

Source: Adapted from Deutschman's which stage of change are you in? "Typical statements" adapted from stages of change: theory and practice by Michael Samuelson, executive director of the National Center for Health Promotion.

visit and moving physicians, nurses, and others to shared locations. After 4 years, patient satisfaction was higher and more received preventive services such as Pap smears or blood pressure checks. Collaboration and teamwork among providers increased. Chreim and colleagues noted that there had been considerable motivation to change and the provincial government supported the change. "What is best for the patient" (p. 227) became a shared value and motivation. There were many difficulties to overcome, including frustration with developing and learning how to use the electronic information system, deciding how to share tasks such as diabetes education, and limited physical space to co-locate care providers. Perseverance when encountering barriers and setbacks and ability to tolerate uncertainty were essential in implementing this large-scale change successfully.

The traditional approach to change is turned on its head: a major change appears easier to accomplish than a minor change, and people are not stressed but feel better making the change. Deutschman's list of five commonly accepted myths about change that have been refuted by new insights from research summarize this approach (Table 9-3).

It remains to be seen whether these new insights on changing behavior are useful outside of these special situations.

Conclusion

Change is an inevitable part of living and working. How people respond to change, the amount of stress it causes, and the amount of resistance it provokes can be influenced by good leadership. Handled well, most changes can become opportunities for professional growth and development rather than just additional stressors with which nurses and their clients have to cope.

table 9-3

Five Myths About Changing Behavior: An Alternative Perspective

Myth	Reality
1. Crisis is a powerful impetus for change.	Ninety percent of patients who have had coronary bypasses do not sustain changes in their unhealthy lifestyles, which worsens their heart disease and threatens their lives.
2. Change is motivated by fear.	It is too easy for people to deny the bad things that might happen to them. Compelling positive visions of the future are a stronger inspiration for change.
3. The facts will set us free.	Our thinking is guided by narratives, not facts. When a fact does not fit people's conceptual "frames"—the metaphors used to make sense of the world—people reject the fact. Change is best inspired by emotional appeals rather than factual statements.
4. Small, gradual changes are easier to make and sustain.	Radical changes may be easier because they yield benefits quickly.
5. People cannot change because the brain becomes "hardwired" early in life.	Brains have extraordinary "plasticity," meaning that people can continue learning throughout life—assuming they remain active and engaged.

Source: Adapted from Deutschman's Fact Take: Five Myths About Changing Behavior. Deutschman, A. (2005/May). Change or die. Fast Company, 94, 52–62.

Study Questions

1. Why is change inevitable? What would happen if no change at all occurred in health care?

2. Why do people resist change? Why do nursing staff seem particularly resistant to change?

3. How can leaders overcome resistance to change?

4. Describe the process of implementing a change from beginning to end. Use an example from your clinical experience to illustrate this process.

Case Study to Promote Critical Reasoning

A large health-care corporation recently purchased a small, 50-bed rural nursing home. A new director of nursing was brought in to replace the former one, who had retired after 30 years. The new director addressed the staff members at the reception held to welcome him. "My philosophy is that you cannot manage anything that you haven't measured. Everyone tells me that you have all been doing an excellent job here. With my measurement approach, we will be able to analyze everything you do and become more efficient than ever." The nursing staff members soon found out what the new director meant by his measurement approach. Every bath, medication, dressing change, episode of incontinence care, feeding of a resident, or trip off the unit had to be counted, and the amount of time each activity required had to be recorded. Nurse managers were required to review these data with staff members every week, questioning any time that was not accounted for. Time spent talking with families or consulting with other staff members was considered time wasted unless the staff member could justify the "interruption" in his or her work. No one complained openly about the change, but absenteeism rates increased. Personal day and vacation time requests soared. Staff members nearing retirement crowded the tiny personnel office, overwhelming the sole staff member with their requests to "tell me how soon I can retire with full benefits." The director of nursing found that shortage of staff was becoming a serious problem and that no new applications were coming in, despite the fact that this rural area offered few good job opportunities.

1. What evidence of resistance to change can you find in this case study?

2. What kind of resistance to change did the staff members exhibit?

3. Why did staff members resist this change?

4. If you were a staff nurse at this facility, how do you think you would have reacted to this change in administration?

5. How do you think the director of nursing handled this change? What could the nurse managers and staff nurses do to improve the situation?

6. How could the new administrator have made this change more acceptable to the staff?

References

Araujo Group. A compilation of opinions of experts in the field of the management of change. Unpublished report.

Berman-Rubera, S. (2008, August 10). Leading and embracing change. *Business/Change-Management.* Retrieved from http://ezinearticles. com/?Leading-And-Embracing-Change&id=1180585

Boyer, D. (2013). Paradigm shift: How ICD-10 will change healthcare. *Health Management Technology, 34*(9), 24.

Braungardt, T., & Fought, S.G. (2008). Leading change during an inpatient critical care unit expansion. *Journal of Nursing Administration, 38*(11), 461–467.

Cameron, K.S., & Quinn, Q.E. (2006). *Diagnosing and changing organizational culture.* New York: Jossey-Bass.

Chreim, S., & Williams, B.E. (2012). Radical change in healthcare organization: Mapping transition between templates, enabling factors, and implementation processes. *Journal of Health Organization and Management, 26*(2), 215–236.

Cornell, P., Riordan, M., & Herrin-Griffith, D. (2010). Transforming nursing workflow, part 2: The impact of technology on nurse activities. *Journal of Nursing Administration, 40*(10), 432–439.

Dent, H.S. (1995). *Job Shock: Four new principles transforming our work and business.* New York: St. Martin's Press.

Deutschman, A. (2005a). Change or die. *Fast Company, 94,* 52–62.

Deutschman, A. (2005b). *What state of change are you in?* Retrieved from www.fastcompany.com/52596/which-stage-change-are-you

Englebright, J.D., & Franklin, M. (2005). Managing a new medication administrative process. *Journal of Nursing Administration, 35*(9), 410–413.

Farrell, K., & Broude, C. (1987). *Winning the change game: How to implement information systems with fewer headaches and bigger paybacks.* Los Angeles: Breakthrough Enterprises.

Fullan, M. (2001). *Leading in a culture of change.* San Francisco: Jossey-Bass.

Guthrie, V.A., & King, S.N. (2004). Feedback-intensive programs. In McCauley, C.D., & Van Velson, E. (eds.), *The center for creative leadership handbook of leadership development.* San Francisco: Jossey-Bass.

Hansten, R.I., & Washburn, M.J. (1999). Individual and organizational accountability for development of critical thinking. *Journal of Nursing Administration, 29*(11), 39–45.

Hart, L.B., & Waisman, C.S. (2005). *The leadership training activity book.* N.Y.: AMACOM.

Heifetz, R.A., & Linsky, M. (June 2002). A survival guide for leaders. *Harvard Business Review,* 65–74.

Heller, R. (1998). *Managing change.* New York: DK Publishing.

Hempel, J. (2005). Why the boss really had to say goodbye. *Business Week,* July 4, p. 10.

Hossainian, N., Slot, D.E., Afennich, F., & Van der Weijden, G.A. (2011). The effects of hydrogen peroxide mouthwashes on the prevention of plaque and gingival inflammation: A systematic review. *International Journal of Dental Hygiene, 9,* 171–181.

Johnston, G. (2008, March 8). Change management—Why the high failure rate. *Business/Change-Management.* Retrieved from http://ezinearticles.

com/?Change-Management—Why-the-High-Failure-Rate?&id=1028294

Kalisch, B.J. (2007). Don't like change? Blame it on your strategic style. *Reflections on Nursing Leadership, 33*(3). Retrieved from http://nursingsociety.org/RNL/3Q_2007/features/feature5.html

Kotter, J.P. (1999). Leading change: The eight steps to transformation. In Conger, J.A., Spreitzer, G.M., & Lawler, E.E. (eds.), *The Leader's Change Handbook: An Essential Guide to Setting Direction and Taking Action.* San Francisco: Jossey-Bass.

Lapp, J. (May 2002). Thriving on change. *Caring Magazine,* 40–43.

Leonard, D. (2012/October 15). Obamacare is not an epithet. *Bloomberg Business Week,* 98–100.

Lewin, K. (1951). *Field theory in social science: Selected theoretical papers.* New York: Harper & Row.

Lindberg, C., & Clancy, T.R. (2010). Positive deviance: An elegant solution to a complex problem. *Journal of Nursing Administration, 40*(4), 150–153.

MacDavitt, K. (2011). Implementing small tests of change to improve patient satisfaction. *The Journal of Nursing Administration, 41*(1), 5–9.

Maslow, A.H. (1970). *Motivation and personality.* New York: Harper & Row.

Maurer, R. (2008, August 13). The 4 reasons why people resist change. *Business/Change-Management.* Retrieved from http://ezinearticles.com/?The-7-Reasons-Why-People-Resist-Change&id=1053595

Parker, M., & Gadbois, S. (2000). Building community in healthcare workplace. Part 3: Belonging and satisfaction at work. *Journal of Nursing Administration, 30,* 466–473.

Pearcey, P., & Draper, P. (1996). Using the diffusion of innovation model to influence practice: A case study. *Journal of Advanced Nursing, 23,* 724–726.

Porter-O'Grady, T. (1996). The seven basic rules for successful redesign. *Journal of Nursing Administration, 26*(1), 46–53.

Rodts, M.F. (2011). Technology changes healthcare. *Orthopedic Nursing, 30*(5), 292

Safian, R. (2012/November). Secrets of the flux leader. *Fast Company, 170,* 96–106, 136.

Schein, E.H. (2004, August 1). Kurt Lewin's change theory in the field and in the classroom: Notes toward a model of managed learning. Retrieved from www.a2zpsychology.com/articles/kurt_lewin's_change_theory.htm

Shirey, M.R. (2011). Establishing a sense of urgency for leading transformational change. *Journal of Nursing Administration, 41*(4), 145–148.

Shirey, M.R. (2012). Stakeholder analysis and mapping as targeted communication strategy. *Journal of Nursing Administration, 42*(9), 399–403.

Staren, E.D., Braun, D.P., & Denny, D.S. (2010/March-April). Optimizing innovation in health care organization. *Physicians Executive Journal,* 54–62.

Suddath, C. (2012/December 3-9). Business by the bard. *Bloomberg Business Week,* 83–85.

Tappen, R.M. (2001). *Nursing leadership and management: concepts and practice.* Philadelphia: F.A. Davis.

Tombes, M.B., & Gallucci, B. (1993). The effects of hydrogen peroxide rinses on the normal oral mucosa. *Nursing Research, 42,* 332–337.

Webb, J.A.K., & Marshall, D.R. (2010). Healthcare reform and nursing. *Journal of Nursing Administration, 49*(9), 345–349.

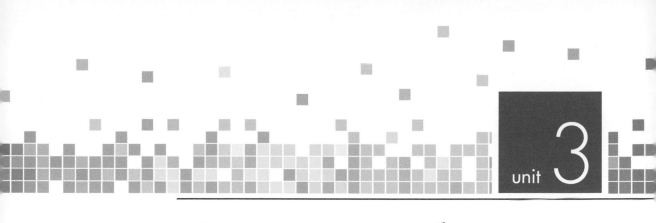

unit 3

Career Considerations

chapter 10

Issues of Quality and Safety

OBJECTIVES

After reading this chapter, the student should be able to:

- Discuss the history of quality and safety within the U.S. health-care system.
- Analyze historical, social, political, and economic trends affecting the nursing profession and the health-care delivery system.
- Explain the importance of quality improvement (QI) for the nurse, patient, organization, and health-care delivery system.
- Discuss the role of the nurse in continuous quality improvement (CQI) and risk management.
- Examine factors contributing to medical errors and evidence-based methods for the prevention of medical errors.
- Explain the use of technology to enhance and promote safe patient care, educate patients and consumers, evaluate health-care delivery, and enhance the nurse's knowledge base.
- Describe the effects of communication on patient-centered care, interprofessional collaboration, and safety.
- Promote the role of the nurse in the delivery of safe, effective quality care in today's health-care environment.

OUTLINE

Overview

You are entering professional nursing at a time when issues pertaining to quality and safety of the U.S. health-care system have come to the forefront in the delivery of health care. Considering the complexity of the decisions nurses make every day in managing patient care at the bedside, it may seem natural that these decisions would be based on safe and effective care. However, often this is not the case. As a professional registered nurse (RN), you will participate daily in activities necessary to support quality and safety initiatives at the bedside, within your organization, and as part of the health-care system. Patients place their lives in nurses' hands and trust them to be knowledgeable and to use good judgment when making decisions about care. As nurses we need to understand that we work within a system, and whenever there is a breakdown somewhere within the system, the risk for error increases. This chapter discusses quality and safety in health care, presents reasons for errors, and offers ways nurses can help to create a culture of safety.

Historical Trends and Issues

Many forces drive the rapidly changing health-care delivery system (Baldwin, Conger, Maycock, & Abegglen, 2002; Davis, 2001; Elwood, 2007; Ervin, Bickes, & Schim, 2006; Menix, 2000; Milton, 2011). In this time of global health-care reform, regulation at the global, national, state, and local levels has taken on a new significance (Milton,

2011). The impetus to decrease costs and improve outcomes influences the current movement toward improved quality and safety. These forces include economics, societal demographics and diversity, regulation and legislation, technology, health-care delivery and practice, and environment and globalization.

Economics. Many economic trends and issues affect the U.S health-care delivery system. Businesses, government, and the media criticize the cost of health care within the United States when compared with that of other developed nations (Jackson, 2006; Kersbergen, 2000; Milton, 2011). The costs of research and the costs to develop new treatments and technology continue to rise. Educated consumers expect safe, quality care with associated satisfaction and positive health outcomes. Nurses need to be prepared to support consumers with a thorough knowledge of quality, accountability, and cost-effectiveness (AACN, 2008, 2012). This means that they must have the knowledge to educate patients regarding the technology used in their treatments and explain the rationale behind the treatment selection. While initial expenses may increase, improvements in quality and safety will reduce costs in the long term (Aiken et. al., 2012; Cronenwett et al, 2007; Institute of Medicine [IOM], 2003a; Weiss, Yakusheva, & Bobay, 2011).

Societal demographics and diversity. Increased numbers of racial and ethnic groups influence health-care delivery (Billings & Halsted, 2011; Davis, 2010; Elwood 2007; Health and Human Services [HHS], 2011; Heller, Oros, & Durney-Crowley, 2000; World Health Organization, 2009). Increased numbers of the elderly, longer life expectancy, and improvements in technology result in an emphasis on specialized geriatric care. Both the elderly and ethnic minorities are at-risk populations who suffer disadvantages in access to care, payment for care, and quality of care (Affordable Care Act, 2010; Anderson, Scrimshaw, Fullilove, Fielding, & Normand, 2003). It is hoped that the passage of the Affordable Care Act (ACA) will minimize these disparities as more of these individuals will have access to health-care services (Davis, 2010).

Regulation and legislation. The diverse interests of consumers, insurance companies, government, and regulation affect health-care legislation. For health-care leaders and providers of care, unprec- edented challenges continue despite the attention that quality and safety have received during the evolution of the existing health-care system. The ACA now provides health care to individuals who previously lacked coverage. This access to care will increase the numbers of individuals who will need providers as well as force changes in regulation and cost management.

Technology. The use of technology and the incorporation of the electronic health record are projected to decrease costs and improve clinical outcomes, quality, and safety (IOM, 2003a; Poon et al., 2010). Nursing practice must adjust to these health-care delivery trends with the inclusion of concepts in interprofessional collaboration, patient-focused systems, and information literacy (Booth, 2006; Sargeant, Loney, & Murphy, 2008). Additionally, nurses must utilize technology and informatics to incorporate evidenced-based practices for improved quality and safety in the health-care delivery system (Hunter, 2011).

Technology also produces advancements in disease treatments, especially in the areas of genetics and genomics, and all professionals must integrate these advancements into practice (Calzone, Cashion, Feetham, Jenkins, Prows, Williams, & Wung, 2010; Lea, Skirton, Read, & Williams, 2011). The current advances in genetics and genomics continue to allow the redesign of treatments for a variety of genetic disorders, quality improvement (QI), and outcomes in clinical practice often related to pharmacotherapeutics (Trossman, 2006; Lea, Skirton, Read, & Williams, 2011).

Health-care delivery and practice. Health-care professionals should be prepared to provide safe, quality care in all settings, including acute care and community settings. Nurses and other health-care professionals need the knowledge, skills, attitudes, and competencies to function in a variety of settings and the ability to support the needs of the increasingly diverse population (Anderson et al., 2003; Ervin, Bickes, & Schim, 2006; Heller, Oros, & Durney-Crowley, 2000).

The integration of evidenced-based practice serves to improve quality and safety for patients, and improves collaboration and interprofessional teamwork (IOM, 2003a; O'Neill, 1998). Both the IOM (2003a) and the Pew Health Professions Commission (PEW, 1998) identified the need for the health-care delivery system and its professionals to improve collaboration and to work in an interprofessional team to improve quality and safety.

Environment and globalization. The emergence of a global economy, the ease of travel, and advances in communication technology affect the movement of people, money, and disease (Heller, Oros, & Durney-Crowley, 2000; Kirk, 2002). Global warming and climate change have been linked to the emergence of new drug-resistant organisms and an increase in vector-borne and waterborne disease as warmer temperatures promote changes in organism structure and increase the growth rate of bacteria. Increased ease of travel allows for migration of affected populations. Safe, quality health care will need to confront the challenges of increasing multiculturalism, potential for pandemic, and the effect of climate change and pollution on health.

In addition, many health-care professionals, government agencies, and supporting organizations have contributed to the evolution of quality and safety within the health-care system. The Historical Timeline (Table 10-1) highlights significant organizations and initiatives of importance to quality and safety.

table 10-1

Historical Timeline

Year	Event
1896	Nurses Associated Alumnae of the United States and Canada formed, later called the American Nurses Association (ANA)
1906	Food and Drug Act signed, which began the regulation of food and drugs to protect consumers
1918	American College of Surgeons founded, which initiated minimum standards for hospitals and on-site hospital inspections for adherence to standards
1930s	Employers began offering *health benefits*, and the first commercial insurance companies arose
1945	Quality management principles developed by Edward Deming were applied successfully to industries such as manufacturing, government, and health care
1951	Joint Commission on Accreditation of Healthcare Organizations (JCAHO) founded; currently referred to as The Joint Commission (JC)
1955	Social Security Act passed; hospitals that had volunteered for accreditation by JCAHO were approved for participation in Medicare and Medicaid
1966	*Quality of health-care services* defined in the literature
1970	IOM established as a nonprofit adviser to the nation to improve health in the national academies
1979	National Committee on Quality Assurance (NCQA) established
1986	National Center of Nursing Research founded at the National Institutes of Health (NIH)
1989	Agency for Healthcare Research and Quality (AHRQ) established
1990	NCQA began accrediting managed care organizations by using data from Health Plan Employer Data and Information Set (HEDIS)
1990	Institute of Healthcare Improvement (IHI) founded
1991	Nursing's Agenda for Health Care Reform published by the ANA
1996	National Patient Safety Foundation (NPSF) founded; JC established Sentinel Event Policies
1996	IOM launched three-part initiative to study health-care system quality
1998	IOM National Roundtable on Health Care Quality released *Consensus Statement*
1999	IOM published *To Err is Human: Building a Safer Health System*
2001	IOM published *Crossing the Quality Chasm: A New Health System for the 21st Century*
2001	IOM published *Envisioning the National Health Care Quality Report*
2001	ANA's National Database for Nursing Quality Indicators (NDNQI) demonstrated the positive impact of the appropriate mix of nursing staff on patient outcomes
2001	JC mandated hospital-wide patient safety standards
2003	IOM published *Priority Areas for National Action: Transforming Health Care Quality*, which established priority areas for national action to improve quality of care and outcomes (Box 10-1)
2003	JC established first set of National Patient Safety Goals (NPSG)
2003	IOM published *Health Professions Education: A Bridge to Quality*
2004	IOM published *Keeping Patients Safe: Transforming the Work Environment of Nurses*
2004	IOM published *Patient Safety: Achieving a New Standard of Care*
2005	ANA updated its Health Care Agenda, urging system reform
2006	IOM published *Preventing Medication Errors: Quality Chasm Series*
2014	JC updated National Patient Safety Goals

Institute of Medicine Priority Areas (IOM, 2003b)

- Asthma
- Cancer screening
- Care coordination
- Children with special care needs
- Diabetes
- End-of-life issues
- Frail elderly
- Health literacy
- Hypertension
- Immunizations
- Ischemic heart disease
- Major depression
- Nosocomial infections
- Obesity
- Pain control in advanced cancer
- Pregnancy and childbirth
- Self-management
- Severe, persistent mental illness
- Stroke
- Tobacco dependence in adults

The Institute of Medicine and the Committee on the Quality of Health Care in America

The Institute of Medicine (IOM) is a private, non-profit organization chartered in 1970 by the U.S government. The IOM's role is to provide unbiased, expert health and scientific advice for the purpose of improving health. The result of the IOM's work supports government policy making, the health-care system, health-care professionals, and consumers (Box 10-1).

In 1998 the IOM National Roundtable on Health Care Quality released *Statement on Quality of Care* (Donaldson, 1998), which urged health-care leaders to make urgent changes in the U.S. health-care system. The Roundtable reached consensus in four areas regarding the U.S. health-care system:

1. Quality can be defined and measured;
2. Quality problems are serious and extensive;
3. Current approaches to quality improvement (QI) are inadequate; and
4. There is an urgent need for rapid change.

This IOM statement launched today's movement to improve quality and safety for the 21st century U.S. health-care system.

In 1998 the IOM charged the Committee on the Quality of Health Care in America to develop a strategy to improve health-care quality in the coming decade (IOM, 2000). The Committee completed a systematic review and critique of literature that highlighted and quantified severe shortcomings in the heath-care system. Its work led to the series of reports that serves as the foundation and strategy for health system reform (Box 10-2). Two in particular, *To Err is Human: Building a Safer Health System* (IOM, 2000) and *Crossing the Quality Chasm: A New Health System for the 21st Century* (IOM, 2001), provide a framework upon which the 21st-century health-care system is being built. In 2011 the IOM released a report on *The Future of Nursing: Leading Change, Advancing Health* (IOM, 2011). This report describes the changes needed in nursing practice and nursing education to promote nursing's role in the new era of health-care delivery.

To Err is Human, discussed later in this chapter, quantified unnecessary death in the U.S. health-care system and placed emphasis on system failures as the foundation for errors and mistakes. According to the report, it is the flawed systems in patient care that often leave the door open for human error. The report made a series of eight recommendations in four areas (Box 10-3) that aimed to decrease errors by at least 50% over 5 years. The goal of the

IOM Quality Reports (IOM, 2006)

- *Crossing the Quality Chasm: The IOM Quality Health Care Initiative* (1996)
- *To Err Is Human: Building a Safer Health System* (2000)
- *Crossing the Quality Chasm: A New Health System for the 21st Century* (2001)
- *Envisioning the National Health Care Quality Report* (2001)
- *Priority Areas for National Action: Transforming Health Care Quality* (2003b)
- *Leadership by Example: Governmental Roles* (2003)
- *Health Professions Education: A Bridge to Quality* (2003a)
- *Patient Safety: Achieving a New Standard of Care* (2003)
- *Keeping Patients Safe: Transforming the Work Environment for Nurses* (2004)
- *Academic Health Centers: Leading Change in the 21st Century* (2004)
- *Preventing Medication Errors: Quality Chasm Series* (2006)

Focus Areas of *To Err is Human* Recommendations (IOM, 2000)

- Enhance knowledge and leadership regarding safety.
- Identify and learn from errors.
- Set performance standards and expectations for safety.
- Implement safety systems within health-care organizations.

Ten Rules to Govern Health-Care Reform for the 21st Century (IOM, 2001, p. 61)

1. Care is based on a continuous healing relationship.
2. Care is provided based on patient needs and values.
3. Patient is source of control of care.
4. Knowledge is shared and free-flowing.
5. Decisions are evidence-based.
6. Safety is a system property.
7. Transparency is necessary; secrecy is harmful.
8. Anticipate patient needs.
9. Waste is continually decreased.
10. Cooperation is needed between health-care providers.

recommendations was "for the external environment to create sufficient pressure to make errors costly to health-care organizations and providers, so they are compelled to take action to improve safety" (IOM, 2000, p. 4). The recommendations sparked public interest in health-care quality and safety and caused prompt responses by the government and national quality organizations.

Crossing the Quality Chasm addressed broad quality issues in the U.S. health-care system. The report indicated that the health-care system is fundamentally flawed with "gaps," and it proposed a system-wide strategy and action plans to redesign the health-care system. The report stated that the gaps between actual care and high-quality care could be attributed to four key inter-related areas in the health-care system: the growing complexity of science and technology, an increase in chronic conditions, a poorly organized delivery system of care, and constraints on exploiting the revolution in information technology. With the overarching goal of improving the health-care system by closing identifiable gaps, the report made 13 recommendations, some of which are in Box 10-4. Additionally, the report addressed the importance of aligning and designing health-care payer systems, professional education, and the health-care environment for quality enhancements, improved outcomes in care, and use of best practices.

The Future of Nursing: Leading Change, Advancing Health discusses the role of nursing in the 21st century. This document recognizes that the nursing profession confronts many challenges in the changing health-care system. It identifies recommendations for an "action-oriented blueprint for the future of nursing" (RWJF, 2008, p. s-2).

As a professional nurse, you have a responsibility to acknowledge the complexity and deficits of the health-care system. In managing patient care, you must continually consider the impact of the system on the care you provide and participate in the quality and safety initiatives at the bedside, in your unit, and within your organization to promote quality and safety within the system.

Quality in the Health-Care System

The IOM defines quality as "the degree to which health services for individuals and populations increase the likelihood of desired health outcomes and are consistent with current and professional knowledge" (IOM, 2001, p. 232). This definition is used by U.S. organizations and many international health-care organizations, and it is the basis for nursing management of patient care. Box 10-5 elaborates on this definition by outlining six primary aims of health care.

Quality Improvement (QI)

QI activities have been part of nursing care since Florence Nightingale evaluated the care of soldiers during the Crimean War (Nightingale & Barnum, 1992). To achieve quality health care, QI activities use evidence-based methods for gathering data and achieving desired results.

Before the 1980s, health-care institutions focused on quality assurance (QA) rather than QI. QA outlined an inspection process to guarantee that hospitals continued to follow minimum

Six Aims for Improving Quality in Health Care (IOM, 2001, p. 39).

Health care should be:
1. **Safe:** Avoiding injuries to patients from the care that is intended to help them
2. **Effective:** Providing services based on scientific knowledge to all who could benefit and refraining from providing services to those not likely to benefit (avoiding underuse and overuse)
3. **Patient-centered:** Providing care that is respectful of and responsive to individual patient preferences, needs, and values and ensuring that patient values guide all clinical decisions
4. **Timely:** Reducing waits and sometimes harmful delays for those who receive and those who give care
5. **Efficient:** Avoiding waste, in particular that of equipment, supplies, ideas, and energy
6. **Equitable:** Providing care that does not vary in quality because of characteristics such as gender, ethnicity, geographic location, and socioeconomic status

standards of patient care quality. This approach used retrospective chart audits and fixed errors after problems were found. QA places very little emphasis on change or assuming a proactive approach. In contrast, QI infers a system-wide approach to maintaining quality. The Joint Commission (2010) vision identifies the core of quality improvement as "All people should always experience the safest, highest quality, best value health care across all settings" (para. 1).

QI usually involves the following common characteristics (McLaughlin & Kaluzny, 2006, p. 3):

- A link to key elements of the organization's strategic plan
- A quality council consisting of the institution's top leadership
- Training programs for all levels of personnel
- Mechanisms for selecting improvement opportunities
- Formation of process improvement teams
- Staff support for process analysis and redesign
- Personnel policies that motivate and support staff participation in process improvement

Several terms, such as QI, total quality management (TQM), Six Sigma, and Continuous Quality Improvement (CQI), are used to describe quality improvement. QI may be accomplished through a variety of approaches and models such as the Focus, Analyze, Develop, and Execute Model (FADE) (http://patientsafetyed.duhs.duke.edu/module_a/methods/fade.html) or the Plan Do Study Act cycle (PDSA). Regardless of the term used, QI provides a structured organizational process for involving the health-care team in planning and executing a continuous flow of improvements to provide quality care that meets or exceeds expectations (McLaughlin & Kaluzny, 2006, p. 3). The following sections focus on CQI.

Using CQI to Monitor and Evaluate Quality of Care

Continuous quality improvement (CQI) is a process. It includes: (a) identifying areas of concern (indicators), (b) continuously collecting data on these indicators, (c) analyzing and evaluating the data, and (d) implementing needed changes. When one indicator is no longer a concern, another indicator is selected. Common indicators include the number of falls, frequency of medication errors, and infection rates. Indicators can be identified by the accrediting agency or by the facility itself. The purpose of CQI is to continuously improve the capability of everyone involved in providing care, including the organization itself. CQI aims to act proactively and avoid a blaming environment. The process attempts to provide a means to improve the entire system.

CQI relies on collecting information and analyzing it. The time frame used in a CQI program can be retrospective (evaluating past performance, often called *quality assurance*), concurrent (evaluating current performance), or prospective (future-oriented, collecting data as they come in). The procedures used to collect data depend on the purpose of the program. Data may be obtained by observation, performance appraisals, patient satisfaction surveys, statistical analyses of length-of-stay and costs, surveys, peer reviews, and chart audits (Ajjawi & Higgs, 2008; Lantham & Maxson-Cooper, 2003).

In the CQI framework, data collection is everyone's responsibility. Collecting comprehensive, accurate, and representative data is the first step in the CQI process. You may be asked to brainstorm your ideas with other nurses or members of the interprofessional team, complete surveys or checklists, or keep a log of your daily activities. How do you administer medications to groups of patients? What steps are involved? Are the medications always available at the right time and in the right dose, or do you have to wait for the pharmacy to bring them to the floor? Is the pharmacy technician delayed by emergency orders that must be processed? Looking at the entire process and mapping it out on paper in the form of a flowchart may be part of the CQI process for your organization (Fig. 10.1).

QI at the Organizational and Unit Levels

Strategic Planning

Leaders and managers are so often preoccupied with immediate issues that they lose sight of their ultimate objectives. To stay on track, an organization needs a strategic plan. A **strategic plan** is a short, visionary, conceptual document that:

- Serves as a framework for decisions or for securing support/approval
- Provides a basis for more detailed planning

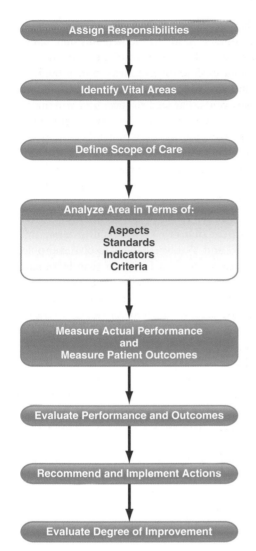

Figure 10.1 Unit level QI process. *Adapted from Hunt, D.V. (1992). Quality in America: How to implement a competitive quality program. Homewood, IL: Business One Irwin; and Duquette, A.M. (1991]). Approaches to monitoring practice: Getting started. In Schroeder, P. [ed.]. Monitoring and Evaluation in Nursing. Gaithersburg, MD: Aspen.*

- Explains the business to others in order to inform, motivate, and involve
- Assists benchmarking and performance monitoring
- Stimulates change and becomes the building block for the next plan (http://www.planware .org/strategicplan.htm).

During the strategic planning process, the organization develops or reviews its vision, mission statement, and corporate values. A group develops business objectives and key strategies to meet these objectives. In order to do this, a SWOT analysis is done—a review of the organization's Strengths, Weaknesses, Opportunities, and Threats. Key strategies are identified, and action plans are developed. The organization's mission, goals, and strategic plan ultimately drive the outcomes and QI plan for that organization. Be proactive, and ask your nurse manager if there are opportunities for the staff to participate in the planning process.

Issues related to QI may also come out of the strategic planning process. Quality issues are not often apparent to senior managers. Staff members at the unit level can often identify quality issues because they are the ones who can feel the impact when quality is lacking. Once a process needing improvement is identified, an interprofessional team is organized consisting of members who have knowledge of the identified process. The team members meet to identify and analyze problems, discuss solutions, and evaluate changes. The team clarifies the current knowledge of the process; it identifies causes for variations in the process and works to unify the process. Box 10-6 identifies questions that team members should ask as they work on the QI plan.

Structured Care Methodologies

Most agencies have tools for tracking outcomes. These tools are called *structured care methodologies* (SCMs). SCMs are interprofessional tools to

---

box 10-6

Questions the Team Needs to Ask

1. Who are our customers, stakeholders, markets?
2. What do they expect from us?
3. What are we trying to accomplish?
4. What changes do we think will make an improvement?
5. How and when will we pilot-test our predicted improvement?
6. What do we expect to learn from the pilot test?
7. What will we do with negative results? Positive results?
8. How will we implement the change?
9. How will we measure success?
10. What did we learn as a team from this experience?
11. What changes would we make for the future?

Adapted from McLaughlin, C., & Kaluzny, A. (2006). Continuous Quality Improvement in Health Care: Theory, Implementations, and Applications. 3rd ed. Massachusetts: Jones & Bartlett.

"identify best practices, facilitate standardization of care, and provide a mechanism for variance tracking, quality enhancement, outcomes measurement, and outcomes research" (Cole & Houston, 1999, p. 53). SCMs include guidelines, protocols, algorithms, standards of care, and critical pathways. In line with this idea is the development of a Nursing Care Performance Framework (NCPF) that identifies core aspects of nursing performance. The framework incorporates many of these other tools and offers decision-makers a conceptual instrument that acts to define performance, create a shared and stable set of performance indicators for a given segment of nursing care, and develop benchmarks to measure the outcomes (Dubois, D'Amour, Pomey, Girard, & Brault, 2013).

- **Guidelines.** Guidelines first appeared in the 1980s as statements to assist health-care providers and patients in making appropriate health-care decisions. Guidelines are based on current research strategies and are often developed by experts in the field. The use of guidelines is seen as a way to decrease variations in practice.
- **Protocols.** Protocols are specific, formal documents that outline how a procedure or intervention should be conducted. Protocols have been used for many years in research and specialty areas but have been introduced into general health care as a way to standardize approaches to achieve desired outcomes. An example in use in many facilities is a chest pain protocol.
- **Algorithms.** Algorithms are systematic procedures that follow a logical progression based on additional information or patient responses to treatment. They were originally developed in mathematics and are frequently seen in emergency medical services. Advanced cardiac life support algorithms are now widely used in health-care agencies.
- **Standards of care.** Standards of care are often discipline-related and help to operationalize patient care processes and provide a baseline for quality care. Lawyers often refer to a discipline's standards of care in evaluating whether a patient has received appropriate services.
- **Critical (or clinical) pathways.** A critical pathway outlines the expected course of treatment for patients who have similar

diagnoses. The critical pathway should orient the nurse easily to the patient's outcomes for the day. In some institutions, nursing diagnoses with specific time frames are incorporated into the critical pathway, which describes the course of events that lead to successful patient outcome within the diagnosis-related group (DRG)–defined time frame. For the patient with an uncomplicated myocardial infarction (MI), a proposed course of events leading to a successful patient outcome within the 4-day DRG-defined time frame might be as follows (Doenges, Moorhouse, & Murr, 2009): (1) Patient states that chest pain is relieved; (2) ST- and T-wave changes resolve and pulse oximeter reading is greater than 90%; patient has clear breath sounds; (3) Patient ambulates in hall without experiencing extreme fatigue or chest pain; (4) Patient verbalizes feelings about having an MI and future fears; (5) Patient identifies effective coping strategies; (6) Ventricular dysfunction, dysrhythmia, or crackles resolved.

Different types of SCMs may be used alone or together. A patient who is admitted for an MI may have care planned using a critical pathway for an acute MI, a heparin protocol, and a dysrhythmia algorithm. In addition, the nurses may refer to the standards of care in developing a traditional nursing care plan.

The use of SCMs can improve physiological, psychological, and financial outcomes. Services and interventions are sequenced to provide safe and effective outcomes at designated times and with the most effective use of resources. They also give an interprofessional perspective that is not found in the traditional nursing care plan. Computer programs allow health-care personnel to track variances (differences from the identified standard) and use these variances in planning QI activities.

SCMs do not take the place of expert nursing judgment. The fundamental purpose of the SCM is to assist health-care providers in implementing practices identified with good clinical judgment, research-based interventions, and improved patient outcomes. Data from SCMs allow comparisons of outcomes, development of research-based decisions, identification of high-risk patients, and identification of issues and problems before they escalate into disasters. Do not be afraid to learn and understand the different SCMs.

Critical Pathways

Critical pathways are clinical protocols involving all disciplines. They are designed for tracking a planned clinical course for patients based on average and expected lengths of stay. Financial outcomes can be evaluated from critical pathways by assessing any variances from the proposed length of stay (Haddad, 2010). The health-care agency can then focus on problems within the system that extend the length of stay or drive up costs because of overutilization or repetition of services. For example:

> *Mr. J. was admitted to the telemetry unit with a diagnosis of MI. He had no previous history of heart disease and no other complicating factors such as diabetes, hypertension, or elevated cholesterol levels. His DRG-prescribed length of stay was 4 days. He had an uneventful hospitalization for the first 2 days. On the third day, he complained of pain in the left calf. The calf was slightly reddened and warm to the touch. This condition was diagnosed as thrombophlebitis, which increased his length of hospitalization. The case manager's review of the events leading up to the complaints of calf pain indicated that, although the physician had ordered compression stockings for Mr. J., the stockings never arrived, and no one followed through on the order. The variances related to his proposed length of stay were discussed with the team providing care, and measures were instituted to make sure that this oversight would not occur again.*

Critical pathways provide a framework for communication and documentation of care. They are also excellent teaching tools for staff members from various disciplines. Institutions can use critical pathways to evaluate the cost of care for different patient populations (Haddad, 2010; Rotter, Kinsman, James, Machotta, Gothe, Willis, Snow, & Kugler, 2010).

Most institutions have adopted a chronological, diagrammatic format for presenting a critical pathway. Time frames may range from daily (day 1, day 2, day 3) to hourly, depending on patient needs. Key elements of the critical pathway include discharge planning, patient education, consultations, activities, nutrition, medications, diagnostic tests, and treatment). Table 10-2 is an example of a critical pathway.

Although originally developed for use in acute care institutions, critical pathways can be developed for home care and long-term care. The patient's nurse is usually responsible for monitoring and recording any deviations from the critical pathway. When deviations occur, the reasons are discussed with all members of the health-care team, and the appropriate changes in care are made. The nurse must identify general trends in patient outcomes and develop plans to improve the quality of care to reduce the number of deviations. Through this close monitoring, the health-care team can avoid last-minute surprises that may delay patient discharge and can predict lengths of stay more effectively.

Aspects of Health Care to Evaluate

A CQI program can evaluate three aspects of health care: the structure within which the care is given, the process of giving care, and the outcome of that care. A comprehensive evaluation should include all three aspects (Brook, Davis, & Kamberg, 1980; Donabedian, 1969, 1977, 1987). When evaluation focuses on nursing care, the independent, dependent, and interdependent functions of nurses may be added to the model (Irvine, 1998). Each of these dimensions is described here, and their interrelationship is illustrated in Table 10-3.

Structure

Structure refers to the setting in which the care is given and to the resources (human, financial, and material) that are available. The following structural aspects of a health-care organization can be evaluated:

- **Facilities.** Comfort, convenience of layout, accessibility of support services, and safety
- **Equipment.** Adequate supplies, state-of-the-art equipment, and staff ability to use equipment
- **Staff.** Credentials, experience, absenteeism, turnover rate, staff-patient ratios
- **Finances.** Salaries, adequacy, sources

Although none of these structural factors alone can guarantee quality care, they make good care more likely. A larger number of nurses each shift and a higher proportion of RNs are associated with shorter lengths of stay; higher proportions of RNs are also related to fewer adverse patient outcomes (Lichtig, Knauf, & Milholland, 1999; Rogers et al., 2004).

table 10-2

Sample Critical Pathway: Heart Failure, Hospital; ELOS 4 Days Cardiology or Medical Unit

ND and Categories of Care	Day 1 _____	Day 2 _____	Day 3 _____	Day 4 _____
Decreased cardiac output R/T: Decreased myocardial contractility, altered electrical conduction, structural changes	Goals: Participate in actions to reduce cardiac workload	Display VS within acceptable limits; dysrhythmias controlled; pulse oximetry within acceptable range Meet own self-care needs with assistance as necessary	Dysrhythmias controlled or absent Free of signs of respiratory distress Demonstrate measurable increase in activity tolerance	
Fluid volume excess R/T compromised regulatory mechanisms: hypertension, sodium/water retention	Verbalize understanding of fluid/food restrictions	Verbalize understanding of general condition and health-care needs Breathing sounds clearing Urinary output adequate Weight loss (reflecting fluid loss)	Plan for lifestyle/ behavior changes Breath sounds clear Balanced I&O Edema resolving	Plan in place to meet postdischarge needs Weight stable or continued loss if edema present
Referrals	Cardiology Dietitian	Cardiac rehabilitation Occupational therapist (for ADLs) Social services Home care	Community resources	
Diagnostic studies	ECG, echo, Doppler ultrasound, stress test, cardiac scan CXR ABGs/pulse oximeter Cardiac enzymes ANP, BNP BUN/Cr CBC/electrolytes, MG++ PT/aPTT Liver function studies Serum glucose Albumin/total protein Thyroid studies Digoxin level (as indicated) UA	Echo-Doppler (if not done day 1) or other cardiac scans Cardiac enzymes (if ≠) BUN/Cr Electrolytes PT/aPTT (if taking anticoagulants)	CXR BUN/Cr Electrolytes PT/aPTT (as indicated) Repeat digoxin level (if indicated)	
Additional assessments	Apical pulse, heart/breath sounds q8h Cardiac rhythm (telemetry) q4h BP, P, R q2h until stable, q4h Temp q8h I&O q8h Weight qAM Peripheral edema q8h Peripheral pulses q8h Sensorium q8h DVT check qd Response to activity Response to therapeutic interventions	q8h	bid D/C bid bid bid	D/C qd D/C D/C

table 10-2

Sample Critical Pathway: Heart Failure, Hospital; ELOS 4 Days Cardiology or Medical Unit —cont'd

ND and Categories of Care	Day 1 _____	Day 2 _____	Day 3 _____	Day 4 _____
Medication allergies	IV diuretic ACEI, ARB, vasodilators, beta blocker IV/PO potassium Digoxin PO/cutaneous nitrates Morphine sulfate Daytime/hs sedation PO/low-dose anticoagulant Stool softener/laxative	PO	D/C D/C PO or D/C	D/C
Patient education	Orient to unit/room Review advance directives Discuss expected outcomes, diagnostic tests/results Fluid/nutritional restrictions/needs	Cardiac education per protocol Review medications: Dose, times, route, purpose, side effects Progressive activity program Skin care	Signs/symptoms to report to health-care provider Plan for home-care needs	Provide written instructions for home care Schedule for follow-up appointments
Additional nursing actions	Bed/chair rest Assist with physical care Pressure-relieving mattress Dysrhythmia/angina care per protocol Supplemental O$_2$ Cardiac diet	BPR/ambulate as tolerated, cardiac program	Up ad lib/graded program D/C if able	(send home)

CP = critical path; ELOS = estimated length of stay; ND = nursing diagnosis.
Source: Doenges, M.E., Moorhouse, M.F., and Geissler, A.C. (2010). Nursing care plans: Guidelines for individualizing patient care, ed. 8. Philadelphia: F.A. Davis, with permission.

table 10-3

Dimensions of QI in Nursing: Examples

	Independent Function	Dependent Function	Interdependent Function
Structure	Pressure ulcer risk assessment form available	High-speed automatic dial-up system puts nurses in touch with physicians rapidly	Nursing case management model of care adopted on rehabilitation unit
Process	Assesses risk for development of pressure ulcer and implements preventive measures	Order to increase dosage of pain medication obtained and processed within 1 hour	Communicates with therapists about need for customized wheelchair
Outcome	Skin intact at discharge	Relief from pain	Able to enter narrow doorway to bathroom unassisted

Source: Adapted from Irvine, D. (1998). Finding value in nursing care: A framework for quality improvement and clinical evaluation. Nursing Economics, 16(3), 110–118.

Process

Process refers to the activities carried out by the health-care providers and all the decisions made while a patient is interacting with the organization (Irvine, 1998). Examples include:

- Setting an appointment
- Conducting a physical assessment
- Ordering a radiograph and magnetic resonance imaging scan
- Administering a blood transfusion
- Completing a home environment assessment

- Preparing the patient for discharge
- Telephoning the patient post-discharge

Each of these processes can be evaluated in terms of timeliness, appropriateness, accuracy, and completeness (Irvine, 1998). Process variables include psychosocial interventions such as teaching and counseling, and physical care measures. Process also includes leadership activities such as interprofessional team conferences. When process data are collected, a set of objectives, procedures, or guidelines is needed to serve as a standard or gauge against which to compare the activities. This set can be highly specific, such as listing all the steps in a catheterization procedure, or it can be a list of objectives, such as offering information on breastfeeding to all expectant parents or conducting weekly staff meetings.

The American Nurses Association (ANA) Standards of Care are process standards that answer the question: What should the nurse be doing, and what process should the nurse follow to ensure quality care?

Outcome

An *outcome* is the result of all the health-care providers' activities. Outcome measures evaluate the effectiveness of nursing activities by answering such questions as: Did the patient recover? Is the family more independent now? Has team functioning improved? Outcome standards address indicators such as physical and mental health; social and physical function; health attitudes, knowledge, and behavior; utilization of services; and customer satisfaction. Evidence-based practice is linked to outcomes in that outcomes research findings guide the formation of appropriate strategies in the delivery of safe, effective, and quality patient care (PCORI, 2012).

The outcome questions asked during an evaluation should measure observable behavior, such as the following:

- **Patient:** Wound healed; blood pressure within normal limits; infection absent
- **Family:** Increased time between visits to the emergency department; applied for food stamps
- **Team:** Decisions reached by consensus; attendance at meetings by all team members

Some of these outcomes, such as blood pressure or time between emergency department visits, are easier to measure than other, equally important outcomes, such as increased satisfaction or changes in attitude. Although the latter cannot be measured as precisely, it is important to include the full spectrum of biological, psychological, and social aspects (Strickland, 1997). For this reason, considerable effort has been put into identifying the patient outcomes that are affected by the quality of nursing care.

According to Benner, Sutphen, Leonard, and Day (2010), patient care outcomes can be improved by employing a better educated nursing workforce. Although 60% of the nation's nurses hold associate degrees in nursing (ADN), the research supports that better patient outcomes occur when nurses hold baccalaureate degrees (Orsolini-Hain, 2008). The American Association of Nurse Executives (AONE) recommends that the educational preparation of the nurse be at the BSN level as this educational level will "prepare the nurse of the future to function as an equal partner" (AONE, 2005). The research and recommendations do not negate the value of the associate degree nurse, but promote the concept of lifelong learning and the need to continue and obtain a baccalaureate degree.

The ANA identified 10 quality indicators in acute care that relate to the availability and quality of professional nursing services in hospitals. Across the United States, data are being collected from nursing units using these quality indicators. The National Database for Nursing Quality Indicators (NDNQI) is continuously updated (www.nursingworld.org).

A major problem in using and interpreting outcome measures is that outcomes are influenced by many factors. For example, the outcome of patient teaching done by a nurse on a home visit is affected by the patient's interest and ability to learn, the quality of the teaching materials, the presence or absence of family support, information (which may conflict) from other caregivers, and the environment in which the teaching is done. If the teaching is successful, can the nurse be given full credit for the success? If it is not successful, who has failed?

In order to determine why an intervention such as patient teaching succeeds or fails, it is necessary to evaluate the process as well as the outcome. A comprehensive evaluation includes all three aspects: structure, process, and outcome. However, it is much more difficult to gather and monitor outcome data than to measure structure or process.

Risk Management

An important part of CQI is **risk management,** a process of identifying, analyzing, treating, and evaluating real and potential hazards. The Joint Commission (JC) recommends the integration of a quality control/risk management program to maintain continuous feedback and communication. To plan proactively, an organization must identify real or potential exposures that might threaten it. As a nurse, it is your responsibility to report adverse incidents to the risk manager, according to your organization's policies and procedures. In many states, this is a legal requirement.

Risk events are categorized according to severity. Although all untoward events are important, not all carry the same severity of outcomes (Benson-Flynn, 2001).

1. **Service occurrence.** A service occurrence is an unexpected occurrence that does not result in a clinically significant interruption of services and that is without apparent patient or employee injury. Examples include minor property or equipment damage, unsatisfactory provision of service at any level, or inconsequential interruption of service. Most occurrences in this category are addressed within the patient complaint process.
2. **Serious incident.** A serious incident results in a clinically significant interruption of therapy or service, minor injury to a patient or employee, or significant loss or damage of equipment or property. Minor injuries are usually defined as needing medical intervention outside of hospital admission or physical or psychological damage.
3. **Sentinel events.** A sentinel event is an unexpected occurrence involving death or serious/permanent physical or psychological injury, or the risk thereof. The phrase "or the risk thereof" includes any process variation for which a recurrence would carry a significant chance of a serious adverse outcome. Such events are called sentinel because they signal the need for immediate investigation and response. When a sentinel event occurs, appropriate individuals within the organization must be made aware of the event; they must

investigate and understand the causes of the event; and they must make changes in the organization's systems and processes to reduce the probability of such an event in the future (jcaho.org/ptsafety_frm.html).

The subset of sentinel events that is subject to review by the JC includes any occurrence that meets any of the following criteria:

■ The event has resulted in an unanticipated death or major permanent loss of function that is not related to the natural course of the patient's illness or underlying condition.
■ The event is one of the following (even if the outcome was not death or major permanent loss of function): suicide of a patient in a setting where the patient receives around-the-clock care (e.g., hospital, residential treatment center, crisis stabilization center), infant abduction or discharge to the wrong family, rape, hemolytic transfusion reaction involving administration of blood or blood products having major blood group incompatibilities, or surgery on the wrong patient or wrong body part (jcaho.org/ptsafety_frm.html).

Adhering to nursing standards of care as well as the policies and procedures of the institution greatly decreases the nurse's risk. Common risk areas for nursing include:

■ Medication errors
■ Documentation errors and/or omissions
■ Failure to perform nursing care or treatments correctly
■ Errors in patient safety that result in falls
■ Failure to communicate significant data to patients and other providers (Kalisch, Landstrom, & Williams, 2009; Swansburg & Swansburg, 2002)

Risk management programs also include attention to areas of employee wellness and injury prevention. Latex allergics, repetitive stress injuries, carpal tunnel syndrome, barrier protection for tuberculosis, back injuries, and the rise of antibiotic-resistant organisms all fall under the area of risk management.

Adhering to standards of care and exercising the amount of care that a reasonable nurse would demonstrate under the same or similar circumstances can protect the nurse from litigation. Understanding what actions to take when something goes wrong is imperative. The main goal is patient safety. Reporting and remediation must occur quickly.

Once an incident has occurred, you must complete an incident report immediately. The incident report is used to collect and analyze data for determination of future risk. The report should be accurate, objective, complete, and factual. If there is future litigation, the plaintiff's attorney can subpoena the report. The report should be prepared in only a single copy and never placed in the medical record (Swansburg & Swansburg, 2002). It is kept with internal hospital correspondence.

Nurses have a responsibility to remain educated and informed and to become active participants in understanding and identifying potential risks to their patients and to themselves. Ignorance of the law is no excuse. Maintaining a knowledgeable, professional, and caring nurse-patient relationship is the first step in decreasing your own risk.

The Nursing Shortage and Patient Safety

The value of registered nurses to the health-care system cannot be minimized. Nurses provide client care within multiple settings. Operationally, nurses have a pivotal role in ensuring patient safety and positive patient outcomes (Dunton, Gajewski, Klaus, & Pierson, 2007).

Factors Contributing to the Nursing Shortage

▪ **Increased demand for nurses.** As health care moves to a variety of community settings, only the most acutely ill patients remain in the hospital. The transfer of less acute patients to nursing homes and community settings creates additional job opportunities. Research supporting improved patient outcomes when patient care is provided by RNs as opposed to unlicensed personnel will also increase demand for RNs. According to Buerhaus (2013), "People are coming into nursing at the same rate as the baby-boom generation; more have earned baccalaureate degrees than have earned associate degrees." Between 2001 and 2012, the number of RN grads more than doubled, from 74,000 in 2002 to 181,000 (Auerbach, Staiger, Muench, & Buerhaus, 2013). Buerhaus attributes this increase to initiatives driven by Johnson & Johnson's "Campaign for Nursing's Future,"

and reinforced by the Robert Wood Johnson Foundation and state workforce centers.

▪ **Reduction in and shortage of nursing faculty.** As fewer younger nurses choose to become educators and current faculty members retire, the shortage of faculty continues to affect the number of students admitted to nursing programs. The American Association of Colleges of Nursing (AACN) report on 2011–2012 Enrollment and Graduations in Baccalaureate and Graduate Programs in Nursing stated 1,181 faculty vacancies existed across the nation and that U.S. nursing schools turned away 75,587 qualified applicants from baccalaureate and graduate nursing programs in 2011 due to an insufficient number of faculty, clinical sites, classroom space, clinical preceptors, and budget constraints.

▪ **Job dissatisfaction.** Staffing levels, heavy workloads, high patient acuity along with lack of sufficient support staff, increased use of overtime, and salary discrepancies between nurses and other health-care professionals have contributed to growing dissatisfaction and lower retention of nurses. Many facilities are now using workplace issues and incentives as a retention strategy.

The need to control spiraling health-care costs, along with the issues of supply and demand for nursing services will continue. According to the ANA, more than 60% of nurses graduate initially from associate-degree nursing programs. You, personally, will be affected by trends in health-care delivery, but you can also be a major voice in decision making. In his closing remarks at the University of Wisconsin, Buerhaus (2013) challenged nurses to "Become a student of health care reform. Make sure your skills sets offer value to an emerging delivery system that will be on the hunt for and will reward those who provide value." As in the past, cost control and demand for nursing services will most likely involve changing nurse staffing, the model of care, and professional nursing practice (Shekelle, 2013).

Safety in the U.S. Health-Care System

Patient safety is the prevention of harm caused by errors. The IOM defines errors as "the failure of a planned action to be completed as intended (e.g., error of execution) or the use of a wrong plan to achieve an aim (e.g., error of planning) (IOM, 2000, p. 57). It is important to note that errors are unintentional and that not all errors lead to an adverse event causing harm or death.

In the United States, medical errors account for approximately 98,000 deaths per year (Pham, Aswani, Rosen, Lee, Huddle, Weeks, & Pronovost, 2012). These include medication errors, falls, handoff errors, diagnostic and surgical errors, and health-care–acquired (nosocomial) infections. The IOM indicates that 1.5 million adverse drug events (ADEs) occur annually in the United States. Hospital acquired infections (HAIs) may result in death, increased financial costs, and extended hospital stays. The most common HAIs include urinary tract infections, surgical site infections, pneumonia, and bacteremia (Pham et al., 2012).

Falls account for a large number of adverse events in hospitals and nursing homes. Injuries from falls are associated with an increase in mortality, extended lengths of stay, and a decrease in the ability of the individual to revert back to his/her previous health status (Haines, Hill, & Hill, 2011; Oliver, Healy, & Haines, 2010). Most falls are the result of unrecognized cognitive impairment, failure of health-care personnel to institute safety measures, and impaired mobility.

Handoff errors involve a break in continuity of care when different providers in one care area assume responsibility of the patient or the patient moves from one care area to another. These are most commonly the result of communication errors. If the responsibility for the patient is not clearly transferred, necessary information to make informed decisions may not be communicated (Raduma-Tomas, Flin, Yule, & Williams, 2011; Raduma-Tomas, Flin, Yule, & Close, 2012).

Approximately 40,000–80,000 deaths per year occur because of diagnostic errors. Diagnostic errors occur more often in certain specialties such as oncology, neurology, and cardiology. According to Brown, McCarthy, Kelen, & Lew, (2010), they are also the greatest source of errors in emergency departments.

Types of Errors

To Err is Human (2000) relied on the work of Leape et al. (1993) to categorize types of errors (Box 10-7). After categorizing types of errors,

---

box 10-7

Types of Errors (IOM, 2000, p. 36)

Diagnostic
Error or delay in diagnosis
Failure to employ indicated tests
Use of outmoded tests or therapy
Failure to act on results of monitoring or testing
Treatment
Error in the performance of an operation, procedure, or test
Error in administering the treatment
Error in the dose or method of using a drug
Avoidable delay in treatment or in responding to an abnormal test
Inappropriate (not indicated) care
Preventive
Failure to provide prophylactic treatment
Inadequate monitoring or follow-up of treatment
Other
Failure of communication
Equipment failure
Other system failure

Leape, L., Lawthers, A.G., Brennan, T.A., et al. (1993). Preventing medical injury. Qual Rev Bull. 19(5):144–149.

Leape and colleagues found that 70% of all errors were preventable.

Human errors can occur for many reasons. *Skill-based errors* occur when slips or lapses in the actions taken by the provider were not what was intended (Duke University Medical Center, 2005). Rule-based errors are those that occur when a standard or "rule" is violated. An example of rule-based error is an experienced nurse administering the wrong medication by picking up the wrong syringe.

Studying events and identifying how each occurred offers data that may be used to improve safety.

- **Near miss.** A near miss is an error or mishap that results in no harm or very minimal patient harm (IOM, 2000, p. 87). Near misses are useful in identifying and remedying vulnerabilities in a system before harm can occur. An example of a near miss is catching a medication error before the medication is administered.
- **Adverse event.** An adverse event is injury to a patient caused by medical management rather than an underlying condition of the patient (IOM, 2000). The IOM reports have highlighted the prevalence of errors, especially preventable adverse events. Adverse events have been classified into four types (see Box 10-7).

- **Accident.** An accident is an event that involves damage to a defined system that disrupts the ongoing or future output of that system. Accidents occur when multiple systems fail and tend to be unplanned or unforeseen. Accidents provide information about systems.
- **Medication error.** A medication error is a preventable incident that occurs during the medication use process that could or did lead to patient harm.

Error Identification and Reporting

Nurses are on the front line in identifying and reporting errors. In the past, individuals involved in medical errors suffered punitive consequences; thus, many errors went unreported. Providers and organizations may fear blame or punishment for mistakes or errors. This culture of blame prevents or discourages individuals from coming forward.

Developing a Culture of Safety

To achieve safe patient care, a *culture of safety* must exist. Organizations and senior leadership must drive change to develop a culture of safety—a blame-free environment in which reporting of errors is promoted and rewarded. A culture of safety promotes trust, honesty, openness, and transparency. In general, hospitals that practice a culture of safety tend to show fewer reported cases of adverse safety events (Mardon, Khanna, Sorra, Dyer, & Famolaro, 2010).

Teamwork and involvement of the patient contribute to promoting a culture of safety. When a culture of safety exists, individual providers do not fear reprisal and are not blamed for identifying or reporting errors. Reported errors provide data and information necessary to understand why or how the error occurred, thus improving care and preventing harm.

Event-reporting systems hold organizations accountable and lead to improved safety. Mandatory reporting systems are operated by regulatory agencies and have a strong focus on errors associated with serious harm or death. In addition, the Food and Drug Administration (FDA) mandates reporting of serious harm or death (adverse events) related to drugs and medical devices. Failure to report mandatory requirements may lead to fines, withdrawal of participation in clinical trials, or loss of licensure to operate.

The Joint Commission relies on *root cause analysis* from each sentinel event. Root cause analysis is the process of learning from consequences. The consequences can be desirable, but most root cause analyses deal with adverse consequences. An example of a root cause analysis is a review of a medication error, especially one resulting in a death or severe complications. Principles of root cause analysis include:

1. Determine what influenced the consequences, i.e., determine the necessary and sufficient influences that explain the nature and the magnitude of the consequences.
2. Establish tightly linked chains of influence.
3. At every level of analysis, determine the necessary and sufficient influences.
4. Whenever feasible, drill down to root causes.
5. Know that there are always multiple root causes.

The Joint Commission also developed the International Center for Patient Safety, which establishes National Patient Safety Goals each year and publishes Sentinel Event Strategies. Box 10-8 summarizes the work of the International Center for Patient Safety. These tools developed by the Joint Commission offer health-care organizations goals and strategies to prevent harm and death based on what has been learned from sentinel events.

---

box 10-8

Joint Commission International Center for Patient Safety

1. Sets patient safety standards
2. Implements and oversees sentinel event policy and advisory group
3. Publishes *Sentinel Event Alert* newsletter and quality check reports
4. Sets yearly national patient safety goals
5. Developed the universal protocol related to surgical procedures
6. Evaluates organizations' monitoring of quality of care issues
7. Conducts patient safety research
8. Provides patient safety resources
9. Supports the Speak Up program
10. Involved with patient safety coalitions and legislative efforts

---

Adapted from Joint Commission on Accreditation of Healthcare Organizations (JCAHO), accessed November 26, 2005, from jcpatientsafety.org

Organizations, Agencies, and Initiatives Supporting Quality and Safety in the Health-Care System

The ongoing movement to improve quality and safety has led to the development of governmental and private organizations (Box 10-9) in addition to those mentioned in the historical perspective at the beginning of this chapter. These organizations and agencies currently monitor, evaluate, accredit, influence, research, finance, and advocate for quality within the health delivery system. Each organization works inside and outside the system to drive change leading to improved health outcomes and improved system quality. Each organization works within its mission to address various characteristics of the health-care system or to address patient needs. Some organizations serve multiple roles beyond their primary mission.

Government Agencies

Federal and state-level government agencies provide tools and resources for improving quality and safety within the U.S. health-care system. Government agencies also oversee regulation, licensure, and mandatory and voluntary reporting programs.

Within the U.S. Department of Health and Human Services (HHS) reside multiple agencies that support quality and safety. HHS is the U.S. government's principal agency for protecting the health of all Americans and providing essential human services, including health care (HHS, 2011). HHS works closely with state and local governments to meet the nation's health and human needs.

In addition to administering Medicare and Medicaid, the Centers for Medicare and Medicaid Services (CMS) administers quality initiatives intended "to assure quality health care for all Americans through accountability and public exposure" (CMS, 2008). Initiatives include:

- **MedQIC.** This initiative aims to ensure each Medicare recipient receives the appropriate level of care. MedQIC is a community-based QI program that provides tools and resources to encourage changes in processes, structures, and behaviors within the health-care community.
- **Post–Acute Care Reform Plan.** CMS is examining post-acute transfers with the aim of reducing care fragmentation and unsafe transitions.

---

box 10-9

Organizations and Agencies Supporting Quality and Safety

Government Agencies
- U.S. Department of Health and Human Services, www.hhs.gov/
- Food and Drug Administration (FDA), www.fda.gov/
- Initiatives: Medwatch and Sentinel Initiative
- Health Resources and Services Administration (HRSA), www.hrsa.gov/
- Initiatives: Health Information Technology and National Practitioner Database
- Centers for Medicare and Medicaid Services (CMS), www.cms.hhs.gov/
- Initiatives: Hospital Quality Initiative, MedQIC, American Health Quality Association (AHQA)
- Agency for Healthcare Research and Quality (AHRQ), www.ahrq.gov/
- Initiatives: Health IT, Improving Health Care Quality, Medical Errors and Patient Safety, Measuring Quality
- VA National Center for Patient Safety, www.va.gov/ncps/

Health-Care Provider Professional Organizations
- American Nurses Association, http://nursingworld.org/
- Initiative: National Database of Nursing Quality Indicators (NDNQI)
- Association of Perioperative Registered Nurses (AORN), https://www.aorn.org/

- Initiative: Patient Safety First and AORN Toolkits
- American Hospital Association (AHA), www.aha.org/
- Initiative: AHA Quality Center
- Association of Academic Health Centers, www.aahcdc.org/index.php
- Priorities: Health Profession Workforce and Health Care Reform

Nonprofit Organizations, Foundations, and Research
- The Leapfrog Group, www.leapfroggroup.org/
- Kaiser Family Foundation, www.kff.org/
- Markel Foundation-Connecting for Health, www.connectingforhealth.org/aboutus/index.html#
- Robert Wood Johnson Foundation-Quality Equality in Healthcare, www.rwjf.org/qualityequality/index.jsp
- National Patient Safety Foundation, www.npsf.org/
- The Commonwealth Fund, www.commonwealthfund.org/aboutus/

Quality Organizations
- Institute for Healthcare Improvement (IHI), www.ihi.org/ihi
- The Joint Commission, www.jointcommission.org/
- National Committee for Quality Assurance (NCQA), http://web.ncqa.org/
- National Quality Forum, www.qualityforum.org/

■ **Hospital Quality Initiative.** This is a major initiative aimed at improving quality of care at the provider and organization level. It creates a uniform set of quality measurements by which consumers can compare organizations and by which organizations can benchmark progress toward achieving goals in specified areas of care, such as acute myocardial infarct, congestive heart failure, pneumonia, and postsurgical infections. Organizations provide data to CMS through public reporting of quality measures. These data feed the *Hospital Compare* Web site (www.hospitalcompare.hhs.gov). Organizations are incentivized to participate with an offering of increased reimbursement.

Also under the HHS is the Agency for Healthcare Research and Quality (AHRQ), which is the lead federal agency charged with improving the quality, safety, efficiency, and effectiveness of health care for all Americans (HHS, 2008). Through multiple initiatives, the support of research, and evidence-based decision-making, the AHRQ aims to fulfill its mission:

■ **Health IT.** A multifaceted initiative that includes (a) research support of $260 million in grants and contracts to support and stimulate investment in health information technology (IT); (b) the newly created AHRQ National Resource Center, which provides technical assistance and research funding to aid technology implementation within communities; and (c) learning laboratories at more than 100 hospitals nationwide to develop and test health IT applications
■ **National Quality Measures Clearinghouse (NQMC).** Web-accessible database provides access to evidence-based quality measures and measure sets; NQMC provides access for obtaining detailed information on quality measures and to further their dissemination, implementation, and use in order to inform health-care decisions
■ **Medical Errors and Patient Safety.** Web site providing access to evidence-based tools and resources for consumers and providers
■ **AHRQ Quality Indicators.** Set of quality indicators used by organizations to highlight potential quality concerns, identify areas that need further study and investigation, and track changes over time

The U.S. Department of Defense (DoD) and the Veterans Health Administration (VHA) have taken leadership positions in developing tools, resources, and programs aimed at improving safety, promoting change, and promoting a culture of safety within the DoD and VHA. The VHA National Center for Patient Safety developed a toolkit for fall prevention and management, tools for escape and elopement management, and cognitive aids for root cause analysis and health failure mode and effect analysis.

Health-Care Provider Professional Organizations

Professional organizations directly address the missions and concerns regarding quality and safety of the professionals they represent. Each organization offers programs, access to evidence-based practices, toolkits, and newsletters to aid their members in driving quality within their own practice and organization.

The vital quality and safety initiative of the ANA is the National Database of Nursing Quality Indicators (NDNQI), a database of unit-specific nurse-sensitive information collected at hospitals. Data are collected and evaluated to improve quality. The indicators reflect the structure, process, and outcomes of nursing care and lead to improved quality and safety at the bedside. The ANA also has a strong focus on safe nurse staffing levels to promote safe, quality patient care.

Many specialty organizations within nursing have also placed safe, quality patient care on their agendas and part of their strategic plans. By developing and implementing standards of care, these organizations outline nursing care standards to obtain positive patient outcomes. Many health-care institutions promote and require implementation of these specialized standards within their own patient care units (www.aacn.org; www.aann.org; www. apna.org).

Nonprofit Organizations and Foundations

With few exceptions, nonprofit organizations and foundations are generally focused on consumer education, policy development, and research to improve quality and safety within the health-care system. Many organizations serve multiple missions. The Kaiser Family Foundation (2005) has a strong emphasis on U.S. and international nonpartisan health policy and health policy research. Self-funded research and public opinion polling on topics related to quality and safety in the health-care system contribute to policy and legislation development.

Also having a multifaceted mission, the renowned Robert Wood Johnson Foundation (RWJF) serves multiple missions and seeks to improve health and health care for all Americans. RWJF's success comes from leveraging partnerships and its endowment to "building evidence and producing, synthesizing and distributing knowledge, new ideas and expertise" (RWJF, 2008, 2011) in eight program areas. RWJF is responsible for successfully funded projects and research that improve quality and safety for all Americans.

The Leapfrog Group is a nonprofit organization interested in improving safety, quality, and affordability of health care through incentives and rewards to those who use and pay for health care (Leapfrog Group, 2007, 2011). With a focus on reducing preventable medical mistakes, the Leapfrog Group touted their benefits to improve safety and quality to consumers and business owners with three *leaps:* (a) improve transparency by reporting hospital survey results addressing quality and safety indicators; (b) incentivize better quality and safety performance; and (c) collaborate with other organizations to improve quality and safety. To date, there is limited evidence that the Leapfrog Group has effectively improved quality or safety. Limitations to success may be in part because too few hospitals have participated in the surveys and too few consumers have used the available information to make health decisions; however, there is an indication that, with time, participation could improve with adjustments in strategy by the Leapfrog Group (Galvin, Delbanco, Milstein, & Belden, 2005).

Quality Organizations

Each of the quality organizations strives to improve system-wide quality for Americans through a variety of programs and methods.

The National Committee for Quality Assurance (NCQA) was established in 1990 to accredit health plans and certify organizations. Its success in supporting quality and safety resides in its Health Effectiveness Data and Information Set (HEDIS). Over 90% of U.S. health plans use HEDIS to measure performance. HEDIS allows consumers and employers to evaluate health plans using data from HEDIS as a report card of the plan's success.

The Joint Commission was established in 1951 with a focus on structural measures of quality, assessment of the physical plant, number of patient beds per nurse, credentialing of service providers, and other standards for each department. This system of evaluation has given way to a more process- and outcome-focused model: CQI. Today, The JC accredits more than 19,000 health-care organizations. Evaluation of nursing services is an important part of the accreditation. JC–accredited agencies are measured against national standards set by health-care professionals. Hospitals, health-care networks, long-term care facilities, ambulatory care centers, home health agencies, behavioral health-care facilities, and clinical laboratories are among the organizations seeking JC accreditation. Although accreditation by the JC is voluntary, Medicare and Medicaid reimbursement cannot be sought by organizations not accredited by the JC.

Integrating Initiatives and Evidenced-Based Practices Into Patient Care

As you familiarize yourself with each of these organizations and their respective initiatives, consider how they will affect the management of patient care. Your responsibility as a professional RN is to acknowledge their presence, understand and value their importance, and participate in your facility-adopted initiatives and evidence-based practices. Additionally, as a leader and manager, you will be expected to drive changes based upon endeavors of many of these organizations, agencies, and initiatives ensuring that quality and safety continue to improve.

The IOM report proposed five core competencies (Box 10-10) in which all health-care professionals need to be effective as providers and leaders in the 21st-century health-care system. Nurses are key to improving patient safety (RWJF, 2011). The IOM's report *The Future of Nursing: Leading Change Advancing Health* (2011) focused on nursing education, research, and leadership as ways to improve patient safety. Nurses need to be full partners with physicians and other members of the interprofessional team in the delivery of health care.

By integrating these competencies into 21st-century health profession education, you can begin to support health-care reform while engaging in safe and effective patient care. As a practicing professional, you can use the competencies to guide

box 10-10

Core Competencies for Health Professionals (IOM, 2003a, p. 4)

Provide patient-centered care. Identify, respect, and care about patients' differences, values, preferences, and expressed needs; relieve pain and suffering; coordinate continuous care; listen to, clearly inform, communicate with, and educate patients; share decision making and management; and continuously advocate disease prevention, wellness, and promotion of healthy lifestyles, including a focus on population health.
Work in interprofessional teams. Cooperate, collaborate, communicate, and integrate care in teams to ensure that care is continuous and reliable.
Employ evidence-based practice. Integrate best research with clinical expertise and patient values for

optimum care, and participate in learning and research activities to the extent feasible.
Apply quality improvement. Identify errors and hazards in care; understand and implement basic safety design principles, such as standardization and simplification; continually understand and measure quality of care in terms of structure, process, and outcomes in relation to patient and community needs; and design and test interventions to change processes and systems of care with the objective of improving quality.
Utilize informatics. Communicate, manage knowledge, mitigate error, and support decision making using information technology.

future professional development and ensure a positive impact on health-care reform while improving quality and safety.

Influence of Nursing

Nurses are empowered through self-determination, meaning, competence, and impact (Whitehead, Weiss, & Tappen, 2010). Additionally, nurses play vital roles in collective bargaining and decision making within their organizations, empowered through professional organization such as the ANA (see Chapter 8). It is through these organizations that nurses can promote safety and quality in nursing practice. Working within organizations and health-care institutions to create guidelines for safe staffing, develop systems that measure patient acuity by nursing time and expertise, and encouraging shared decision making promote safe practice (Aiken et al., 2012; Pham et al., 2012).

Nurses are respected and trusted health-care professionals. To influence change in the health-care system, professional nurses must first acknowledge power within the profession and recognize their central role in health care. To be effective, nurses must leverage their professional expertise and the trust and respect they have garnered. Nurses need to act, not stand on the sidelines, and raise the volume of their collective voice. It is critical that nurses speak up and seek an active role in shaping health-care reform:

■ **Become informed.** Research topics of interest to *you* and your practice. Rely on appropriate Internet sites and your professional organizations as resources for current policy and legislative topics.

■ **Plan.** After selecting a topic, prepare your plan: gather facts and figures that will support your ideas and position. Outline them, and address your audience in person, on paper, or via the Web. The most influential people are prepared and believe in their topic.

■ **Take action.** Shape public opinion by the method of your choice. Start small, and build your impact. (1) Write a letter to your representative (local, state, federal), ANA leadership or state-level delegate, the editor of your local newspaper, or to the editor of your favorite nursing journal/magazine. (2) Attend a meeting where your topic will be addressed in a public forum or at a professional gathering. Meet the people who are influential, and share your ideas or learn from others. (3) Vote for candidates and officers in your professional organizations and within the government. (4) Visit your representative (local, state, federal) or ANA leadership or state-level delegate to share your ideas. (5) Volunteer. Ask what you can do to help. (6) Testify before decision-making bodies. (7) Educate yourself on the Affordable Care Act so that you can educate others.

Conclusion

Pressure from quality organizations, consumers, payers, and providers has shifted the focus in the health-care system from patient care to issues of cost and quality. Experts indicate that quality promotes decreased costs, increased satisfaction, and better patient outcomes. This is an opportunity for nurses to become more professional and empowered to organize and manage patient care so that it is safe, efficient, and of the highest quality. Begin early in your career to participate actively in QI initiatives and familiarize yourself with the causes of medical errors. Participate on committees to create policies that promote safety and quality. Focus attention on the following in patient care delivery (Hansten & Washburn, 2001, p. 24D):

1. **Think critically.** Use your creative, intuitive, logical, and analytical processes continually in working with patients and their families.
2. **Plan and report outcomes.** Emphasizing results is a necessary part of managing resources in today's cost-conscious environment. Focusing on the outcomes moves the nurse and other members of the interprofessional team away from tasks.
3. **Make introductory rounds.** Begin each shift with the interprofessional team members introducing themselves, describing their roles, and providing patient updates.
4. **Plan in partnership with the patient.** In conjunction with the introductory rounds, spend a few minutes early in the shift with each patient, discussing care objectives and long-term goals. This event becomes the center of the nursing process for the shift and ensures that the patient, nurse, and other members of the interprofessional team are working toward the same outcomes.
5. **Communicate the plan.** Avoid confusion among members of the interprofessional team by communicating the intended outcomes and the important role that each member plays in the plan.
6. **Evaluate progress.** Schedule time during the shift quickly to evaluate outcomes and the progress of the plan and to make revisions as necessary.

Study Questions

1. How have historical, social, political, and economic trends affected nursing practice? Give specific examples and their implications.

2. What problems have you identified during your clinical experiences that could be considered issues to be addressed using CQI?

3. What SCMs have you seen implemented in practice? Which ones might you use to assist you in planning care? If you have not seen any, ask the nurse manager what is used on the unit.

4. How do nursing organization care models affect quality and safety outcomes?

5. Discuss the role of the nurse in CQI and risk management.

6. Based on patient safety goals for the current year, what will you do to ensure adherence to these goals?

7. What are evidence-based practices that promote quality and safety within the health-care system?

8. Describe how regulatory agencies and accrediting agencies affect patient care and outcomes at the bedside.

9. Review the nonprofit organizations and government agencies that influence and advocate for quality and safety in the health-care system. What do the organizations or agencies do that supports the hallmarks of quality? What have been the results of their efforts for patients, facilities, the health-care delivery system, and the nursing profession? How have the organizations or agencies affected your facility and professional practice?

10. Explain how technology enhances and promotes safe patient care, educates patients and consumers, evaluates health-care delivery, and enhances the nurse's knowledge base in your practice and at your organization.

11. How would you begin discussion on quality and safety issues with the nurse manager or colleague?

12. What issues may arise when the care delivery system is changed? What does the RN need to consider when implementing these changes?

Case Study to Promote Critical Reasoning

The director of CQI has called a meeting of all the interprofessional team members on your floor. Based on last quarter's statistics, the readmission rate of patients who have infections after hip replacements for osteoarthritis is twice that of patients for the first half of the year. The director has requested that the staff identify members who wish to be CQI team members investigating this problem. You, the staff nurse, have volunteered to be a member of the team. The team will consist of the physical therapist on the unit, a physician's assistant who works with the hospital orthopedic surgeons, the clinical educator, the nursing case manager, and you.

1. Why were these people selected for the team?

2. What data need to be collected to evaluate this situation?

3. What are the potential outcomes for patients with who have had hip replacements?

4. Develop a flowchart of a typical hospital discharge and readmission rate for patients who have had hip replacements.

References

Affordable Care Act. 2010. Retrieved on February 3, 2014, from www.hhs.gov/healthcare/rights

Aiken, L.H., Sermeus, W., Van den Heede, K., Sloan, D.M., Russe, R., McKee, M., Bruyneel, L., Rafferty, A.M., Griffiths, R., & Moreno-Casbas, M.T. (2012). Patient safety, satisfaction, and quality of hospital care: Cross sectional surveys of nurses and patients in 12 countries in Europe and the United States. *British Medical Journal,* 2012:344:e1717. doi: 10.1136/bmj.e1717. Retrieved October 4, 2013, from www.bmj.com/content/344/bmj.e1717

Ajjawi, R., & Higgs, J. (2008). Learning to reason: A journey of professional socialization. *Advances in Health Sciences Education, 13*(2), 133–150.

American Association of Colleges of Nursing. (2008). Essentials of baccalaureate education. Retrieved October 4, 2013, from www.aacn.nche.edu/

American Association of Colleges of Nursing. (2012). Nursing shortage fact sheet. Retrieved October 4, 2013, from www.aacn.nche.edu/media-relations/FacultyShortageFS.pdf

American Association of Colleges of Nursing (AACN). (2012). Creating a more qualified nursing workforce. Retrieved October 4, 2013, from www.aacn.nche.edu/Media/FactSheets/ImpactEdNP.htm

American Association of Nurse Executives (2005). BSN level nursing resources. Retrieved from http://www.anoe.org/resources/leadership%20tools/BSN.shtml

American Nurses Association. (2008). ANA's health care agenda. Retrieved October 3, 2013, from www.nursingworld.org/Content/HealthcareandPolicyIssues/Agenda/ANAsHealthSystemReformAgenda.pdf

Anderson, L.M., Scrimshaw, S.C., Fullilove, M.T., Fielding, J.E., & Normand, J. (2003). Culturally competent healthcare systems: A systematic review. *American Journal of Preventive Medicine, 24*(3S), 68–79.

Auerbach, D.I., Staiger, D.O., Muench, U., & Buerhaus, P.I. (2013). The nursing workforce in an era of health care reform. *New England Journal of Medicine, 368*(16), 1470–1472.

Baldwin, J.H., Conger, C.O., Maycock, C., & Abegglen, J.C. (2002). Health care delivery system influences changes in nursing educational materials. *Public Health Nursing, 19*(4), 246–254.

Benner, P., Sutphen, M., Leonard, V., & Day, L. (2010). *Educating nurses: A call for radical transformation.* San Francisco: Jossey-Bass.

Benson-Flynn, J. (2001). Incident reporting: Clarifying occurrences, incidents, and sentinel events. *Home Healthcare Nurse, 19,* 701–706.

Billings, D.M., & Halstead, J.A. (2011). *Teaching in nursing: A Guide for Faculty* (4th ed.). St. Louis: Elsevier Saunders.

Booth, R.G. (2006). Educating the future health professional nurse. *International Journal of Nursing Education Scholarship, 3*(1), 1–10.

Brook, R.H., Davis, A.R., & Kamberg, C. (1980). Selected reflections on quality of medical care evaluations in the 1980s. *Nursing Research, 29*(2), 127.

Brown, T.W., McCarthy, M.L., Kelen, G.D., and Lew, F. (2010). An epidemiologic study of closed emergency department malpractice claims in a national database of physician malpractice insurers. *Academic Emergency Medicine, 17*(5), 553–560.

Buerhaus, P.I. (2013). This era's health care reform built on quality/cost ratio. University of Wisconsin School of Nursing, Retrieved October 5, 2013, from www.son.wisc.edu/buerhaus-health-care-reform-2013-littlefield-leadership-lecture.htm

Calzone, K.A., Cashion, A., Feetham, S., Jenkins, J., Prows, C.A., Williams, J.K., & Wung, S.F. (2010). Nursing transforming healthcare using genetics and genomics. *Nursing Outlook, 58*(5). 26–35.

Centers for Medicare and Medicaid Services (CMS). (2008). Retrieved February 3, 2014, from www.cms.gov

Cole, L., & Houston, S. (1999). Linking outcomes management and practice improvement. structured care methodologies: Evolution and use in patient care delivery. *Outcomes Management for Nursing Practice, 3*(2), 53.

Cronenwett, L., Sherwood, G., Barnsteiner, J., Disch, J., et al. (2007). Quality and safety education for nurses. *Nursing Outlook, 55*(3), 122–131.

Davis, K. (2001). Preparing for the future: A 2020 vision for American health care. *Academic Medicine, 76*(4), 304–306.

Davis, K. (2010). *A new era in American health care: Realizing the potential of reform.* New York: The Commonwealth Fund.

Donabedian, A. (1969). A guide to medical care administration. In *Medical care appraisal: Quality and Utilization,* vol. II. New York: American Public Health Association.

Donabedian, A. (1977). Evaluating the quality of medical care. *Milbank Memorial Fund Quarterly, 44* (part 2), 166.

Donabedian, A. (1987). Some basic issues in evaluating the quality of health care. In Rinke, L.T. (ed.). *Outcome measures in home care.* New York: National League of Nursing.

Donaldson, M.S. (ed.). (1998). Statement on quality of care. Washington, DC: National Academy Press. Retrieved August 1, 2008, from www.nap.edu/

Doenges, M.E., Morrhouse, M., & Murr, A. (2009). Nursing care plans (8th ed.). Philadelphia: F.A. Davis. Co.

Dubois C.A., D'Amour D., Pomey M.P., Girard F., & Brault I. (2013). Conceptualizing performance of nursing care as a prerequisite for better measurement: A systematic and interpretive review. *Biomed Central Nursing, 12*(7). doi: 10.1186/1472-6955-12-7.

Duke University Medical Center. (2005). Anatomy of an error: Basic tenet of human error. Retrieved August 7, 2008, from http://patientsafetyed.duhs.duke.edu/index.html

Dunton, N., Gajewski, B., Klaus, S., & Pierson, B., (2007). "The Relationship of Nursing Workforce Characteristics to Patient Outcomes" OJIN: The Online Journal of Issues in Nursing. 12 (3). Retrieved on June 19, 2014 from http://www.nursingworld.org/MainMenuCategories/ANAMarketplace/ANAPeriodicals/OJIN/TableofContents/Volume122007/No3Sept07/NursingWorkforceCharacteristics.html

Elwood, T.W. (2007). The future of health care in the United States. *Journal of Allied Health, 36*(1), 3–10.

Ervin, N.E., Bickes, J.T., & Schim, S.M. (2006). Environments of care: A curriculum model for preparing a new generation of nurses. *Journal of Nursing Education, 45*(2), 75–80.

Galvin, R.S., Delbanco, S., Milstein, A., & Belden, G. (2005, Jan/Feb). Has the Leapfrog Group had an impact on the health care market? *Health Affairs, 24*(1), 228–233.

Haddad, S.M. (2010). Clinical pathways: Effects on professional practice, patient outcomes, length of stay and hospital costs: RHL commentary. WHO. Retrieved October 5, 2013, from http://apps.who.int/rhl/effective_practice_and_organizing_care/cd006632_haddadsm_com/en/.

Haines, T.P., Hill, A.M., & Hill, K.D. (2011). Patient education to prevent falls among older hospital inpatients: A randomized controlled trial. *Archives of Internal Medicine, 171*(6), 516–524.

Hansten, R., & Washburn, M. (2001). Outcomes-based care delivery. *American Journal of Nursing, 101*(2), 24A–D.

Heller, B.R., Oros, M.T., & Durney-Crowley, J. (2000). The future of nursing education: 10 trends to watch. *Nursing and Health Care Perspectives, 21*(1), 9.

Hunt, D.V. (1992). *Quality in America: How to implement a competitive quality program.* Homewood, IL: Business One Irwin.

Hunter, K.M. (2011). Implementation of an electronic medication administration record and bedside verification system. *Online Journal of Nursing Informatics, 15*(2), 672–678. Retrieved October 5, 2013, from http://ojini.org/issues/?p=672

Institute of Medicine. (2000). *To err is human: Building a safer health system.* Kohn, L.T., Corrigan, J.M., & Donaldson, M.S. (eds.). Washington, DC: National Academy Press.

Institute of Medicine. (2001). *Crossing the quality chasm: A new health system for the 21st century.* Washington, DC: National Academy Press.

Institute of Medicine. (2003a). *Health professions education: A bridge to quality.* Washington, DC: National Academy Press.

Institute of Medicine. (2003b). *Priority areas for national actions: Transforming health care quality. Quality Chasm Series.* Washington, DC: National Academies Press.

Institute of Medicine. (2004). *Keeping patients safe: Transforming the work environment for nurses.* Washington, DC: National Academy Press.

Institute of Medicine. (2006). *Crossing the quality chasm: The IOM quality health care initiative.* Retrieved August 8, 2008, from www.iom.edu/CMS/8089.aspx

Institute of Medicine. (2011). *The future of nursing: Leading change, advancing health.* Washington: DC: National Academies Press.

Irvine, D. (1998). Finding value in nursing care: A framework for quality improvement and clinical evaluation. *Nursing Economics, 16*(3), 110–118.

Jackson, S.E. (2006). The influence of managed care on U.S. baccalaureate nursing education programs. *Journal of Nursing Education, 45*(2), 67–74.

Joint Commission. (2010). Retrieved February 3, 2014, from www.jointcommission.org/quality_improvement_tools.aspx

Joint Commission. (2008). Sentinel event. Retrieved October 2, 2013, from www.jointcommission.org/SentinelEvents/

Joint Commission on Accreditation of Healthcare Organizations (JCAHO). (2005). Retrieved November 26, 2005, from http://jcpatientsafety.org

Kaiser Family Foundation. (2005). Trends and indicators in the changing health care marketplace. Retrieved June 14, 2008, from www.kff.org/insurance/7031/index.cfm

Kalisch, B., Landstrom, G., & Williams, R.A. (2009). Missed nursing care: Errors of omission, *Nursing Outlook, 57*(1), 3–9.

Kersbergen, A.L. (2000). Managed care shifts health care from an altruistic model to a business framework. *Nursing & Health Care Perspectives, 21*(2), 81–83.

Kirk, M. (2002). The impact of globalization and environmental change on health: Challenges for nurse education. *Nurse Education Today, 22*(1), 60–71.

Lantham, B., & Maxson-Cooper, P. (2003). Is six sigma the answer for nursing to reduce medical errors and enhance patient safety? *Nursing Economics, 21*(1).

Lea, D.H., Skirton, H., Read, C.Y., & Williams, J.K. (2011). Implications for educating the next generation of nurses on genetics and genomics in the 21st century. *Journal of Nursing Scholarship, 43*(4), 3–12.

Leape, L.L., Bates, D.W., & Petrycki, S. (1993). Incidence and preventability of adverse drug events in hospitalized adults. *Journal of Internal Medicine, 8,* 289–294.

Leapfrog Group. (2007). About us. Retrieved August 20, 2008, from www.leapfroggroup.org/about_us

Leapfrog Group. (2011). About us. Retrieved December 7, 2013, from www.leapfroggroup.org/about_us

Lichtig, L.K., Knauf, R.A., & Milholland, D.K. (1999). Some impacts of nursing on acute care hospital outcomes. *Journal of Nursing Administration, 29*(2), 25–33.

Mardon, R.E., Khanna, K., Sorra J., Dyer, N., & Famolaro, T. (2010). Exploring relationships between hospital patient safety culture and adverse event. *Journal of Patient Safety, 6*(4). 226–232.

McLaughlin, C., & Kaluzny, A. (2006). *Continuous quality improvement in health care: theory, implementations, and applications,* 3rd ed. Sudbury, MA: Jones and Bartlett.

Menix, K.D. (2000). Educating to manage the accelerated change environment effectively: Part 1. *Journal for Nurses in Staff Development, 16*(6), 282–288.

Milton, C.L. (2011). An ethical exploration of quality and safety initiatives in nurse practice. *Nursing Science Quality, 24*(2), 107–110.

Nightingale, F., & Barnum, B.S. (1992). *Notes on nursing: What it is, and what it is not,* commemorative ed. Philadelphia: Lippincott-Raven.

Oliver, D., Healey, F., & Haines, T.P. (2010). Preventing falls and fall-related injuries in hospitals. *Clinical Geriatric Medicine, 26*(4), 645–692.

O'Neill, E.H., & Pew Health Professions Commission. (1998). *Recreating health professional practice for a new century.* San Francisco: Pew Health Professions Commission.

Orsolini-Hain, L.M. (2008). *An interpretive phenomenological study on the influences on associate Degree Prepared Nurses to Return to School to Earn a higher degree in nursing.* San Francisco: University of California, San Francisco.

Patient-Centered Outcomes Research Institute (PCORI). (2012). Improving health care systems. Retrieved October 4, 2013, from www.pcori.org/assets/PFA-Improving-Healthcare-Systems-05222012.pdf

PEW Health Commission. (1998). Fourth report of the Pew health professions commission. Retrieved February 3, 2014, from http://Fourth_report_of_the_Pew_Health_Professi.htm

Pham, J.C., Aswani, M.S., Rosen, M., Lee, H.W., Huddle, M., Weeks, K., & Pronovost, P.J. (2012). Reducing medical errors and adverse events. *Annual Review of Medicine, 63,* 447–463. Retrieved October 5, 2013, from www.annualreviews.org

Plan to reduce racial and ethnic health disparities. Retrieved October 5, 2013, from minorityhealth.hhs.gov/npa/files/Plans/HHS/HHS_Plan_complete.pdf.

Poon, E.G., Keohane, C.A., Yoon, C.S., Ditmore, M., Bane, A., Levtzion-Korach, O., & Moniz, T. (2010). Effect of bar-code technology on the safety and medication administration. *The New England Journal of Medicine, 362*(18), 1698–1707.

Raduma-Tomas, M.A., Flin, R., Yule, S.J., & Close, S. (2012). The importance of preparation for doctors' handovers in an acute medical assessment unit: A hierarchal task analysis. *Quality and Safety in Health Care, 21,* 211–217.

Raduma-Tomas, M.A., Flin, R., Yule, S.J., & Williams, D. (2011). Doctors' handovers in hospitals: A literature review. *Quality and safety in health care, 20,* 128–133.

Robert Wood Johnson Foundation. (2008). About us. Retrieved August 20, 2008, from www.rwjf.org/about/

Robert Wood Johnson Foundation (2011). Nurses are key to improving patient safety. Retrieved from http://www.rwjf.org/en/about-rwjf/newsroom/newsroom-content/2011/04/nurses-are-key-to-improving-patient-safety.html

Rogers, A.E., Hwang, W., Scott, L.D., Aiken, L.H., et al. (2004). The working hours of hospital staff nurses and patient safety: Both errors and near errors are more likely to occur when hospital staff nurses work twelve or more hours at a stretch. *Health Affairs, 23*(4), 202–212.

Rotter, T., Kinsman, L., James, E.L., Machotta, A., Gothe, H., Willis, J., Snow, P., & Kugler, J. (2010). Clinical pathways: Effects on professional practice, patient outcomes, length of stay and hospital costs. *The Cochrane Library, 7.* Retrieved October 2, 2013, from http://thecochranelibrary.com

Sargeant, J., Loney, E., and Murphy, G. (2008) Effective interprofessional teams. *Journal of Continuing Education in the Health Professions, 28*(4), 228–234.

Schroeder, P., ed. *Monitoring and Evaluation in Nursing.* Gaithersburg, MD: Aspen.

Shekelle, P.G. (2013). Nurse–patient ratios as a patient safety strategy: A systematic review. *Annals of Internal Medicine, 158*(5), 404–409.

Strickland, O. (1997). Challenges in measuring patient outcomes. *Nursing Clinics of North America, 32,* 495–512.

Swansburg, R., & Swansburg, R. (2002). *Introduction to management and leadership for nurse managers,* 3rd ed. Boston: Jones and Bartlett.

Trossman, S. (2006). Issues update. It's in the genes: The ANA and nurse leaders want RNs and students to practice with genetics and genomics in mind. *American Journal of Nursing, 106*(2), 74–75.

U.S. Department of Health and Human Services. (2008). About HHS. Retrieved August 20, 2008, from www.hhs.gov/

U.S. Department of Health and Human Services (HHS). (2011). http://www.hhs.gov/

Weiss, M.E., Yakusheva, O., & Bobay, K.L. (2011). Quality and cost analysis of nurse staffing, discharge preparation and postdischarge utilization. *Health Service Research, 46*(5), 1–22.

Whitehead, D.K., Weiss, S.A., & Tappen, R.M. (2010). *Essentials of nursing leadership and management,* 5th ed. Philadelphia: F.A. Davis.

World Health Organization (WHO). (2009). "World health statistics 2009." Retrieved October 4, 2013, from www.who.itl

Chapter 11

Promoting a Healthy Work Environment

OBJECTIVES

After reading this chapter, the student should be able to:

- Recognize threats to safety in the workplace.
- Identify agencies responsible for overseeing workplace safety.
- Describe methods for dealing with violence in the workplace.
- Identify the role of the nurse in dealing with catastrophes including terrorism threats.
- Recognize situations that may reflect sexual harassment.
- Make suggestions for improving the physical and social work environment.
- Identify signs and symptoms of stress, reality shock, and burnout.
- Describe the impact of stress, reality shock, and burnout on the individual and the health-care team.
- Discuss the factors that affect job satisfaction.
- Develop strategies to manage personal and professional stresses.

OUTLINE

Almost half of our waking hours are spent in the workplace. Yet, the quality of the workplace environment is neglected to a surprising extent in many health-care organizations. It is neglected by administrators who would never allow peeling paint or poorly maintained equipment but who leave their staff, their most costly and valuable resource, unmaintained and unrefreshed. The current "do more with less" attitude places additional pressure on staff and management alike (Chisholm, 1992).

Many nurses are still struggling to achieve healthy environments where they work (Bylone, 2011).

Much of the responsibility for enhancing the workplace rests with the people who have the authority and resources to encourage organization-wide improvements. Nurses, however, have begun to take more responsibility for identifying workplace issues and advocating improvement. This chapter focuses on these many issues.

Workplace Safety

Threats to Safety

A health-care facility may be one of the most dangerous work environments in the United States. Health and safety threats include infectious diseases, physical violence, ergonomic injuries related to the movement and repositioning of patients, exposure to hazardous chemicals and radiation, and sharps injuries (ANA, 2007). Consider the following two examples:

In spring 2001, a Florida nurse with 20 years' psychiatric nursing experience died of head and face trauma. Her assailant, a former wrestler, had been admitted involuntarily in the early morning to the private mental health-care facility. An investigation found that the facility did not have procedures for handling workplace violence and no method of summoning help in an emergency (Arbury, 2002).

Somewhere between 600,000 and 1,000,000 needlestick injuries occur annually in the United States. Why is this a concern? Percutaneous exposure is the principal route for human immunodeficiency virus (HIV) infection as well as hepatitis B and C and other blood-borne pathogens.

The American Nurses Association (ANA) surveyed 4,614 nurses to learn about their primary concerns related to workplace safety. Their top concerns were stress and overwork (74%) and ergonomic injury (62%). An encouraging finding was that more nurses reported the availability of devices for patient transfers and for reducing sharps injuries, fewer assaults, and less illness due to work environment (ANA, 2012). When surveyed about factors considered essential to a healthy workplace environment, employees listed collaborative work relationships, good communication, empowerment, recognition, opportunities for growth, effective leadership, adequate staffing, and workplace safety (Lindberg &Vingard, 2012).

Threats to safety in the workplace vary from one setting to another and from one individual to another. A pregnant staff member may be more vulnerable to risks from radiation; staff members working in the emergency room are at more risk for HIV and tuberculosis exposure than are the staff in the newborn nursery. All staff members have the right to be made aware of potential risks and be provided with as much protection as possible. No worker should feel uncomfortable or unsafe in the workplace.

Addressing Threats to Safety

The modern movement for safety in the workplace began near the end of the Industrial Revolution. The National Council for Industrial Safety (now the National Safety Council) was formed in 1913. The Occupational Safety and Health Act of 1970 created both the National Institute of Occupational Safety and Health (NIOSH) and the Occupational Safety and Health Administration (OSHA). OSHA, part of the U.S. Department of Labor, is responsible for developing and enforcing workplace safety and health regulations. NIOSH, part of the U.S. Department of Health and Human Services, supports research, education, and training. The National Safety Council (NSC) partners with OSHA to provide training. The NSC maintains that safety in the workplace is the responsibility of both the employer and the employee. The employer must ensure a safe, healthful work environment, and employees are accountable for knowing and following safety guidelines and standards (National Safety Council, 1992). The journey to "world-class safety," says the NSC, is a process of continuous assessment and improvement (National Safety Council, 2013).

OSHA

The goal of OSHA is to prevent injuries and illness and save the lives of employees across the United States (OSHA, 2013a). Employers must comply with OSHA regulations for providing a safe, healthful work environment. They are also required to keep records of all occupational (job-related) illnesses and accidents such as chemical exposures, lacerations, hearing loss, respiratory exposure, musculoskeletal injuries, and exposure to infectious diseases. Workplace inspections may be conducted with or without prior notification to the employer. Catastrophic or fatal accidents and employee complaints may trigger an OSHA inspection. OSHA encourages employers and employees to work together to identify and remove workplace hazards before contacting OSHA. If the employer has not been able to resolve the safety or health issue, however, the employee may file a formal complaint, and an inspection will be ordered (U.S. Department of Labor, 1995). Any violations found are posted where all employees can view them. The employer has the right to contest the OSHA decision. The law also states that the employer cannot punish or discriminate against employees for exercising their rights related to job safety and health hazards or participating in OSHA inspections (U.S. Department of Labor, 1995).

OSHA inspections of health-care facilities have focused especially on blood-borne pathogens, lifting and ergonomic (proper body alignment) guidelines, confined-space regulations, respiratory guidelines, and workplace violence. OSHA added protecting the work site against terrorism after the September 11, 2001 attacks (www.osha.gov).

Centers for Disease Control and Prevention (CDC)

The CDC partners with other agencies to investigate health problems, conduct research, implement prevention strategies, and promote safe and healthy environments. CDC publishes continuous updates of recommendations for prevention of HIV transmission in the workplace and universal precautions related to blood-borne pathogens and other infectious diseases. CDC also targets public health emergency preparedness and response related to biological and chemical agents and threats (CDC, 1992; www.cdc.gov/). CDC recommendations can be found in the Mortality and Morbidity Weekly Report (MMWR), on the Internet (www.cdc.gov/health/diseases), or at its toll-free phone number (800-311-3435).

American Nurses Association (ANA)

The ANA Web site (www.nursingworld.org) provides up-to-date information related to workplace advocacy and safety for all nurses. In 1999, ANA established its Commission on Workplace Advocacy, which addresses issues such as collective bargaining, workplace violence, mandatory overtime, staffing ratios, conflict management, delegation, ethical issues, compensation, needlestick safety, latex allergies, pollution prevention, and ergonomics.

The Joint Commission

To maintain Joint Commission (JC) accreditation, organizations must have an extensive on-site review, including workplace safety, by a team of JC health-care professionals at least once every 3 years.

Institute of Medicine (IOM)

The Institute of Medicine (IOM) is a private, non-governmental organization whose mission is to improve the health of people everywhere; thus, the topics it studies are very broad (www.iom.edu). In 1996 the IOM began a quality initiative to assess the nation's health-care system. One result was the 2004 report, "Keeping Patients Safe: Transforming the Work Environment of Nurses." The report identified concerns related to organizational management, workforce deployment practices, work design, and organizational culture (Beyea, 2004). Box 11-1 lists the most important federal laws enacted to protect individuals in the workplace.

Developing Workplace Safety Programs

Workplace safety programs should protect staff members from harm and the organization from any liability that could result.

1. The first step in development of a workplace safety program is to *recognize a potential hazard.* OSHA (U.S. Department of Labor, 1995) requires employers to inform employees of any potential health hazards and provide as much protection from these hazards as possible. In many cases, initial warnings come from the CDC, NIOSH, and other federal, state, and local agencies. For example, employers must provide tuberculosis testing and hepatitis B vaccine; protective equipment such as gloves, gowns, and masks; and immediate treatment after exposure for all staff members who may have contact with blood-borne pathogens. They are expected to remove hazards, educate employees, and establish institution-wide policies and procedures to protect their employees (Herring, 1994; Roche, 1993). If not provided with protective gloves, for example, employees may refuse to participate in any activities involving blood or blood products. Reasonable accommodations must also be made. For example, a nurse with latex allergies may be placed in an area such as patient

---

box 11-1

Federal Laws Enacted to Protect the Worker in the Workplace

- **Equal Pay Act of 1963:** Employers must provide equal pay for equal work, regardless of gender.
- **Title VII of Civil Rights Act of 1964:** Employees may not be discriminated against on the basis of race, color, religion, sex, or national origin.
- **Age Discrimination in Employment Act of 1967:** Private and public employers may not discriminate against persons 40 years of age or older except when a certain age group is a bona fide occupational qualification.
- **Pregnancy Discrimination Act of 1968:** Pregnant women cannot be discriminated against in employment benefits if they are able to perform job responsibilities.
- **Fair Credit Reporting Act of 1970:** Job applicants and employees have the right to know of the existence and content of any credit files maintained on them.
- **Vocational Rehabilitation Act of 1973:** An employer receiving financial assistance from the federal government may not discriminate against individuals with disabilities and must develop affirmative action plans to hire and promote individuals with disabilities.
- **Family Education Rights and Privacy Act—Buckley Amendment of 1974:** Educational institutions may not supply information about students without their consent.
- **Immigration Reform and Control Act of 1986:** Employers must screen employees for the right to work in the United States without discriminating on the basis of national origin.
- **Americans with Disabilities Act of 1990:** Persons with physical or mental disabilities or who are chronically ill cannot be discriminated against in the workplace. Employers must make "reasonable accommodations" to meet the needs of the disabled employee. These include such provisions as installing foot or hand controls; readjusting light switches, telephones, desks, tables, and computer equipment; providing access ramps and elevators; offering flexible work hours; and providing readers for blind employees.
- **Family Medical Leave Act of 1993:** Employers with 50 or more employees must provide up to 13 weeks of unpaid leave for family medical emergencies, childbirth, or adoption.
- **Needlestick Safety and Prevention Act of 2001:** This act directed OSHA to revise the blood-borne pathogens standard to establish in greater detail requirements that employers identify and make use of effective and safer medical devices.
- **Lilly Ledbetter Fair Pay Act of 2009:** This act supports fair pay and provides protection against discrimination in compensation based upon race, color, religion, sex, or national origin.

Adapted from Strader, M., & Decker, P. (1995). *Role transition to patient care management.* Norwalk, CT: Appleton and Lange; osha.gov/needlesticks/needlefact; Lilly Ledbetter Fair Pay Act of 2009, S.181, 123 Stat. 5 and General Industry Regulations Book, Subpart Z Occupational Safety and Health Standards, Title 29 *Code of Federal Regulations*, Part 1910.

---

education where exposure to blood-borne pathogens is unlikely (Strader & Decker, 1995; U.S. Department of Labor, 1995).

2. The second step in a workplace safety program is a *thorough assessment of the amount of risk entailed.* For example:

Nancy Wu is the nurse manager on a busy geriatric unit. Most patients require total care: bathing, feeding, and positioning. She observed that several of the staff members working on the unit use poor body mechanics when lifting and moving the patients. In the last month, several went to Employee Health complaining of back pain. This week, she noticed that the patients seemed to remain in the same position for long periods and were rarely out of bed or left in a chair for the entire day. When she confronted the staff, the response was the same from all of them: "I have to work for a living. I can't afford to risk a back injury for someone who may not live past the end of the week." Nancy was concerned about the care of the patients as well as the apparent lack of information her staff had about prevention of back injuries. She decided to

seek assistance from the nurse practitioner in Employee Health to develop a back injury prevention program.

Assessment of the workplace may require considerable data gathering. Formal committees are often formed to assess these risks. Staff from various levels and departments should be included.

3. The third step is to *create a plan* to provide optimal protection for staff members without interfering with the provision of quality patient care. For example, some devices that are worn to prevent transmission of tuberculosis interfere with communication with the patient. Some attempts have been made to limit visits or withdraw home health-care nurses from high-crime areas, but this leaves homebound patients without care (Nadwairski, 1992). These are not acceptable solutions. Developing a safety plan includes the following:
   - Distinguish real from imagined risks
   - Consult federal, state, and local regulations and experts on work safety

- Seek evidence-based practices related to the problem
- Develop a plan to reduce risks
- Calculate the costs of the program/plan
- Seek administrative support for the plan

4. The fourth and final stage in developing a workplace safety program is *implementing the plan.* Educating the staff, providing the necessary safety supplies and equipment, and modifying the environment may be necessary.

Violence

Workplace violence includes physical assault, threats of assault, and verbal abuse. Nurses' frequent and close contact with individuals in distress makes them a potential target (Magnavita & Heponiemi, 2011). The overall private sector rate for assault resulting in injury is 2 per 10,000 full-time workers; compare this to the rate for health service workers at 9.3. The incidence rate for social service workers is 15, and the rate for nurses and personal care workers is 25 per 10,000 (www.bls.gov/news.release/archives/osh2_02242010.pdf). Most of the incidents involve patients (McPhaul & Lipscomb, 2004). Some of the circumstances surrounding health-care work contribute to workers' susceptibility (Edwards, 1999; www.nursingworld.org/dlwa/osh/wp5; www.cdc.gov/niosh/pdfs/2002-101.pdf; www.osha.gov/) in the following:

- Units for treating violent individuals
- Patients needing seclusion or restraint
- Increased numbers of acute and chronic mentally ill patients being released without effective follow-up
- Working late or until very early morning hours
- Working in high-crime areas
- Working in buildings with poor security
- Treating weapons-carrying patients and families
- Inexperienced staff who have not been trained to manage crises or handle volatile situations
- Long wait times for service
- Overcrowded, uncomfortable waiting areas

To assess the risk of violence, nurses must know their workplace. Ask the following:

- How frequently do assaultive incidents, threats, and verbal abuse occur in your facility? Where? Who is involved? Are incidents reported?

- Are current emergency response systems effective?
- Are staffing patterns sufficient? Is the staff experienced in handling these situations (http://www.nursingworld.org/MainMenu Categories/ANAMarketplace/ANAPeriodicals/OJIN/TableofContents/Vol-18-2013/No1-Jan-2013/Measurement-and-Monitoring-Worker-Aggression-Exposure.html)?
- Are post-assaultive treatment and support available to staff?

Although assaults that result in severe injury or death usually receive media coverage, most assaults on nurses by patients or coworkers are not even reported by the nurse. For example:

Robert Jones works on the evening shift in the emergency department (ED) at a large urban hospital that frequently receives victims of gunshot wounds, stabbings, and other gang-related incidents. Many are high on alcohol or drugs. Robert has just interviewed a 21-year-old male patient awaiting treatment for injuries resulting from a fight after an evening of heavy drinking. Because his injuries have been determined not to be life-threatening, he had to wait to see a physician. "I'm tired of waiting. Let's get this show on the road," he screamed as Robert walked by. "I'm sorry you have to wait, Mr. P., but the doctor is busy with another patient and will get to you as soon as possible." He handed him a cup of juice he had been bringing to another patient. The patient grabbed the cup, threw it in Robert's face, and then grabbed his arm. Slamming him against the wall, the patient jumped off the stretcher and yelled obscenities at him. He continued to scream until a security guard intervened.

Be aware of clues that may indicate a potential for violence (Box 11-2). These behaviors may occur in patients, family members, visitors, or even other staff members.

Not only are episodes of violence underreported, there are persistent misperceptions that assaults are part of the job and that the victim somehow caused the assault. Underreporting may also be due to a lack of institutional reporting policies or employee fear that the assault was a result of negligence or poor job performance (U.S. Department of Labor, 1995). Box 11-3 lists some of the faulty reasoning that leads to placing blame on the victim of the assault.

Behaviors Indicating a Potential for Violence

- History of violent behavior
- Delusional, paranoid, or suspicious speech
- Aggressive, threatening statements
- Rapid speech, angry tone of voice
- Pacing, tense posture, clenched fists, tightening jaw
- Alcohol or drug use
- Policies that set unrealistic limits

Adapted from Kinkle, S. (1993). Violence in the ED: How to stop it before it starts. American Journal of Nursing, 93(7), 22–24; Carroll, C., & Sheverbush, J. (September 1996). Violence assessment in hospitals provides basis for action. The American Nurse, 18.

Actions to address violence in the workplace include (1) identifying the factors that contribute to violence and controlling as many as possible, and (2) preparing staff to prevent and manage violence (Carroll & Sheverbush, 1996; Collins, 1994; Mahoney, 1991).

Preventing Violent Behavior

Preventing an incident is better than having to intervene after violence has occurred. The following are suggestions to nurses about how to participate in workplace safety related to prevention of violence (www.nursingworld.org/osh/wp5/htm):

- *Participate in or initiate regular workplace assessments.* Identify unsafe areas and factors within the organization that contribute to assaultive behavior, such as inadequate staffing, high-activity times of day, invasion of personal space, seclusion or restraint activities, and lack

of experienced staff. Work with management to make and monitor changes.

- *Be alert for behaviors that precede violence* such as verbal expressions of anger and frustration, threatening body language, signs of drug or alcohol use, or presence of a weapon. Evaluate each situation for potential violence. Have an exit strategy.
- *Know your patients.* Be aware of any history of violent behaviors, diagnoses suggesting potential for violent behavior, and alcohol or drug intoxication.
- *Maintain behavior that helps to defuse anger.* Present a calm, caring attitude. Do not match threats, give orders, or present with behaviors that may be interpreted as aggressive. Acknowledge the person's feelings.
- *If you cannot defuse the situation,* then remove yourself from it quickly, call security, and report the situation to management.

Box 11-4 lists some additional actions that can be taken to protect staff members and patients from violence in the workplace.

If Violent Behavior Occurs

What if, in spite of all precautions, violence occurs? What should you do? You should:

- Report to your supervisor. Report threats as well as actual violence. Include a description of the situation, names of victims, witnesses, and perpetrators, and any other pertinent information.

When an Assault Occurs: Placing Blame on Victims

- **Victim gender:** Women receive more blame than men.
- **Subject gender:** Female victims receive more blame from women than from men.
- **Severity:** The more severe the assault, the more often the victim is blamed.
- **Beliefs:** The world is a just place, and therefore the person deserves the misfortune.
- **Age of victim:** The older the victim, the more he or she is held to blame.

Adapted from Lanza, M.L., & Carifio, J. (1991). Blaming the victim: Complex (nonlinear) patterns of causal attribution by nurses in response to vignettes of a patient assaulting a nurse. Journal of Emergency Nursing, 17(5), 299–309.

Steps Toward Increasing Protection From Workplace Violence

- Security personnel and escorts
- Panic buttons in medication rooms, stairwells, activity rooms, and nursing stations
- Bulletproof glass in reception, triage, and admitting areas
- Locked or key-coded access doors
- Closed-circuit television
- Metal detectors
- Use of beepers and/or cellular phones
- Handheld alarms or noise devices
- Lighted parking lots
- Escort or buddy system
- Enforce wearing of photo identification badges

Adapted from Simonowitz, J. (1994). Violence in the workplace: You're entitled to protection. RN, 57(11), 61–63; nursingworld.org/dlwa/osh/wp6.

- Call security. Nurses are entitled to the same protections as anyone else who has been assaulted.
- Get medical attention. This includes medical care, counseling, and evaluation.
- Contact your collective bargaining unit, your state nurses association, or OSHA if the problems persist.
- Be proactive. Get involved in policy making (Gilmore-Hall, 2001; www.nursingcenter.com).

Horizontal Violence

Horizontal violence among employees may also occur. Although very disturbing, it rarely leads to physical violence. Also called *incivility* or *bullying,* it may include verbal abuse, punishment, humiliating comments, and malicious gossip. Bullies in the workplace may be coworkers, superiors, or subordinates. Regardless of their place on the organizational chart, they can cause a great deal of distress to others in the workplace. In fact, The Joint Commission characterizes horizontal violence as a sentinel event because it may pose a threat to patient safety (Kear, 2012). In a sample of 2,659 RNs from 19 facilities in New York state, 22% reported they were expected to do other's work, 9% had been reprimanded in front of others, 9.8% reported attempts to destroy their credibility, 9.2% reported being constantly criticized, and 6% had been threatened with negative consequences (Sellers & Millenbach, 2012).

A study of new graduates in Canada found that the majority had noted at least some incivility in their workplace, more from their coworkers than their supervisors (Smith, Andrusyszyn, & Spence-Laschinger, 2010). Nursing managers in Canada have noted an increase in the reporting of horizontal violence as staff has become more aware of their rights and protections as employees (Rocker, 2012). Although lower in intensity than physical violence, the long-term effects of incivility are far from benign and need to be addressed. The following are a few ways in which these behaviors can be addressed (Kear, 2012; Lewis & Malecha, 2011):

- Establish a zero tolerance policy for these behaviors
- Develop a code of conduct
- Administrators, supervisors, and managers can model appropriate behavior

- Discuss strategies for handling such behavior in staff meetings
- Report bullying behavior to your nurse manager
- Confront bullying and belittling behavior, and express your concerns objectively

Kear (2012) provides an objective response to this behavior: "When you call me incompetent, I feel angry. Instead, I would like you to teach me what I may not know ..." (p. 1). It requires courage to confront these behaviors directly but failing to do so encourages them.

Sexual Harassment

After months of interviewing, a new supervisor was hired, a young male nurse whom the staff members jokingly described as "a blond Tom Cruise." The new supervisor was an instant hit with the predominantly female executives and staff members. However, he soon found himself on the receiving end of sexual jokes and innuendoes. He had been trying to prove himself a competent supervisor, with hopes of eventually moving up to a higher management position. He viewed the behavior of the female staff members and supervisors as undermining his credibility, as well as being embarrassing and annoying. He attempted to have the unwelcome conduct stopped by discussing it with his boss, a female nurse administrator. She told him jokingly that it was nothing more than "good-natured fun" and besides, "men can't be harassed by women" (Outwater, 1994).

Sexual harassment is a persistent problem in the workplace. The reasons are complex, but sex-role stereotypes and the unequal balance of power between men and women are major contributors. Unfortunately, underreporting of this problem is common, even though the emotional costs of anger, humiliation, and fear are high (www.nursingworld.org/dlwa/wpr/wp3/htm).

The EEOC issued a statement in 1980 that sexual harassment is prohibited by Title VII of the Civil Rights Act of 1964. Two forms are identified, both based on the premise that the action is unwelcome sexual conduct:

1. **Quid pro quo.** Sexual favors are solicited in exchange for favorable job benefits or

continuation of employment. The employee must demonstrate that he or she was required to endure unwelcome sexual advances to keep the job or job benefits and that rejection of these behaviors would have resulted in deprivation of a job or benefits. Example: An administrator approaches a nurse for a date in exchange for the promise of a promotion.

2. **Hostile environment.** This is the most common sexual harassment claim and the most difficult to prove. The employee making the claim must prove that the harassment is based on gender and that it has affected conditions of employment or created an environment so offensive that the employee could not effectively discharge the responsibilities of the job (Outwater, 1994). If an environment can be shown to be hostile or abusive, there is no further need to establish that it was also psychologically injurious. Although sexual harassment against women is more common, men can be victims as well (Box 11-5).

Do not ignore the issue of sexual harassment in the workplace. If you supervise other employees, review your agency's policies and procedures and seek appropriate guidance from Human Resources if needed. If an employee approaches you with a complaint, a confidential investigation of the charges has to be initiated. Do not dismiss any incidents or charges of sexual harassment involving yourself or others as "just having fun" or respond that "there is nothing anyone can do." Responses such as this can have serious consequences in the workplace (Outwater, 1994).

The ANA cites four tactics to fight sexual harassment (www.nursingworld.org/dlwa/wpr/wp3/htm):

---

box 11-5

Behaviors That Could Be Defined as Sexual Harassment

- Pressure to participate in sexual activities
- Asking about another person's sexual activities, fantasies, preferences
- Making sexual innuendoes, jokes, comments, showing sexual graffiti or visuals
- Continuing to ask for a date after the other person has expressed disinterest
- Making suggestive facial expressions or gestures with hands or body movements
- Making remarks about a person's gender or body

---

1. **Confront.** Indicate immediately and clearly to the harasser that the attention is unwanted. If you are in a unionized facility, ask the nursing representative to accompany you.
2. **Report.** Report the incident immediately to your supervisor. If the harasser is your supervisor, report the incident to a higher authority and file a formal complaint.
3. **Document.** Document the incident immediately while it is fresh in your mind—what happened, when and where it occurred, and how you responded. Name any witnesses. Keep thorough records in a safe place away from work.
4. **Support.** Seek support from friends, relatives, and organizations such as your state nurses association. If you are a student, seek support from a trusted faculty member or advisor. Your employer has a responsibility to maintain a harassment-free workplace. You should expect your employer to demonstrate commitment to creating a harassment-free workplace, provide strong written policies prohibiting sexual harassment and describing how employees will be protected, and educate all employees verbally and in writing.

Discrimination

The laws that prohibit discrimination in the workplace are based on the Fifth and Fourteenth Amendments to the Constitution, mandating due process and equal protection under the law. The federal Equal Employment Opportunity Commission (EEOC) oversees the administration and enforcement of issues related to workplace equality. Although there may be exemptions from any law, it is important that nurses recognize that there is significant legislation that prohibits employers from making workplace decisions based on race, color, sex, age, disability, religion, or national origin. The employer may ask questions related to these issues but cannot make decisions about employment based on them.

Latex Allergy

Since the 1987 recommendations for universal precautions from the CDC, the use of gloves has greatly increased exposure of health-care workers to natural rubber latex (NRL). The two major routes of exposure to NRL are skin and inhalation, particularly when glove powder acts as a carrier for NRL protein (OSHA latex alert: www.cdc.gov/niosh/latexalt). Reactions range from contact dermatitis with scaling, drying, cracking, and blistering skin, to generalized urticaria, rhinitis, wheezing, swelling, shortness of breath, and anaphylaxis.

Allergic contact dermatitis (sometimes called *chemical sensitivity dermatitis*) results from the chemicals added to latex during harvesting, processing, or manufacturing. These chemicals can cause a skin rash similar to that of poison ivy (www.cdc.gov/niosh/docs/98-113/).

Latex allergy should be suspected if an employee develops symptoms after latex exposures. A complete medical history can reveal latex sensitivity, and blood tests approved by the U.S. Food and Drug Administration are available to detect latex antibodies. Skin testing and glove-use tests are also available.

A midwife began experiencing hives, nasal congestion, and conjunctivitis. Within a year, she developed asthma, and 2 years later she went into shock after a routine gynecological examination during which latex gloves were used. The midwife also suffered respiratory distress in latex-containing environments when she had no direct contact with latex products. She was unable to continue working (Bauer et al., 1993).

A physician with a history of seasonal allergies, runny nose, and eczema on his hands suffered severe rhinitis, shortness of breath, and then collapsed minutes after putting on a pair of latex gloves. A cardiac arrest team successfully resuscitated him (Rosen, Isaacson, Brady, & Corey, 1993).

Complete latex avoidance is the most effective approach. Medications may reduce allergic symptoms, and special precautions are needed to prevent exposure during medical and dental care. Employees with a latex allergy should consider wearing a medical alert bracelet.

Many employees in a health-care setting can use alternative gloves of vinyl or nitrile. If an employee must use NRL gloves, gloves with lower protein content and those that are powder-free should be considered. Good housekeeping practices should be used to remove latex-containing dust from the workplace. Those with histories of allergies to pollens, grasses, and certain foods or plants (avocado, banana, kiwi, chestnut) and histories of multiple surgeries may be at greater risk.

The following will help to decrease the potential for latex allergy problems (www.cdc.gov/niosh/docs/98-113/):

- Evaluate any cases of hand dermatitis or other signs of latex allergy.
- Use latex-free procedure trays and crash carts.
- Use nonlatex gloves for activities that do not involve contact with infectious materials.
- Avoid using oil-based creams or lotions, which can cause glove deterioration.
- Seek ongoing training and the latest information related to latex allergy.
- Wash, rinse, and dry hands thoroughly after removing gloves or when changing gloves.
- Use powder-free gloves.

If you develop a latex allergy, be aware of the following precautions (www.cdc.gov/niosh/docs/98-113/):

- Avoid all types of latex exposure.
- Wear a medical alert bracelet.
- Carry an EpiPen with auto-injectable epinephrine.
- Alert your employer and colleagues to your latex sensitivity.
- Carry nonlatex gloves.

The number of new cases of latex allergy has decreased due to improved diagnostic methods, improved education, more accurate labeling, and use of powder-free gloves. Although current research does not demonstrate whether the amount of allergen released during shipping and storage of medications from vials with rubber closures is sufficient to induce a systemic allergic reaction, nurses should take special precautions when patients are identified as high risk for latex allergies. Nursing staff should work closely with the pharmacy staff to follow universal one-stick-rule precautions, which assumes that every pharmaceutical vial may contain a natural rubber latex closure, and the nurse should remain with any patient at the start of medication administration and keep frequent observations and vital signs for 2 hours (Hamilton et al., 2005).

Needlestick (Sharps) Injuries

In 1997 a 27-year-old nurse, Lisa Black, attended an in-service session on post-exposure prophylaxis for needlesticks. A short time later, she was attempting to aspirate blood from a patient's intra-venous line when the patient moved, and the needle went into Lisa's hand. Nine months later she tested positive for HIV and 3 months after that for hepa-titis C (Trossman, 1999a).

There are several legal sources of protection from sharps injuries. The Needlestick Safety and Pre-vention Act went into effect April 18, 2001. The revised OSHA Blood Borne Pathogens Stan-dard obligates employers to consider safer needle devices when they conduct their annual review (Foley, 2012). JC surveyors routinely ask if health-care organization leaders are familiar with the Needlestick Safety and Prevention Act and what action has been taken to comply (www.osha.gov/needlesticks/needlefaq.html; jointcommission.org/sentinel_event_alert_issue_22_preventing_needlestick_and_sharps_injuries/).Althoughmuch progress has been made in preventing sharps injuries, a recent consensus statement from ANA and other groups calls for more attention to (Daley, 2012):

■ Greater safety in surgical settings
■ Sharps safety outside the hospital
■ Including nurses in selection of safety devices
■ Encouraging product design and development to fill existing gaps (e.g., in dentistry, use of longer needles)
■ Increased staff training

Your Employer's Responsibility

All health-care facilities should have a written plan to prevent sharps injuries that is updated annually. Staff should receive annual training during work hours and have a right to be involved in the selec-tion of safety devices. Additional control measures include (Foley, 2012):

■ The employee must be evaluated and treated within 2 hours of a sharps injury, including free hepatitis B vaccine.
■ Safety and efficacy of sharps purchased must be evaluated.
■ Recapping of needles and related practices should be prohibited.
■ Contaminated work surfaces must be cleaned according to established guidelines.
■ Employers must provide personal protective equipment of good quality, including gloves, gowns, and masks in all needed sizes.

The surgical setting presents special challenges to prevention of sharps injuries due to such factors as the intense pressures of the situation, open wounds susceptible to contamination, and extensive use of sharp instruments. Thirty percent of sharps injuries occur here, and the encouraging decline in injuries seen in other areas of the hospital has not yet been seen in the surgical setting. Some recommenda-tions for addressing this risk include (Guglielmi & Ogg, 2012):

■ Use blunt tip suture needles where possible.
■ Use safety scalpels, either sheathed or retractable.
■ Initiate the hands-free technique (HFT) or neutral passing zone (a container or sterile towel) instead of passing instruments hand-to-hand.
■ Double glove to increase protection from punctures.
■ Share information (educate) with staff about sharps injury prevention.

Employee Responsibilities

What are your responsibilities related to preventing sharps injuries? You will need to learn how to use new devices, and make certain that the current safety requirements are enforced. Also: (ANA, 1993; Brooke, 2001; www.osha.gov/Publications/osha3161.pdf):

■ Always use universal precautions.
■ Use and dispose of sharps properly.
■ Obtain immunization against hepatitis B.
■ Get involved in sharps selection.
■ Keep your training up to date.
■ Report all exposures immediately following your facility's protocol.
■ Comply with post-exposure follow-up procedures/policies.

If you have questions about treatment for a needle-stick, you can call the National Clinician's Post-Exposure Prophylaxis (PEPLine) number, 1-888-448-4911 (Handelman, Perry, & Parker, 2012).

Ergonomic Injuries

Poor ergonomics is a safety concern factor for both nurses and patients (Durr, 2004).

Back Injuries

Occupation-related back injuries affect more than 75% of nurses over the course of their careers. Every year, 12% of nurses leave the profession due to back injury, and 52% complain of chronic back pain. Nursing aides, orderlies, and attendants ranked second and registered nurses sixth in a list of at-risk occupations for strains and sprains (U.S. Department of Labor, 2002). The problem with lifting a patient is not just one of overcoming heavy weight but also of overcoming improper lifting technique (OSHA, 2013b). Size, shape, and deformities of the patient as well as the patient's balance, combativeness, uncooperativeness, and contractures must be considered. Any unexpected movement or resistance from the patient can throw the nurse off balance and result in a back injury. Limited space, equipment, beds, chairs, and commodes also contribute to back injury risk (Edlich, Woodard, & Haines, 2001).

OSHA issued an ergonomics guideline for the nursing home industry on March 13, 2003 (www .osha.gov/ergonomics/guidelines/nursinghome/ index.html)

The back injury guide for health-care workers (www.dir.ca.gov/dosh/dosh_publications/backinj .pdf) and the OSHA guidelines for nursing homes (www.osha.gov/ergonomics/guidelines/nursing-home/index.html) are comprehensive resources. Employers must keep their workplaces free from recognized hazards, including ergonomic hazards.

ANA conducted a campaign entitled "Handle With Care" aimed at preventing back and other musculoskeletal injuries. Health-care facilities that have invested in recommended assistive patient handling programs report cost savings in the thousands of dollars both for direct costs of back injuries and for lost workdays (www.nursingworld.org/ MainMenuCategories/WorkplaceSafety/Healthy -Work-Environment/SafePatient/Resources/Handle withCare.pdf). In addition, assistive patient handling equipment improves the quality care of patients, improving patients' comfort, dignity, and safety during transfers.

Repetitive Stress Injuries

The use of computers continues to increase exponentially for all health-care personnel. Repetitive stress injuries (RSIs) affect people who spend long hours at computers, switchboards, and the like where repetitive motions are performed. The most common RSIs are carpal tunnel syndrome and mouse elbow. Badly designed computer workstations present the highest risk of RSIs. Preventive measures include the following (Feiler & Stichler, 2011; Krucoff, 2001):

■ Keep the monitor screen straight ahead of you, about an arm's length away. The top of the screen should be at eye level.
■ Align the keyboard so that your forearms, wrists, and hands are parallel to the floor. Tilt if needed to keep wrists in neutral position.
■ Position the mouse (if used) directly next to you and on the same level as the keyboard.
■ Keep thighs parallel to the floor as you sit on the chair. Feet should touch the floor and the chair back should be ergonomically sound.
■ Vary tasks. Avoid long sessions of sitting. Do not use excessive force when typing or clicking the mouse.

Toxic Environments

Inside air pollution is a more recently identified problem. Dioxin emissions, mercury, and battery waste are often not handled properly in the hospital environment. Disinfectants, chemicals, waste anesthesia gases, and laser plumes that float in the air are other sources of pollution exposure for nurses. Rethinking product choices, such as avoiding the use of polyvinyl chloride or mercury products, providing convenient collection sites for battery and mercury waste, and making waste management education for employees mandatory are starts toward a more pollution-free environment (Slattery, 1998). Better ventilation and air filtration can keep the air cleaner (Feiler & Stichler, 2011). Recycled paper and products, minimizing use of toxic disinfectants, and waste disposal choices that reduce incineration to a minimum are needed. Nurses as professionals need to be aware of the consequences of the medical waste produced by the health sector, supporting continued education for both nurses and patients.

Impaired Workers

Shawna had been a nurse for 20 years. Serious marital problems were affecting her work. To ease the tension one evening, she took a Xanax from a patient's medication drawer and it seemed to ease her tension. She surreptitiously took more patient medications, eventually escalating to narcotic analgesics.

Jorge began weekend binge-drinking in college. Ten years later, he is still drinking almost every weekend. He does not believe he is an alcoholic because he can "control" his drinking. But after he began showing up at work hung over and making multiple medication errors, he was fired. At the exit interview, no mention was made of his drinking problem because the agency feared a lawsuit for defamation of character.

Joanne has been late for work frequently, often appearing unkempt. She has been overheard making terse remarks to patients such as, "Who do you think I am—your maid?" and spends longer and longer periods off the unit. The floor has a large number of surgical patients who receive pain medications. Joanne's patients began complaining of pain even after pain medication administration has been charted. Joanne frequently "forgets" to waste her residual intramuscular narcotics in front of another nurse.

In the 1980s, the National Nurses' Society on Addictions (NNSA) and the ANA task forces jointly passed a resolution calling for acknowledgment of substance abuse problems and guidelines for impaired nurse programs (Heise, 2003).

Health-care professionals are not immune to alcoholism or chemical dependency. Various kinds of mental illnesses may also affect a nurse's ability to deliver safe, competent care. The most common signs of impairment are (Blair, 2005; Damrosch & Scholler-Jaquish, 1993):

■ Witnessed consumption of alcohol or controlled substances on the job
■ Changes in dress, appearance, posture, gestures
■ Slurred speech; abusive/incoherent language
■ Reports of impairment or erratic behavior
■ Witnessed unprofessional conduct
■ Significant lack of attention to detail
■ Witnessed theft of controlled substances
■ Assigned patients routinely requesting pain medication within a short period of being medicated

Impaired-nurse programs, which are conducted by state boards of nursing, work with the employer to assist the impaired nurse to remain licensed while receiving help for his or her problem. (Damrosch & Scholler-Jaquish, 1993; Sloan & Vernarec, 2001).

Often coworkers become protective and take on more work to ease the burden of their coworker. Although it is difficult to report a colleague, ignoring the problem or covering for an impaired colleague can pose serious risks for the patient and the nurse. Many state boards make it mandatory for nurses to report suspected impaired coworkers, and they accept anonymous reports. In many states, state law also requires hospitals and health-care providers to report impaired practitioners, but grants immunity from civil liability if the report was made in good faith (Blair, 2005; Sloan & Vernarec, 2001).

Disabled Employees

The Americans with Disabilities Act, enacted in 1990, makes it unlawful to discriminate against a qualified individual with a disability. Employers are required to provide reasonable accommodations for the disabled person. A reasonable accommodation is a modification or adjustment to the job, work environment, work schedule, or work procedures that enables a qualified person with a disability to perform the job. Both you and your employer may seek information from the Equal Employment Opportunity Commission (EEOC) for information (http://www.nursingworld.org/MainMenu Categories/ANAMarketplace/ANAPeriodicals/ OJIN/TableofContents/Volume92004/ No3Sept04/HandleWithCare.html).

Natural Disasters and Terrorism Threats

Since the 2001 anthrax outbreak and attacks on the World Trade Center, concern related to biological and chemical agents has heightened. The ANA provides nurses with valuable information on how they can better care for their patients, protect themselves, and prepare their hospitals and communities to respond to acts of bioterrorism and natural disasters (http://www.nursingworld.org/Main MenuCategories/Policy-Advocacy/Positions-and -Resolutions/Issue-Briefs/Disaster-Preparedness .pdf). Nurses are often called upon when a disaster occurs: Many worked with the ANA to provide support for the victims of Hurricane Katrina. A nurse holding a newborn rescued from the severely damaged NYU Langone Medical Center became a symbol of the rescue efforts following the destruction caused by Super Storm Sandy (2012).

Following are some steps that can be implemented in the workplace to better prepare for these threats: (www.nurses.com/doc.mvc/AWHONN -Takes-Action-Against-Bioterrorism-0001):

- Know the evacuation procedures and routes for your facility.
- Monitor your patient caseload for any unusual disease patterns and notify appropriate authorities as needed.
- Know the backup systems available for communication and staffing in the event of emergencies.
- Become familiar with the disaster policies in your facility.

Enhancing the Quality of Work Life

We turn our attention from safety to quality of the work environment. The American Association of Critical-Care Nurses (AACN) published standards for a healthy work environment noting that "relationship issues are real obstacles" to provision of safe care (2005, p. 188). These standards include skilled communication, real collaboration, effective decision making, adequate staffing, meaningful recognition, and effective leadership. There is evidence that a healthy work environment increases patient satisfaction and reduces nurses' stress and burnout (Kramer & Schmalenberg, 2008).

Shift Work Disorders

Although nurses who work nights permanently often can readjust their sleep-wake cycle from night to day, even permanent night-workers may be subject to continuous sleep deprivation. Those who continuously rotate shifts may seriously disturb their circadian rhythms: A typical night shift worker's scenario is to feel sleepy during work and travel home but have difficulty falling asleep during the day. Symptoms that continue for more than a month indicate the presence of shift work disorder. Those who suffer this disorder have a higher risk of ulcer, heart disease, depression, chronic fatigue, poor work performance, and accidents both on and off work (O'Malley, 2011). Suggestions for nurses who rotate shifts (Shandor, 2012; O'Malley, 2011) include the following:

- Shorter (8-hour) shifts allow you to get at least 7 hours' sleep before returning to work.

- Try to schedule the same shifts for an entire scheduling period instead of rotating different shifts within one scheduling period.
- Try to schedule the same days off consistently.
- If you become sleepy during the shift, try exercise (take a walk or climb stairs), bright light, a brief nap if possible, and a cup of coffee (not near the end of your shift).
- If you work evenings or nights, do not eat a big meal or take caffeine or alcohol at the end of the shift as this interferes with sleep. Try to avoid using sleep medications.
- If driving home in bright morning light, put on sunglasses.
- Try to sleep a continuous block of time at regularly scheduled times instead of catching a few hours here and there.
- Make sure the room you are sleeping in is a comfortable temperature and as dark and noise-free as possible.
- Find time to maintain good nutrition and daily exercise.
- Self-scheduling increases perceived control and may reduce the stress of shift work.

It is evident from this list that there are a number of ways an employer can help reduce the stress of shift work. Making healthy food available around the clock and providing nap facilities can help employees stay healthy and alert during their shifts (Shandor, 2012).

Mandatory Overtime

When nurses are routinely forced to work beyond their scheduled hours, they can suffer a range of emotional and physical effects. As patient acuity and workloads increase, overtime puts both patients and nurses at greater risk. Working overtime should be a choice, not a requirement, but nurses have been threatened with dismissal or charge of patient abandonment if they refuse to participate in mandatory overtime (http://www.nursingworld.org/ MainMenuCategories/ThePracticeofProfessional Nursing/NurseStaffing/OvertimeIssues/Overtime .pdf).

The ANA opposes the use of mandatory overtime, stating that nurses should be allowed to refuse overtime if they believe that they are too fatigued to provide quality care (http://www.nursingworld .org/MainMenuCategories/WorkplaceSafety/ Healthy-Work-Environment/Work-Environment/

NurseFatigue). In a 2006 position statement regarding nurses working when fatigued, the ANA takes the position that, regardless of the number of hours worked, each registered nurse has an ethical responsibility to carefully consider her/his level of fatigue when deciding whether to accept any assignment extending beyond the regularly scheduled workday or week, including a mandatory or voluntary overtime assignment (ANA, 2006). Rogers et al. (2004) found that nurses' error rates increase significantly during overtime, after 12 hours or after working more than 60 hours per week. Currently, half of staff nurses are scheduled routinely to work 12-hour shifts, and 85% of staff nurses routinely work longer than scheduled hours.

Staffing Ratios

Findings from 12 key studies cite specific effects of low nurse staffing on patient outcomes: incidences of failure to rescue, inpatient mortality, pneumonia, urinary tract infections, and pressure ulcers. Effects on the nurses themselves include needlestick injuries and eventual burnout (Aiken et al., 2002). Hospital length of stay and finances are affected as well.

The ANA recommends moving staffing decisions away from the industrial model of measuring time and motion to a professional model that examines the factors needed to provide quality care. The effect of changes in staffing levels should be evaluated on the basis of nursing-sensitive indicators (http://www.nursingworld.org/MainMenu Categories/ANAMarketplace/ANAPeriodicals/ OJIN/TableofContents/Volume122007/No3 Sept07/MandatoryNursetoPatientRatios.html).

Is this important? In 2002, Dr. Linda Aiken and her colleagues identified a relationship between staffing, mortality, nurse burnout, and job dissatisfaction (Aiken et al., 2002). With each additional patient assigned to a nurse, the following occurred:

■ A 30-day mortality increase of 7%
■ Failure-to-rescue rate increase of 7%
■ Nursing job dissatisfaction increase of 15%
■ Burnout rate increase of 23%
■ 43% of nurses surveyed suffering from burnout

A survey of 820 nurses and 621 patients in 20 hospitals across the United States (Vahey et al., 2004) showed that units characterized by nurses as having adequate staff, good administrative support

for nursing care, and good relations between physicians and nurses were twice as likely as other units to report high satisfaction with nursing care.

Reporting Questionable Practices

Most employers have policies that encourage the reporting of behavior that may adversely affect the workplace environment, including but not limited to (ANA, 1994):

1. Endangering a patient's health or safety
2. Abusing authority
3. Violating laws, rules, regulations, or standards of professional ethics
4. Grossly wasting funds

The Code for Nurses (ANA, 2001) is very specific about nurses' responsibility to report questionable behavior that may affect the welfare of a patient. If you become aware of inappropriate or questionable practices in the provision of health care, concern should be expressed to the person carrying out the questionable practice and attention called to the possible detrimental effect on the patient's welfare. Use official channels if it becomes necessary to report these practices. ANA's Code of Ethics further states that

> *When incompetent, unethical, illegal, or impaired practice is not corrected within the employment setting and continues to jeopardize patient well-being and safety, the problem should be reported to appropriate authorities such as practice committees of the pertinent professional organizations, the legally constituted bodies concerned with licensing of specific categories of health workers and professional practitioners, or the regulatory agencies concerned with evaluating standards or practice (ANA, 2001).*

Protection should be afforded to both the accused and the person doing the reporting, but this is not always the case:

Two Texas nurses not only lost their jobs but also were charged with misuse of official information when they reported a physician to the medical board for patient safety concerns. The charges against one were dropped eventually and the other was found not guilty in court. The Texas Nurses Association (TNA) Legal Defense Fund helped pay their legal expenses and the nurses won a civil judgment of $750,000 against the county. The physician was placed on 4 years' probation. "Nurses need to be able to advocate for patient safety," said Cindy Zolnierek, TNA Director of Practice, "and anything that stands in the way is not good for patients or nurses" (Trossman, 2011b, p. 11). For more information about related legislation in Texas, go to www.texasnurses.org.

Whistleblower is the term used for an employee who reports employer violations to an outside agency. You cannot assume that doing the right thing will protect you. Speaking up could get you fired unless you are protected by a union contract or other formal employment agreement. Your professional organization (the ANA) may also be able to support you. In May 1994, the U.S. Supreme Court ruled that nurses who direct the work of other employees may be considered supervisors and therefore may not be covered by the protections guaranteed under the National Labor Relations Act. This ruling may cause nurses to have no protection from retaliation if they report illegal practices in the workplace (ANA, 1995b). The 1995 brochure from the ANA (1995a), *Protect Your Patients—Protect Your License*, states, "Be aware that reporting quality and safety issues may result in reprisals by an employer." Does this mean that you should never speak up? Case law, federal and state statutes, and the federal False Claims Act may afford a certain level of protection. Some states have whistleblower laws, but they often apply only to state employees or to certain types of workers. Although these laws may offer some protection, the most important point is to work through the employer's chain of command and internal procedures. You may also (a) make sure that whistleblowing is addressed at your facility, either through a collective bargaining contract or workplace advocacy program; (b) contact your state nurses association to find out if your state offers whistleblower protection or has such legislation pending; (c) be politically active by contacting your state legislators and urging them to support a pending bill or by educating your elected state officials on the need for such protection for all health-care workers; and (d) contact your U.S. congressional representatives and urge them to support the Patient Safety Act (http://www.nursingworld.org/MainMenuCategories/Policy-Advocacy/Expired Content-GOVA/2006/whistle12768.html).

Social Environment

Working Relationships

Many aspects of the social environment received attention in earlier chapters. Team building, communicating effectively, and developing leadership skills are essential to the development of working relationships.

The day-to-day interactions with one's peers and supervisors have a major impact on the quality of the workplace environment. Most employees feel keenly the difference between a supportive and a nonsupportive environment. For example:

Ms. B. came to work already tired. Her baby was sick and had been awake most of the night. Her team expressed concern about the baby when she told them she had a difficult night. Each team member voluntarily took an extra patient so that Ms. B. could have a lighter assignment that day. When Ms. B. expressed her appreciation, her team leader said, "We know you would do the same for us." Ms. B. worked in a supportive environment.

Ms. G. came to work after a sleepless night. Her young son had been diagnosed with leukemia, and she was very worried about him. When she mentioned her concerns, her team leader interrupted her, saying, "Please leave your personal problems at home. We have a lot of work to do, and we expect you to do your share." Ms. G. worked in a nonsupportive environment.

In a supportive environment, people are willing to make difficult decisions, take risks, and "go the extra mile" for team members and the organization. In a non-supportive environment, members are afraid to take risks, avoid making decisions, and usually limit their commitment. Incivility, discussed earlier in this chapter, contributes to a nonsupportive environment.

Involvement in Decision Making

Having a voice in the decisions made about one's work and patients is very important to health-care professionals. Many actions can be taken to empower nurses: remove barriers to their participation in decision making, publicly express confidence in their capability and value, reward initiative and assertiveness, and provide role models who demonstrate confidence and competence. The following illustrates the difference between empowerment and powerlessness:

Soon after completing orientation, Nurse A heard a new nurse aide scolding a patient for soiling the bed. Nurse A did not know how incidents of potential verbal abuse were handled in this institution, so she reported it to the nurse manager. The nurse manager asked Nurse A several questions and thanked her for the information. The new aide was counseled immediately after their meeting. Nurse A noticed a positive change in the aide's manner with patients after this incident. Nurse A felt good about having contributed to a more effective patient care team. Nurse A felt empowered and will take action again when another occasion arises.

A colleague of Nurse B was an instructor at a community college. This colleague asked Nurse B if students would be welcome on her unit. "Of course," replied Nurse B. "I'll speak with my head nurse about it." When Nurse B did so, the response was that the unit was too busy to accommodate students. In addition, Nurse B received a verbal reprimand from the supervisor for overstepping her authority by discussing the placement of students. "All requests for student placement must be directed to the education department," she said. The supervisor directed Nurse B to write a letter of apology for having made an unauthorized commitment to the community college. Nurse B was afraid to make any decisions or public statements after this incident. Nurse B felt alienated and powerless.

Professional Growth and Innovation

The difference between a climate that encourages staff growth and creativity and one that does not can be quite subtle. In fact, many people are only partly aware, if at all, whether they work in an environment that fosters professional growth and learning. Yet the effect on the quality of the work done is pervasive, and it is an important factor in distinguishing the merely good health-care organization from the excellent health-care organization.

The increasingly rapid accumulation of knowledge in health-care mandates continuous learning for safe practice. Much of the responsibility for staff development and promotion of innovation lies with upper-level management. Some of the ways in which first-line managers can develop and support a climate of professional growth are to encourage

critical thinking, provide opportunities to take advantage of educational programs, encourage new ideas and projects, and reward professional growth.

Encourage New Ideas and Critical Thinking

Intellectual curiosity is a hallmark of the professional. An inquisitive frame of mind is relatively easy to suppress in a work environment. Patients and staff quickly perceive a nurse's impatience or defensiveness when too many questions are raised. Their response will be to simply give up asking these questions. But if you are a critical thinker and support other critical thinkers, you can contribute to an open-minded work environment.

Participating in brainstorming sessions, group conferences, and discussions encourages the generation of new ideas. Although new nurses may think they have nothing to offer, this is rarely the case. It is important for them to participate in activities that encourage them to contribute fresh, new ideas.

Reward Professional Growth

A primary source of discontent in the workplace is lack of recognition. Everyone enjoys praise and recognition. A smile, a card or note, or a verbal "thank you" goes a long way with coworkers in recognizing a job well done. Staff recognition programs have also been identified as a means of increasing self-esteem, social gratification, morale, and job satisfaction (Hurst, Croker, & Bell, 1994).

Cultural Diversity

Ms. V. is beginning orientation as a new staff nurse. She has been told that part of her orientation will be a morning class on cultural diversity. She says to the Human Resources person in charge of orientation, "I don't think I need to attend that class. I treat all people as equal. Besides, anyone living in our country has an obligation to learn the language and ways of those of us who were born here, not the other way around."

Mr. M. is a staff nurse on a medical-surgical unit. A young man with HIV infection has been admitted. He is scheduled for surgery in the morning and has requested that his significant other be present for the preoperative teaching. Mr. M. reluctantly agrees but mumbles under his breath to a coworker, "It wouldn't be so bad if they didn't flaunt their homosexuality and act like a married couple. Why can't he act like a man and get his own pre-op instructions?"

Diversity in health-care organizations includes ethnicity, race, culture, gender, sexual orientation, lifestyle, primary language, age, physical capabilities, and career stages of employees. Working with and caring for people who have different customs, traditions, communication styles, and beliefs can be rewarding as well as challenging. An organization that fosters diversity encourages respect and understanding of human characteristics and acceptance of the similarities and differences that make us human.

Consider these factors in understanding cultural diversity (Davidhizar, Dowd, & Giger, 1999):

1. **Communication.** Communication and culture are closely bound. Not only is culture transmitted through communication, it influences how people express themselves. Vocabulary, voice qualities, intonation, rhythm, speed, silence, touch, body postures, eye movements, and pronunciation differ among cultural groups and vary among persons from similar cultures. Using respect as a central core to a relationship, everyone needs to assess communication preferences of others in the workplace.
2. **Space.** Personal space is the area that surrounds a person's body. The amount of personal space individuals prefer varies from person to person and from situation to situation. Cultural beliefs also influence a person's perception of personal space. In the workplace, an understanding of coworkers' comfort related to personal space is important. Often, this comfort or discomfort is relayed in nonverbal rather than verbal communication.
3. **Social organization.** For some people, the importance of family supersedes that of other personal, work, or national causes. For example, caring for a sick child may override the importance of being on time or even coming to work, regardless of staffing needs or policies.
4. **Time.** Time orientation is often related to culture. Some cultures are more past-oriented, emphasizing traditions. People from cultures with a future orientation may be more likely to forego current pleasure for later rewards,

returning to school for a higher degree or earning certification, for example. Working with people who have different time orientations may cause difficulty in managing rotating shifts, planning schedules, setting deadlines, and even defining what "on time" means.
5. **Internal or external control.** Individuals with an external locus of control believe in the primacy of fate or chance. People with an internal locus of control believe they can influence, even determine, outcomes. In the workplace, nurses are expected to operate from an internal locus of control. This approach may be different from what a person has grown up with.

Indications of an organization's diversity "fitness" include the following (Mitchell, 1995):

- Minorities are represented at all levels of personnel.
- Individual cultural preferences pertaining to issues of social distance, touching, voice volume and inflection, silence, and gestures are respected.
- There is awareness of special family and holiday celebrations important to people of different cultures.

You can be a culturally competent practitioner and a role model for others by becoming:

- Aware of and sensitive to your own culture-based preferences
- Willing to explore your own biases and values
- Knowledgeable about other cultures
- Respectful of and sensitive to diversity among individuals
- Skilled using culturally sensitive intervention strategies

Physical Environment

The use of lighting, colors, and music to improve the workplace environment is increasing. Computer workstations are designed to promote efficiency in the patient care unit. When well designed, health information technologies are generally found by nurses to be useful and supportive of quality care (Waneka & Spetz, 2010). Relocation of supplies and substations closer to patient rooms to reduce the number of steps; improved visual and auditory scanning of patients from the nurses' station or decentralized workstations; better light and ventilation, especially in medication preparation areas; a unified information system; and reduced need for patient transport are all possible with changes in the physical environment (Feiler & Stichler, 2011).

Stress, Burnout, and Job Satisfaction

Stress

In the workplace, stress is related to a mismatch between an individual's perception of the demands being made and his or her perception of the ability to meet those demands. An individual's stress threshold also depends on the individual's characteristics, experiences, coping mechanisms, and the circumstances of the event (McVicar, 2003).

Sources of Stress

The nature of nurses' work creates the potential for experiencing stress (McGibbon, Peter, & Gallop, 2010), especially for younger, less experienced nurses (Purcell, Keitash, & Cobb, 2011). Some settings seem to generate more stressful situations than others. In the emergency department, for example, nurses reported several sources:

- Inadequate staffing, shift work, and overcrowding
- Aggression and violence on the part of patients and their families
- The death of a young patient
- High-acuity patients, especially those needing resuscitation (Healy & Tyrrell, 2011)

Nurses in a pediatric intensive care unit reported some additional sources:

- Bodily caring, especially when it was necessary to inflict pain on a child
- Being "tethered" (p. 1360) to their patients continuously for 12 hours
- Dealing with inexperienced medical residents
- Taking on others' work (e.g., therapy on the weekend, double-checking doctors' orders) without credit for it
- Malfunctioning equipment (McGibbon, Peter, & Gallop, 2010)

Additional sources of stress, including risk of infection, inadequate pay, and emotionally intensive work, were reported by a group of Latvian nurses (Circenis & Millere, 2012). Outside demands such as family caregiving can also be a source (Tucker, Weymiller, Cutshall, Rhudy, & Lohse, 2012). Small stressors can accumulate with negative effects on one's health (Evans, Becker, Zahn, Bilotta, & Keesee, 2011).

However, although most discussions emphasize the stressful nature of nurses' work, a study of over 2,000 staff nurses from a Midwestern medical center actually found they reported an average level of perceived stress (Tucker et al., 2012), suggesting most nurses learn how to manage these stresses.

Why Is Health Care a Stressful Occupation?

Job-related stress is broadly defined by the National Institute for Occupational Safety and Health as the "harmful physical and emotional responses that occur when the requirements of the job do not match the capabilities, resources, or needs of the worker." Much of the stress experienced by nurses is related to the nature of their work: continued intensive, intimate contact with people who often have serious physical, mental, emotional, and/or social problems and sometimes fatal diseases. Efforts to save patients or help them achieve a peaceful ending to their lives are not always successful. Some patients return to their destructive behaviors. The continued loss of patients alone can lead to burnout.

Health-care providers experiencing burnout may become cynical and even hostile toward their coworkers and colleagues (Carr & Kazanowski, 1994; Dionne-Proulx & Pepin, 1993; Goodell & Van Ess Coeling, 1994; Stechmiller & Yarandi, 1993; Tumulty, Jernigan, & Kohut, 1994).

In some instances, human service professionals also experience lower pay, longer hours, and more extensive regulation than do professionals in other fields. Inadequate advancement opportunities for women and minorities in lower-status, lower-paid positions may also contribute to job dissatisfaction.

The often unrealistic and sometimes sexist image of nurses in the media adds to the problem. Neither the school ideal nor the media image is realistic, but either may make nurses feel dissatisfied with themselves and their jobs, keeping stress levels high (Corley et al., 1994; Fielding & Weaver, 1994; Grant, 1993; Kovner, Hendrickson,

Knickman, & Finkler, 1994; Malkin, 1993; Nakata & Saylor, 1994; Pines, 2004; Skubak, Earls, & Botos, 1994).

Responses to Stress

"Whether the stress you experience is the result of major life changes or the cumulative effect of minor everyday hassles, it is how you respond to these experiences that determines the impact stress will have on your life" (Davis, Eshelman, & McCay, 2000).

Some people manage potentially stressful events more effectively than others (Crawford, 1993; Teague, 1992). A patient situation that one nurse considers stressful may not seem at all stressful to a coworker. The following is an example:

A new graduate was employed on a busy telemetry floor. Often, when patients were admitted, they were in acute distress, with shortness of breath, diaphoresis, and chest pain. Family members were distraught and anxious. Each time the new graduate had to admit a patient, she experienced a "sick-to-the-stomach" feeling, tightness in the chest, and difficulty concentrating.

She was afraid that she would miss something important and that the patient would die during admission. The more experienced nurses seemed to handle each admission with ease, even when the patient's physical condition was severely compromised.

Managing Stress

Psychologists noted over 100 years ago (1908) that too little stress can cause a lackadaisical attitude, while too much hurts performance and eventually one's health. A moderate amount can stimulate high performance without deleterious effects (Beck, 2012, p. 72) (see Box 11-6 for signs that your work-related stress level is too high).

There are some actions you can take to manage your stress; others need to be initiated by your

---

box 11-6

Signs That Your Stress Level Is Too High

- Dreading going to work
- Thinking frequently about mistakes, failures
- Avoiding patients, colleagues, assignments
- Using alcohol or drugs to relax after work
- Worrying about all of the above

Adapted from Beck, M. (2012/June 19). Anxiety can bring out the best. Wall Street Journal, D1.

---

employer. A health-promoting lifestyle, including attention to exercise, adequate sleep, and spiritual concerns is fundamental to caring for oneself (Johnson, 2011; Tucker et al., 2012). Riahi (2011, p. 729) suggests the following to maintain a healthy work life: self-reflect on your perceived role, develop hardiness through use of positive coping styles, and embrace various forms of prevention and stress-reduction actions.

Recent research suggests that mindfulness-based stress reduction (e.g., noting your physical response to stress) and cognitive behavioral training (screening out negative thoughts) are more helpful than earlier relaxation approaches, but they do require a substantial investment of time (Shellenbarger, 2012).

Realistic expectations of yourself and your new profession will also reduce stress related to unrealistic goals.

There is much that your employer can do as well to reduce workplace stress and mitigate its effects. These include:

- Provision of well-prepared preceptors and mentors for newly employed nurses
- Sufficient staffing so employees can take breaks and vacation time
- Peer support groups
- Debriefing after critical events have occurred
- Well-developed employee-assistance programs (EAPs) for counseling when needed
- Stress reduction training and workshops
- On-site exercise rooms
- On-site relaxation rooms

Hoolahan and Greenhouse (2012) describe a "restoration room" that was created from a conference room for use by nursing staff as a safe place to go and to calm themselves. Staff called this "chair time" and occasionally used it for family members as well after critical incidents occurred.

Ultimately, you are in control. Every day you are faced with choices. By gaining power over your choices and the stress they cause, you empower yourself.

Instead of being preoccupied with the past or the future, acknowledge the present moment and say the following to yourself (Davidson, 1999):

- I choose to relish my days.
- I choose to enjoy this moment.
- I choose to be fully present to others.

Questions for Self-Assessment

- What does the term *health* mean to me?
- What prevents me from living this definition of health?
- Is health important to me?
- Where do I find support?
- Which coping methods work best for me?
- What tasks cause me to feel pressured?
- Can I reorganize, reduce, or eliminate these tasks?
- Can I delegate or rearrange any of my family responsibilities?
- Can I say no to less important demands?
- What are my hopes for the future in terms of (1) career, (2) finances, (3) spiritual life and physical needs, (4) family relationships, (5) social relationships?
- What do I think others expect of me?
- How do I feel about these expectations?
- What is really important to me?
- Can I prioritize in order to have balance in my life?

- I choose to fully engage in the activity at hand.
- I choose to proceed at a measured, effective pace.
- I choose to acknowledge all I have achieved so far.
- I choose to focus on where I am and what I am doing.
- I choose to acknowledge that this is the only moment in which I can take action.

People cannot live in a problem-free world, but they can learn how to handle stress. Using the suggestions in this chapter, you will be able to adopt a healthier personal and professional lifestyle. The self-assessment questions in Box 11-7 can help you manage stress and help you understand your responses better. Boxes 11-8, 11-9, and 11-10 offer some guidelines for dealing with stress in the workplace.

Burnout

The ultimate result of unmediated job stress is burnout. The term *burnout* was a favorite buzzword of the 1980s and continues to be part of today's vocabulary. Herbert Freudenberger formally identified it as a leadership concern in 1974. The literature on job stress and burnout continues to grow as new books, articles, workshops, and videos regularly appear. A useful definition of *burnout* is the "progressive deterioration in work and other performance resulting from increasing difficulties in coping with high and continuing levels of job-related stress and professional frustration" (Paine, 1984, p. 1).

Much of the burnout experienced by nurses has been attributed to the frustration that arises because care cannot be delivered in the ideal manner. For those whose greatest satisfaction comes from caring for patients, anything that interferes with providing the highest quality care causes work stress and feelings of failure.

People who expect to derive a sense of significance from their work enter their professions with high hopes and motivation and relate to their work as a calling. When they feel that they have failed, that their work is meaningless, that they make no difference in the world, they may start feeling helpless and hopeless and eventually burn out (Pines, 2004, p. 67).

Stages of Burnout

Goliszek (1992) identified four stages of burnout:

1. **High expectations and idealism.** At the first stage, the individual is enthusiastic, dedicated,

Useful Relaxation Techniques

- Guided imagery
- Yoga
- Tai chi
- Meditation
- Relaxation tapes or music
- Exercise
- Favorite sports or hobbies
- Quiet corners or favorite places

Coping With Daily Work Stress

- Spend time on outside interests and take time for yourself.
- Increase your professional knowledge.
- Identify problem-solving resources.
- Identify realistic expectations for your position. Make sure you understand what is expected of you; ask questions if anything is unclear.
- Assess the rewards your work can realistically deliver.
- Develop good communication skills and treat coworkers with respect.
- Join rap sessions with coworkers. Be part of the solution, not part of the problem.
- Do not exceed your limits—you do not always have to say yes.
- Deal with other people's anger by asking yourself, "Whose problem is this?"
- Recognize that you can teach other people how to treat you.

---

box 11-10

Ten Daily De-Stressors

1. Express yourself! Communicate your feelings and emotions to friends and colleagues to avoid isolation and share perspectives. Sometimes, another opinion helps you see the situation in a different light.
2. Take time off. Taking breaks, or doing something unrelated to work, will help you feel refreshed as you begin work again.
3. Understand your individual energy patterns. Are you a morning or an afternoon person? Schedule stressful duties during times when you are most energetic.
4. Do one stressful activity at a time. Although this may take advanced planning, avoiding more than one stressful situation at a time will make you feel more in control and satisfied with your accomplishments.
5. Exercise! Physical exercise builds physical and emotional resilience. Do not put physical activities "on the back burner" as you become busy.

6. Tackle big projects one piece at a time. Having control of one part of a project at a time will help you to avoid feeling overwhelmed and out of control.
7. Delegate if possible. If you can delegate and share in problem solving, do so. Not only will your load be lighter, but others will be able to participate in decision making.
8. It's okay to say no. Do not take on every extra assignment or special project.
9. Be work-smart. Improve your work skills with new technologies and ideas. Take advantage of additional job training.
10. Relax. Find time each day to consciously relax and reflect on the positive energies you need to cope with stressful situations more readily.

Adapted from Bowers, R. (1993). Stress and your health. National Women's Health Report, 15(3), 6.

---

and committed to the job and exhibits a high energy level and a positive attitude.

2. **Pessimism and early job dissatisfaction.** In the second stage, frustration, disillusionment, or boredom with the job develops, and the individual begins to exhibit the physical and psychological symptoms of stress.
3. **Withdrawal and isolation.** As the individual moves into the third stage, anger, hostility, and negativism are exhibited. The physical and psychological stress symptoms worsen. Up through this stage, simple changes in job goals, attitudes, and behaviors may reverse the burnout process.
4. **Detachment and loss of interest.** As the physical and emotional stress symptoms become severe, the individual exhibits low self-esteem, chronic absenteeism, cynicism, and total negativism. Once the individual has moved into this stage and remains there for any length of time, burnout is inevitable.

Sharon had wanted to be a nurse for as long as she could remember. She married early, had three children, and put her dreams of being a nurse on hold. Now her children are grown, and she finally realized her dream by graduating last year from the local community college with a nursing degree. However, she has been overwhelmed at work, critical of coworkers and patients, and argumentative with supervisors. She is having difficulty adapting to the restructuring changes at her hospital and goes

home angry and frustrated every day. She cannot stop working for financial reasons but is seriously thinking of quitting nursing and taking some computer classes. "I'm tired of dealing with people. Maybe machines will be more friendly and predictable." Sharon is experiencing burnout.

Box 11-11 lists factors to consider to determine whether you may be experiencing stress or burnout.

Buffers Against Burnout

The idea that personal hardiness provides a buffer against burnout has been explored in recent years. Hardiness includes the following:

- A sense of personal control rather than powerlessness
- Commitment to work and life's activities rather than alienation
- Seeing life's demands and changes as challenges rather than as threats

The hardiness that comes from having this perspective leads to the use of adaptive coping responses, such as optimism, effective use of support systems, and healthy lifestyle habits (Duquette, Sandhu, & Beaudet, 1994; Nowak & Pentkowski, 1994). In addition, letting go of guilt, fear of change, and the self-blaming, "wallowing-in-the-problem" syndrome will help you buffer yourself against burnout (Lenson, 2001).

box 11-11

Assessing Your Risk for Stress and Burnout

- Do you feel more fatigued than energetic?
- Do you work harder but accomplish less?
- Do you feel cynical or disenchanted most of the time?
- Do you often feel sad or cry for no apparent reason?
- Do you feel hostile, negative, or angry at work?
- Are you short-tempered? Do you withdraw from friends or coworkers?
- Do you forget appointments or deadlines? Do you frequently misplace personal items?
- Are you becoming insensitive, irritable, and short-tempered?
- Do you experience physical symptoms such as headaches or stomachaches?
- Do you feel like avoiding people?
- Do you laugh less? Feel joy less often?
- Are you interested in sex?
- Do you crave junk food more often?

- Do you skip meals?
- Have your sleep patterns changed?
- Do you take more medication than usual? Do you use alcohol or other substances to alter your mood?
- Do you feel guilty when your work is not perfect?
- Are you questioning whether the job is right for you?
- Do you feel as though no one cares what kind of work you do?
- Do you constantly push yourself to do better, yet feel frustrated that there is no time to do what you want to do?
- Do you feel as if you are on a treadmill all day?
- Do you use holidays, weekends, or vacation time to catch up?
- Do you feel as if you are "burning the candle at both ends"?

Adapted from Golin, M., Buchlin, M., & Diamond, D. (1991). Secrets of Executive Success. Emmaus, PA: Rodale Press; and Goliszek, A. (1992). Sixty-Six Second Stress Management: The Quickest Way to Relax and Ease Anxiety. Far Hills, NJ: New Horizon.

Job Satisfaction

Job satisfaction encompasses the feelings or attitudes, positive or negative, that an individual has about his or her work. The nature of the work, people with whom one works, and the organization in which this all takes place are usually the focus of job satisfaction studies. Factors found to be important in nurses' satisfaction with their work are the work itself, the health-care team, and the employing organization.

The Work Itself

Ability to provide high-quality patient care is very important to most nurses. In a study of 1,091 medical-surgical nurses, Amendolair (2012) found a positive relationship between perceived ability to express caring behaviors and job satisfaction. Their ability to do so was related to the amount of time available to spend with patients.

The Health-Care Team

Nurses work with and interact with many different people in a day: patients, families, nursing assistants, many kinds of therapists, housekeeping and transport staff, social workers, and physicians, to name a few. How well they all work together, whether cooperatively and collegially or in constant conflict, affects job satisfaction. In a study of 3,675 nursing staff from five hospitals, Kalisch and colleagues (2010) found that higher levels of team-work (trust, cohesiveness, mutual help and understanding, and leadership) and adequate staffing lead to greater job satisfaction.

The Employing Organization

An organization that supports its most valuable asset, its staff members, is one that keeps its experienced nurses. Effective nurse leaders are key to accomplishing the goal of a healthy work environment (Blake, 2012). Higher pay, better benefits, and the means to turn sources of dissatisfaction into actual improvements in the work environment (one could call this empowerment) are elements contributing to retention of experienced nurses (Seago, Spetz, Ash, Herrera, & Keane, 2011).

New Graduates' Concerns

Most employers expect new graduates to come to the work setting able to organize their work, set priorities, and provide leadership to ancillary personnel. Even though nursing programs are designed to help students prepare for the demands of the work setting, new nurses still need to continue to learn and practice their skills on the job. Experienced nurses say that what they learned in school is only the beginning; school provided them with the fundamental knowledge and skills needed to continue to grow and develop as they practiced nursing in various capacities and work settings. Graduation is not the end of learning but the beginning of a journey toward becoming an expert nurse (Benner, 1984).

In most associate degree programs, students are assigned to care for one to three patients a day, working up to six or seven patients under a preceptor's supervision by the end of their program. Compare this with your first real job as a nurse: You may work 7–10 days in a row on 8- to 12-hour shifts, caring for 10 or more patients. You may also have to supervise several licensed practical nurses, technicians, and nursing assistants. These big changes from school to employment cause many new graduates to experience *reality shock* (Kraeger & Walker, 1993; Kramer, 1981).

Initial Concerns

The first few weeks on a new job are the "honeymoon" phase. The new employee is excited and enthusiastic about the new position. Coworkers usually go out of their way to make the new person feel welcome and overlook any problems that arise. But honeymoons do not last forever. The new graduate is soon expected to behave like everyone else and discovers that expectations for a professional employed in an organization are quite different from expectations for a student in school. Behaviors that brought rewards in school, such as crafting detailed care plans, taking extra time to prepare a patient for discharge, or delaying another task to look up the side effects of a new medication, are not necessarily valued by the organization. In fact, some of them are criticized. The new graduate who is not prepared for this change may feel confused, shocked, angry, and disillusioned. The stress can be high if it is not resolved.

Typical concerns of new nurses in their first 3 months of employment are related to skills, professional roles, patient care management, criticism from other staff members, knowledge of unit routine, and competing demands of school, family, and work (Godinez, Schweiger, Gruver, & Ryan, 1999; Heslop, 2001).

Well-supervised orientation programs are very helpful for newly licensed nurses. In some cases, the orientation program may be cut short and the new nurse required to function on his or her own very quickly. One way to minimize initial work stress is to ask questions about the orientation program before accepting a position: How long will it be? With whom will I be working? When will I be on

my own? What happens if at the end of the orientation I still need more assistance?

Differences in Expectations

Regardless of the career one chooses, there is no perfect job. After 2 or 3 months, the new nurse begins to experience a formal separation from being a student to embracing the professional nursing role. To cope with reality, several facts of work life need to be recognized (Goliszek, 1992, pp. 36, 46):

1. Expectations may not be met. You can accept this and react constructively or you can continue to experience disappointment and frustration.
2. To at least some extent, you need to adapt to the demands of your job, not expect the work to be adapted to your needs. Having a positive attitude and a sense of humor helps to maintain flexibility.
3. Feelings of helplessness or powerlessness at work cause frustration and job stress. If you go to work every day feeling that you do not make a difference, it is time to reevaluate your position and your goals. How you perceive your contribution to health care will definitely influence your reality.

When efficiency is the goal, the speed and amount of work done are rewarded rather than the quality of the work. This creates a conflict for the new graduate, who while in school was allowed to take as much time as needed to provide good care. The following is an example:

Brenda, a new graduate, was assigned to give medications to all her team's patients. Because this was a fairly light assignment, she spent some time looking up the medications and explaining their actions to the patients receiving them. Brenda also straightened up the medicine cart and restocked the supplies, which she thought would please her task-oriented team leader. At the end of the day, Brenda reported these activities with some satisfaction to the team leader. She expected the team leader to be pleased with the way she used the time. Instead, the team leader looked annoyed and told her that whoever passes out medications always does the blood pressures as well and that the other nurse on the team, who had a heavier assignment, had to do them. Also, because supplies were always ordered on Fridays for the weekend, it would have to be done again tomorrow, so Brenda had in fact wasted her time. Brenda had encountered differences in expectations and discovered how much more she needed to learn about the routines in her workplace.

Additional Pressures on the New Graduate

The first job a person takes after finishing school is often considered a proving ground where newly gained knowledge and skills are tested. Some new graduates set up mental tests for themselves that they feel must be passed before they can be confident of their ability to function. Passing these self-tests also confirms achievement of identity as a practitioner rather than a student.

At the same time, new graduates are undergoing testing by their coworkers, who are also interested in finding out whether the new graduate can handle the job. Sometimes new graduates are given tasks they are not ready to handle. If this happens, Kramer (1981) recommends that new graduates refuse to take the test rather than fail it. Another opportunity for proving themselves will soon come along.

Easing the Transition

Instead of focusing on the stress, new nurses can meet the transition to professional nursing by adapting to good stress:

- **Develop a professional identity.**
  Opportunities to challenge one's competence and develop an identity as a professional can begin in school. Success in meeting these challenges can immunize the new graduate against the loss of confidence that accompanies reality shock.
- **Learn about the organization.** The new graduate who understands how organizations operate will not be as shocked as the naïve individual. When you begin a new job, it is important to learn as much as you can about the organization and how it really operates.
- **Use your energy wisely.** Much energy goes into learning a new job. You may see many things that you think need to be changed, but

you need to recognize that to implement change requires your time and energy.
- **Communicate effectively.** Confront problems that might arise with coworkers. Use the problem-solving and negotiating skills you've learned in this course.
- **Seek feedback often and persistently.** Seeking feedback pushes the people you work with to be more specific about their expectations of you.
- **Develop a support network.** Identify colleagues who have held onto their professional ideals with whom you can share your problems and the work of improving the organization. Their recognition of your work can keep you going when rewards from the organization are meager. A support network is a source of strength when resisting pressure to give up professional ideals and a source of power when attempting to bring about change.
- **Mentoring.** New graduates need help with organizing their work, time management, communicating with other members of the health-care team, especially with physicians, and recognition of critical changes in their patients. Even experienced nurses, when newly hired or transferred to different positions, usually need to learn the culture of the new organization, their role on the new team, and new skills (Ellisen, 2011). Mentors can provide the support needed to increase new nurses' clinical success, job satisfaction, and retention (Cottingham, DiBartolo, Battistoni, & Brown, 2010; Burr, Stichler, & Poettler, 2011; Weng, Huang, Tsai, Chang, Lin, & Lee, 2010). For example:

At Sharp Mary Birch Hospital for Women and Newborns in San Diego, new graduates, nurses returning to work after some time away, and nurses entering a new specialty area are matched with an experienced mentor for their first year. The program includes a 3-hour orientation for mentors and mentees, quarterly support workshops, and ongoing support. It has not only reduced their new graduate turnover rate but also helps to recruit new nurses (Burr et al., 2011).

A mentor-mentee relationship may be formal as in the example above or it may develop informally

table 11-1	

Mentor and Mentee Responsibilities

Mentor Responsibilities	Mentee Responsibilities
Utilizes excellent communication and listening skills	Demonstrates eagerness to learn
Shows sensitivity to needs of nurses, patients, and workplace	Participates actively in the relationship by keeping all appointments and commitments
Encourages excellence in others	Seeks feedback and uses it to modify behaviors
Shares and provides counsel	Demonstrates flexibility and an ability to change
Exhibits good decision-making skills	Is open in the relationship with mentor
Shows an understanding of power and politics	Demonstrates an ability to move toward independence
Demonstrates trustworthiness	Able to evaluate choices and outcomes

over time. Formal relationships usually include some training for the mentor and mentee, have specific objectives, and often have mentors assigned to mentees, while those in informal mentoring relationships usually choose each other (Harrington, 2011). Either approach can be a valuable and rewarding experience for both mentor and mentee (see Table 11-1)

Ineffective Coping Strategies

Some less successful ways of coping with these problems are listed.

- **Abandon professional ideals.** When faced with reality shock, some new graduates abandon their professional ideals. This may eliminate their conflict but puts the needs of the organization before their needs or the needs of the patient.
- **Leave the profession.** A significant proportion of those who do not want to give up their professional ideals escape these conflicts by leaving their jobs and abandoning their profession. There would probably be fewer shortages of nurses if more health-care organizations met these professional ideals (Kramer & Schmalenberg, 1993).

When you have made it through the first 6 months of employment and are finally starting to feel like a "real" nurse, you are probably beginning to realize that a completely stress-free work environment is almost impossible to achieve. Shift work, overtime, distraught families, staff shortages, and pressure to do more with less continue to contribute to place demands on nurses. An inability to deal with this

continued stress may lead to burnout unless you take steps to prevent it.

Conclusion

Workplace safety is an area of increasing concern for employer and employees alike. Staff members have a right to be informed of any potential risks in the workplace. Employers have a responsibility to provide adequate equipment and supplies to protect employees and to create programs and policies to inform employees about minimizing risks as much as possible. Issues of workplace violence, sexual harassment, impaired workers, ergonomics and workplace injuries, and terrorism should be addressed to protect both employees and patients.

A social environment that promotes professional growth and creativity and a physical environment that offers comfort and maximum work efficiency should be considered in improving the quality of work life. Cultural awareness, respect for the diversity of others, and increased contact between groups should also be addressed.

Many waking hours are spent in the workplace. It can offer a climate of professional growth, excitement, and satisfaction. Everyone is responsible for promoting a safe, healthy work environment for each other.

You already know that the work of nursing is not easy and may sometimes be very stressful. Yet nursing is also a profession filled with a great deal of personal and professional satisfaction. Periodically ask yourself the questions designed to help you assess your stress level and review the stress management techniques described in this chapter to reduce your risk for burnout.

Study Questions

1. Why is it important for nurses to understand the major federal laws and agencies responsible to protect the individual in the workplace?

2. What actions can nurses take if they believe that OSHA guidelines are not being followed in the workplace?

3. What are nurses' responsibilities in dealing with the following workplace issues: transmission of blood-borne pathogens, violence, sexual harassment, and impaired coworkers?

4. What information do you need to obtain from your employer related to disasters or a terrorist threat?

5. What will you look for in the work environment that will support positive patient outcomes?

6. Consider experiences you have had in your clinical rotations: were the environments supportive or nonsupportive? What recommendations would you make for improvement?

7. Discuss the characteristics of health-care organizations that may lead to burnout among nurses. How could they be changed or eliminated?

8. How can a new graduate adequately prepare for the work world? What is your plan to make the transition from student to practicing professional successful?

9. What qualities would you look for in a mentor? What qualities would you try to demonstrate as a mentee? Can you identify someone you know who might become a mentor to you?

10. How are the signs of stress, burnout, and reality shock related?

11. How can you help colleagues deal with substance abuse problems? What if a colleague does not recognize that he/she has a problem? What might you do to help your colleague?

12. Identify the physical and psychological signs and symptoms you exhibit during stress. What sources of stress are most likely to affect you? How do you deal with these signs and symptoms?

Case Studies to Promote Critical Reasoning

Diversity

You have been hired as a new RN on a busy pediatric unit in a large metropolitan hospital. The hospital provides services for a culturally diverse population, including African American, Asian, and Hispanic people. Family members often attempt alternative healing practices specific to their culture and bring special foods from home to entice a sick child to eat. One of the more experienced nurses said to you, "We need to discourage these people from fooling with all this hocus-pocus. We are trying to get their sick kid well in the time allowed under their managed care plans, and all this medicine-man stuff is only keeping the kid sick longer. Besides, all this stuff stinks up the rooms and brings in bugs." You have observed how important these healing rituals and foods are to the patients and families and believe that both the families and the children have benefited from this nontraditional approach to healing.

1. What are your feelings about nontraditional healing methods?

2. How would you respond to the experienced nurse?

3. How can you be a patient advocate without alienating your coworkers?

4. What could you do to assist your coworkers in becoming more culturally sensitive to their patients and families?

5. How can health-care facilities incorporate both Western and nontraditional medicine? Should they do this? Why or why not?

Burnout

Shawna, a new staff member, has been working from 7 a.m. to 3 p.m. on an infectious disease floor since obtaining her RN license 4 months ago. Most of the staff members with whom she works with have been there since the unit opened 5 years ago. On a typical day, the staffing includes a nurse manager, two RNs, an LPN, and one technician for approximately 40 patients. Most patients are HIV-positive with multisystem failure. Many are severely debilitated and need help with their activities of daily living. Although staff members encourage family members and loved ones to help, most of them are unavailable because they work during the day. Several days a week, the nursing students from Shawna's community college program are assigned to the floor.

Tina, the nurse manager, does not participate in any direct patient care, saying that she is "too busy at the desk." Laverne, the other RN, says the unit depresses her and that she has requested a transfer to pediatrics. Lynn, the LPN, wants to "give meds" because she is "sick of the patients' constant whining," and Sheila, the technician, is "just plain exhausted." Lately, Shawna has noticed that the other staff members seem to avoid the nursing students and reply to their questions with annoyed, short answers. Shawna is feeling alone and overwhelmed and goes home at night worrying about the patients, who need more care and attention. She is afraid to ask Tina for more help because she does not want to be considered incompetent or a complainer. When she confided in Lynn about her concerns, Lynn replied, "Get real—no one here cares about the patients or us. All they care about is the bottom line! Why did a smart girl like you choose nursing in the first place?"

1. What is happening on this unit in leadership terms?

2. Identify the major problems and the factors that contributed to these problems.

3. What factors might have contributed to the behaviors exhibited by Tina, Lynn, and Sheila?

4. How would you feel if you were Shawna?

5. Is there anything Shawna can do for herself, for the patients, and for the staff members?

6. What do you think Tina, the nurse manager, should do?

7. How is the nurse manager reacting to the changes in her staff members?

8. What is the responsibility of administration?

9. How are the patients affected by the behaviors exhibited by all staff members?

References

Aiken, L.H., Clarke, S.P., Slane, D.M., Sochalski, J., et al. (2002). Hospital nurse staffing and patient mortality, nurse burnout, and job dissatisfaction. *Journal of the American Medical Association, 288*(16), 1987–1993.

Amendoliar, D. (2012). Caring behaviors and job satisfaction. *Journal of Nursing Administration, 42*(1), 34–39.

American Association of Critical-Care Nurses. (2005). AACN standards for establishing and sustaining healthy work environments: A journey to excellence. *American Journal of Critical Care 14*(3), 187–197.

American Nurses Association. (2012). ANA survey: Improved work environment, more can be done. Available at: www.theamericannurse.org/index .php/2012/02/07/ ana-survey-improved-work-environment-more-can-be-done/

American Nurses Association. (1993). *HIV, hepatitis-B, hepatitis-C: Blood-borne diseases*. Washington, DC: ANA.

American Nurses Association. (1994). *Guidelines on reporting incompetent, unethical, or illegal practices*. Washington, DC: ANA.

American Nurses Association. (1995a). *Protect your patients—Protect your license*. Washington, DC: ANA.

American Nurses Association. (1995b). *The Supreme Court has issued the ultimate gag order for nurses*. Washington, DC: ANA.

American Nurses Association. (2001). *Code for nurses*. Washington, DC: ANA.

American Nurses Association. (2006/December 8). *Assuring patient safety: Registered nurses' responsibility in all roles and settings to guard against working when fatigued*. Washington, DC: ANA.

American Nurses Association. (2007). *Occupational health*. Retrieved July 10, 2009, from www.nursingworld.org/ MainMenuCategories/OccupationalandEnvironmental/ occupationalhealth.aspx

Arbury, S. (2002). Healthcare workers at risk. *Job Safety and Health Care Quarterly, 13*(2), 30–31.

Bauer, X., Ammon, J., Chen z., Beckman, W. et al. (1993). Health risk in hospitals through airborne allergens for patients pre-sensitized to latex. *Lancet, 342*, 1148–1149.

Beck, M. (2012/June 19). Anxiety can bring out the best. *Wall Street Journal*, D1.

Benner, P. (1984). *From novice to expert*. Menlo Park, CA: Addison-Wesley.

Beyea, S. (2004). A critical partnership-safety for nurses and patients. *AORN, 79*(6), 1299–1302.

Blair, D. (2005). Spot the signs of drug impairment. *Nursing Management, 36*(2), 20–21, 52.

Blake, N. (2012). Practical steps for implementing healthy work environments. *Creating a Healthy Workplace, 23*(1), 14–17.

Bowers, R. (1993). Stress and your health. *National Women's Health Report, 15*(3), 6.

Brooke, P. (2001). The legal realities of HIV exposure. *RN, 64*(12), 71–73.

Burr, S., Stichler, J.F., & Poettler, D. (2011). Establishing a mentoring program. *Nursing for Women's Health, 15*(3), 215–224.

Bylone, M. (2011). Healthy work environment 101. *AACN Advanced Critical Care, 22*(1), 10–21.

Carr, K., & Kazanowski, M. (1994). Factors affecting job satisfaction of nurses who work in long-term care. *Journal of Advanced Nursing, 19*, 878–883.

Carroll, C., & Sheverbush, J. (September 1996). Violence assessment in hospitals provides basis for action. *The American Nurse*, 18.

Centers for Disease Control and Prevention (CDC). (1992). Surveillance for occupationally acquired HIV infection—United States, 1981–1992. *MMWR, 41*(43), 823–825.

Chisholm, R.F. (1992). Quality of working life: A crucial management perspective for the year 2000. *Journal of Health and Human Resources Administration, 15*(1), 6–34.

Circenis, K., & Millere, I. (2012). Stress related work environments: Nurses survey result. *International Journal of Collaborative Research on Internal Medicine & Public Health, 4*(6), 1150–1157.

Collins, J. (1994). Nurses' attitudes toward aggressive behavior following attendance at "The Prevention and Management of Aggressive Behavior Programme." *Journal of Advanced Nursing, 20*, 117–131.

Corley, M., Farley, B., Geddes, N., Goodloe, L., et al. (1994). The clinical ladder: Impact on nurse satisfaction and turnover. *Journal of Nursing Administration, 24*(2), 42–48.

Cottingham, S., DiBartolo, M.C., Battistoni, S., & Brown, T. (2010). Partners in nursing: A mentoring initiative to enhance nurse retention. *Nursing Education Perspectives, 32*(4), 250–255.

Crawford, S. (1993). Job stress and occupational health nursing. *American Association of Occupational Health Nurses Journal, 41*, 522–529.

Daley, K.A. (2012/September). Editorial: Moving the sharps agenda forward. *American Nurse Today*, 1.

Damrosch, S., & Scholler-Jaquish, A. (1993). Nurses' experiences with impaired nurse coworkers. *Applied Nursing Research, 6*(4), 154–160.

Davidhizar, R., Dowd, S., & Giger, J. (1999). Managing diversity in the healthcare workplace. *Health Care Supervisor, 17*(3), 51–62.

Davidson, J. (1999). *Managing stress* (2nd ed.). New York: Pearson.

Davis, M., Eshelman, E., & McCay, M. (2000). *The Relaxation and stress reduction workbook*, 5th ed. Oakland, CA: New Harbinger Publications.

Dionne-Proulx, J., & Pepin, R. (1993). Stress management in the nursing profession. *Journal of Nursing Management, 1*, 75–81.

Duquette, A., Sandhu, B., & Beaudet, L. (1994). Factors related to nursing burnout: A review of empirical knowledge. *Issues in Mental Health Nursing, 15*, 337–358.

Durr, L. (2004). Commission on workforce issues: What nurses should expect in the workplace: The ANA Bill of Rights for registered nurses. *Virginia Nurses Today, 12*(2), 17.

Edlich, R., Woodard, C., & Haines, M. (2001). Disabling back injuries in nursing personnel. *Journal of Emergency Nursing, 27*(2), 150–155.

Edwards, R. (1999). Prevention of workplace violence. *Aspen's Advisor for Nurse Executives, 14*(8), 8–12.

Ellisen, K. (2011/August). Recruitment & retention report: Mentoring smart. *Nursing Management, 42*(8), 12–16.

Evans, G.W., Becker, F.D., Zahn, A., Bilotta, E., & Keesee, A.M. (2011). Capturing the ecology of workplace stress with cumulative risk assessment. *Environment and Behavior, 44*(1), 136–154.

Feiler, J.L., & Stichler, J.F. (2011). Ergonomics in healthcare facility design: Part 2. *Journal of Nursing Administration, 41*(3), 97–99.

Fielding, J., & Weaver, S. (1994). A comparison of hospital and community-based mental health nurses: Perceptions of their work environment and psychological health. *Journal of Advanced Nursing, 19*, 1196–1204.

Foley, M. (2012/September). Essential elements of a comprehensive sharps injury-prevention program. *American Nurse Today*, 2–4.

General Industry Regulations Book, Subpart Z Occupational Safety and Health Standards, Title 29 *Code of Federal Regulations*, Part 1910.

Gilmore-Hall, A. (2001). Violence in the workplace. *Issues Update, ANA*, 55–56. Available at: www.nursingcenter .com

Godinez, G., Schweiger, J., Gruver, J., & Ryan, P. (1999). Role transition from graduate to staff nurse: A qualitative analysis. *Journal for Nurses in Staff Development, 15*(3), 97–110.

Golin, M., Buchlin, M., & Diamond, D. (1991). *Secrets of executive success*. Emmaus, PA: Rodale Press.

Goliszek, A. (1992). *Sixty-six second stress management: The quickest way to relax and ease anxiety*. Far Hills, NJ: New Horizon.

Goodell, T., & Van Ess Coeling, H. (1994). Outcomes of nurses' job satisfaction. *Journal of Nursing Administration, 24*(11), 36–41.

Grant, P. (1993). Manage nurse stress and increase potential at the bedside. *Nursing Administration Quarterly, 18*(1), 16–22.

Guglielmi, C., & Ogg, M.J. (2012/September). Practical strategies to prevent surgical sharps injuries. *American Nurse Today*, 0–10.

Guglielmi, C., & Ogg, M.J. (2012/September). Moving the sharps safety agenda forward: Consensus statement and call to action. *American Nurse Today*, 11–16.

Hamilton, R., Brown, R., Veltri, M., Feroli, R., et al. (2005). Administering pharmaceuticals to latex allergy patients from vials containing natural rubber latex closures. *American Journal Health Systems Pharmacy, 62*, 1822–1827.

Handelman, E., Perry, J.L., & Parker, G. (2012/September). Reducing sharps injuries in non-hospital settings. *American Nurse Today*, 5–7.

Harrington, S. (2011). Mentoring new nurse practitioners to accelerate their development as primary care providers: A literature review. *Journal of the American Academy of Nurse Practitioners, 23*, 168–174.

Healy, S., & Tyrrell, M. (2011). Stress in emergency departments: Experiences of nurses and doctors. *Emergency Nurse, 19*(4), 31–37.

Heise, B. (2003). The historical context of addictions within the nursing profession. *Journal of Addictions Nursing, 14*, 117–124.

Herring, L.H. (1994). *Infection control*. New York: National League for Nursing.

Heslop, L. (2001). Undergraduate student nurses: Expectations and their self-reported preparedness for the graduate year role. *Journal of Advanced Nursing, 36*, 626–634.

Hoolahan, S.E., & Greenhouse, P.K. (2012). Energy capacity model for nurses: The impact of relaxation and restoration. *Journal of Nursing Administration, 42*(2), 103–109.

Hurst, K.L., Croker, P.A., & Bell, S.K. (1994). How about a lollipop? A peer recognition program. *Nursing Management, 25*(9), 68–73.

Johnson, L. (2011/August). Easing workplace stressors. *Healthcare Traveler*, 28–34.

Kalisch, B.J., Lee, H., & Rochman, M. (2010). Nursing staff teamwork and job satisfaction. *Journal of Nursing Management, 18*, 938–947.

Kear, M. (2012/December). Caring and civility go hand-in-hand. *The Florida Nurse, 1*, 3.

Kinkle, S. (1993). Violence in the ED: How to stop it before it starts. *American Journal of Nursing, 93*(7), 22–24.

Kovner, C., Hendrickson, G., Knickman, I., & Finkler, S. (1994). Nurse care delivery models and nurse satisfaction. *Nursing Administration Quarterly, 19*(1), 74–85.

Kraeger, M., & Walker, K. (1993). Attrition, burnout, job dissatisfaction and occupational therapy manager. *Occupational Therapy in Health Care, 8*(4), 47–61.

Kramer, M. (January 27–28, 1981). Coping with reality shock. Workshop presented at Jackson Memorial Hospital, Miami, FL.

Kramer, M., & Schmalenberg, C. (1993). Learning from success: Autonomy and empowerment. *Nursing Management, 24*(5), 58–64.

Kramer, M., Schmalenberg, C., & McGuire P. (2008). Essentials of a magnetic environment. *Volume Career Directory. January 2008*, 23–27.

Krucoff, M. (2001). How to prevent repetitive stress injury in the workplace. *American Fitness, 19*(1), 31.

Lanza, M.L., & Carifio, J. (1991). Blaming the victim: Complex (nonlinear) patterns of causal attribution by nurses in response to vignettes of a patient assaulting a nurse. *Journal of Emergency Nursing, 17*(5), 299–309.

Lenson, B. (2001). *Good stress—Bad stress*. New York: Marlowe and Company.

Lewis, P.S., & Malecha, A. (2011). The impact of workplace incivility on the work environment, manager skill and productivity. *Journal of Nursing Administration, 41*(7/8), S17–S24.

Lilly Ledbetter Fair Pay Act of 2009, S.181, 123 Stat. 5

Lindberg, P., & Vingård, E. (2012). Indicators of healthy work environments—a systematic review. *Work: A Journal of Prevention, Assesment and rehabilitation, 41* (Supl 1), 3032–3038.

Magnavita, N., & Heponiemi, T. (2011). Workplace violence against nursing students and nurses: An Italian experience. *Journal of Nursing Scholarship, 43*(2), 203–210.

Mahoney, B. (1991). The extent, nature, and response to victimization of emergency nurses in Pennsylvania. *Journal of Emergency Nursing, 17*, 282–292.

Malkin, K.F. (1993). Primary nursing: Job satisfaction and staff retention. *Journal of Nursing Management, 1*, 119–124.

McGibbon, E., Peter, E., & Gallop, R. (2010). An institutional ethnography of nurses's stress. *Qualitative Health Research, 20*(11), 1353–1378.

McLennan, M. (2005). Nurses' views on work enabling factors. *Journal of Nursing Administration, 35*(6), 311–318.

McPhaul, K. & Lipscomb, J. (September 30, 2004). "Workplace violence in health care: Recognized but not regulated." *Online Journal of Issues in Nursing, 9*(3), Manuscript 6. Available at: www.nursingworld.org/ MainMenuCategories/ANAMarketplace/ ANAPeriodicals/OJIN/TableofContents/Volume92004/ No3Sept04/ViolenceinHealthCare.aspx

McVicar, A. (2003). Workplace stress in nursing: A literature review. *Journal of Advanced Nursing, 44*(6), 633–642.

Mitchell, A. (1995). Cultural diversity: The future, the market and the rewards. *Caring, 14*(12), 44–48.

Nadwairski, J.A. (1992). Inner-city safety for home care providers. *Journal of Nursing Administration, 22*(9), 42–47.

Nakata, J., & Saylor, C. (1994). Management style and staff nurse satisfaction in a changing environment. *Nursing Administration Quarterly, 18*(3), 51–57.

National Institute for Occupational Safety and Health (NIOSH). Accessed July 27, 2002, at www.cdc.gov/niosh/homepage.html

National Safety Council. (1992). *Accident prevention manual for business and industry.* Chicago: National Safety Council.

National Safety Council. (2013). *Continue on a journey to safety excellence.* Available at: www.nsc.org/safety_work/Pages/Home.aspx

Nowak, K., & Pentkowski, A. (1994). Lifestyle habits, substance use, and predictors of job burnout in professional women. *Work and Stress, 8*(1), 19–35.

O'Malley, P. (2011). Staying awake and asleep: The challenge of working nights and rotating shifts. *Clinical Nurse Specialist, 25*(1), 15–17.

OSHA (2013a). OSHA trade news release. Available at: www.osha.gov/pls/oshaweb/owadisp.show_document?p_table= NEWS_RELEASES. . .

OSHA (2013b). OSHA technical manual. Available at: www.osha.gov/dts/osta/otm/otm_vii/otm_vii_1.html

Outwater, L.C. (1994). Sexual harassment issues. *Caring, 13*(5), 54–56, 58, 60.

Paine, W.S. (1984). Professional burnout: Some major costs. *Family and Community Health, 6*(4), 1–11.

Perry, J. (2001). Attention all nurses! New legislation puts safer sharps in your hands. *American Journal of Nursing, 101*(9), 24AA–24CC.

Pines, A. (2004). Adult attachment styles and their relationship to burnout: A preliminary, cross-cultural investigation. *Work & Stress, 18*(1), 66–80.

Purcell, S.R., Keitash, M., & Cobb, S. (2011). The relationship between nurses' stress and nurse staffing factors in a hospital setting. *Journal of Nursing Management, 19,* 714–720.

Riahi, S. (2011). Role stress amongst nurses at the workplace: Concept analysis. *Journal of Nursing Management, 19,* 1721–731.

Roche, E. (23 February 1993). Nurses' risks and their rights. *Vital Signs,* 3.

Rocker, C., (2012/September 24) "Responsibility of a frontline manager regarding staff bullying." *OJIN: The Online Journal of Issues in Nursing, 18*(2).

Rogers, A.E., Hwang, W., Scott, L.D., Aiken, L.H., et al. (2004). The working hours of hospital staff nurses and patient safety: Both errors and near errors are more likely to occur when hospital staff nurses work twelve or more hours at a stretch. *Health Affairs, 23*(4), 202–212.

Rosen, A., Isaacson, D., Brady, M., & Corey J.P. (1993). Hypersensitivity to latex in healthcare workers: Report of five cases. *Otolaryngology—Head and Neck Surgery, 109,* 731–734.

Seago, J.A., Spetz, J., Ash, M., Herrera, C-N., & Keane, D. (2011). Hospital RN job satisfaction and nurse unions. *Journal of Nursing Administration, 41*(3), 109–114.

Sellers, K.F., & Millenbach, L. (2012). The degree of horizontal violence in RNs practicing in New York State. *Journal of Nursing Administration, 42*(10), 483–487.

Shandor, A. (2012/May). The health impacts of nursing shift work. MSN Thesis, Minnesota State University, Mankoto, MN.

Shellenbarger, S. (2012/October 10). To cut office stress, try butterflies and meditation? *The Wall Street Journal,* D2.

Simonowitz, J. (1994). Violence in the workplace: You're entitled to protection. *Registered Nurse, 57*(11), 61–63.

Skubak, K., Earls, N., & Botos, M. (1994). Shared governance: Getting it started. *Nursing Management, 25*(5), 80I-J, 80N, 80P.

Slattery, M. (September/October 1998). Caring for ourselves to care for our patients. *The American Nurse,* 12–13.

Sloan, A., & Vernarec, E. (2001). Impaired nurses: Reclaiming careers. *Medical Economics, 64*(2), 58–64.

Smith, L.M., Andrusyszyn, M.A., & Spence-Laschinger, H.K.S. (2010). Effects of workplace incivility and empowerment on newly-graduated nurses' organizational commitment. *Journal of Nursing Management, 18,* 1004–1015.

Stechmiller, J., & Yarandi, H. (1993). Predictors of burnout in critical care nurses. *Heart Lung, 22,* 534–540.

Strader, M.K., & Decker, P.J. (1995). *Role transition to patient care management.* Norwalk, CT: Appleton & Lange.

Teague, J.B. (1992). The relationship between various coping styles and burnout among nurses. *Dissertation Abstracts International,* 1994.

Trossman, S. (May/June 1999a). When workplace threats become a reality. *The American Nurse,* 1, 12.

Trossman, S. (2011b/May/June). Texas Nurses Association promoting enhanced nurse protection. *The American Nurse,* 11.

Tucker, S.J., Weymiller, A.J., Cutshall, S.M., Rhudy, L.M., & Lohse, C.M. (2012). Stress ratings and health promotion practices among RNs. *Journal of Nursing Administration, 42*(5), 282–292.

Tumulty, G., Jernigan, E., & Kohut, G. (1994). The impact of perceived work environment on job satisfaction of hospital staff nurses. *Applied Nursing Research, 7*(2), 84–90.

U.S. Department of Labor (OSHA). (1995). *Employee workplace rights and responsibilities.* OSHA, 95–35.

U.S. Department of Labor, Bureau of Labor Statistics. (2002). Lost-work time injuries and illnesses: Characteristics and resulting time away from work, 2000. April 10, 2002. Retrieved April 13, 2008, from ftp://ftp.bls.gov/pub/news.release/History/osh2.04102002.news.ftp://ftp.bls.gov/pub/news.release/History/osh2.04102002.news.

Vahey, D., Aiken, L., Sloane, D., Clarke, S., et al. (2004). Nurse burnout and patient satisfaction. *Medical Care, 42*(2), II-57–II-66.

Waneka, R., & Spetz, J. (2010). Hospital information technology systems' impact on nurses and nursing care. *Journal of Nursing Administration, 40*(12), 509–514.

Weng, R-H., Huang, C-Y., Tsai, W-C., Chang, L-P., Lin, S-E., & Lee, M-Y. (2010). Exploring the impact of mentoring functions on job satisfaction and organizational commitment of new staff nurses. *BMC Health Services Research, 10,* 240.

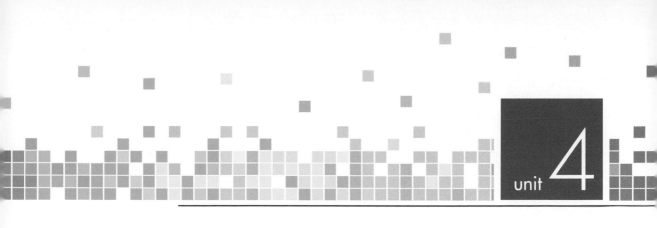

unit 4

Professional Issues

OBJECTIVES

After reading this chapter, the student should be able to:

- Evaluate personal strengths, weaknesses, opportunities, and threats using a SWOT analysis.
- Develop a résumé including objectives, qualifications, skills experience, work history, education, and training.
- Compose job search letters including cover letter, thank-you letter, and acceptance and rejection letters.
- Discuss components of the interview process.
- Discuss the factors involved in selecting the right position.
- Explain why the first year is critical to planning a career.

The National Center for Health Workforce Analysis at the Health Resources and Services Administration has projected a growing shortage of registered nurses (RNs) over the next 15 years, with a 12% shortage by 2010 and a 20% shortage by 2015 (http://bhpr.hrsa.gov/healthworkforce/nursingshortage/tech_report/default.htm). This continued shortage of RNs will allow you to have many choices and opportunities as a professional nurse. By now you have invested considerable time, expense, and emotion into preparing for your new career. Your educational preparation, technical and clinical expertise, interpersonal and management skills, personal interests and needs, and commitment to the nursing profession will contribute to meeting your career goals. Successful nurses view nursing as a lifetime pursuit, not as an occupational stepping stone.

This chapter deals with the most important endeavor: finding and keeping your first nursing position. The chapter begins with planning your initial search; developing a strengths, weaknesses, opportunities, and threats (SWOT) analysis; searching for available positions; and researching organizations. Also included is a section on writing a résumé and employment-related information about the interview process and selecting the first position.

Getting Started

By now at least one person has said to you, "Good career choice. Nurses are always needed and will never be out of a job." This statement is only one of several career myths. These myths include the following:

1. "Good workers do not get fired." They may not get fired, but many good workers have lost their positions during restructuring and downsizing.
2. "Well-paying jobs are available without a college degree." Even if entrance into a career path does not require a college education, the potential for career advancement is minimal without that degree. In many health-care agencies, a baccalaureate degree in nursing is required for an initial management position, and due to the Institute of Medicine (IOM) report (2001), many health-care institutions are encouraging nurses to return for their BSN and MSN degrees in order to maintain employment.
3. "Go to work for a good company, and move up the career ladder." This statement assumes that people move up the career ladder due to longevity in the organization. In reality, the responsibility for career advancement rests on the employee, not the employer.
4. "Find the 'hot' industry, and you will always be in demand." Nursing is projected to continue to be one of the "hottest" industries well into the next decade. However, a nurse who performs poorly will never be successful, no matter what the demand.

Many students attending college today are adults with family, work, and personal responsibilities. On graduating with an associate degree in nursing, you may still have student loans and continued responsibilities for supporting a family. Your focus may be on job security and a steady source of income. The idea of career planning might not be a thought at this time; however, this is a strategic process and requires some thought and personal self-assessment

(Schoessler & Waldo, 2006). The correct goal is to find a job that fits *you*. It is also not too early to begin formal planning of your career. In today's dynamic health-care environment, nursing managers want nurses who consider nursing as a profession, not a just a job. They look for individuals who express a commitment to forming partnerships with the health-care team and institution (Arvidsson, Skarsater, Oijerval, & Friglund, 2008).

SWOT Analysis

New graduates often secure their first position as a staff nurse on a medical-surgical floor. They see themselves as "putting in their year" and then moving on to their dream position as a critical care or mother-baby nurse. However, as the health-care system continues to evolve and reallocate resources, this may no longer be the automatic first step for new graduates. Instead, new graduates should focus on long-term career goals and the different avenues by which they can be reached. Some of you may already have determined your career path knowing that you will need to pursue advanced nursing degrees to achieve your goal.

Consider your past experiences as they may be an asset in presenting your abilities for a particular position. A SWOT analysis, borrowed from the corporate world, can guide you in discovering your internal strengths and weaknesses as well as external opportunities and threats that may help or hinder your job search and career planning. The SWOT analysis is an in-depth look at what will make you happy in your work. Although you have already made the decision to pursue nursing, knowing your strengths and weaknesses can help you select the work setting that will be satisfying personally (Christie, 2012). Your SWOT analysis may include the following factors:

Strengths

■ Relevant work experience
■ Advanced education
■ Product knowledge
■ Good communication and people skills
■ Computer skills
■ Self-managed learning skills
■ Flexibility

Weaknesses

■ Ineffective communication and people skills
■ Inflexibility

- Lack of interest in further education
- Difficulty adapting to change
- Inability to see health care as a business

Opportunities
- Expanding markets in health care
- New applications of technology
- New products and diversification
- Increasing at-risk populations
- Nursing shortage

Threats
- Increased competition among health-care facilities
- Changes in government regulation

Take some time to strategically plan your career and personalize the preceding SWOT analysis. What are *your* strengths? What skills do *you* need to improve? What weaknesses do *you* need to minimize, or what strengths do *you* need to develop as you begin your job search? What opportunities and threats exist in the health-care community *you* are considering? Doing a SWOT analysis will help you make an initial assessment of the job market. It can be used again after you narrow your search for that first nursing position.

Many graduates find using the SMART acronym helpful to determine career goals. SMART represents specific (S), measurable (M), achievable (A), realistic (R), and timely (T) (www.health .mo.gov/living/families/wic/wicupdates/. . ./Goal Setting-SMART.doc). SMART helps you specify what you want to accomplish during your career. For example, perhaps you desire to work as a perinatal nurse. Many health-care institutions promote certification as part of a clinical ladder. You would include obtaining certification as part of your plan (www. ancc.org).

In addition to completing a SWOT analysis, there are several other tools that can help you learn more about yourself. Two of the most common are the Strong Interest Inventory (SII) and the Myers-Briggs Type Indicator (MBTI). The SII compares the individual's interests with the interests of those who are successful in a large number of occupational fields in the areas of (1) work styles, (2) learning environment, (3) leadership style, and (4) risk-taking/adventure. Completing this inventory can help you discover what work environment might be best suited to your interests.

The MBTI is a widely used indicator of personality patterns. This self-report inventory provides information about individual psychological-type preferences on four dimensions:

1. Extroversion (E) or Introversion (I)
2. Sensing (S) or Intuition (N)
3. Thinking (T) or Feeling (F)
4. Judging (J) or Perceiving (P)

Although many factors influence behaviors and attitudes, the MBTI summarizes underlying patterns and behaviors common to most people. Both tools should be administered and interpreted by a qualified practitioner. Most university and career counseling centers are able to administer them. If you are unsure of where you fit in the workplace, consider exploring these tests with your college or university or take the MBTI online at www.myersbriggs.org/.

Beginning the Search

Even with a nationwide nursing shortage, hospital mergers, emphasis on increased staff productivity, budget crises, staffing shifts, and changes in job market availability affect the numbers and types of nurses employed in various facilities and agencies. Instead of focusing on long-term job security, the career-secure employee focuses on becoming a career survivalist or developing resilience. Resilience requires that an individual develop the ability to recover or adapt to changes (Jackson, Firtko, & Edinborough, 2007). A career survivalist or resilient individual focuses on the person, not the position. Consider the following career survivalist strategies (Morgan, 2013):

- **Be engaged.** Your career belongs to you. Define your values and determine what motivates you. Be the lookout for opportunities to break from the status quo. Opportunities for nurses are growing every day.
- **Stay informed.** Health care is dynamic and changing daily. Go out there, stay informed, and start thinking about your options for riding the waves of change.
- **Learn for employability.** Take personal responsibility for your career success. Continue to be a "work in progress." Employability in health care today means learning technology tools, job-specific technical skills, and people

skills such as the ability to negotiate, coach, work in interprofessional teams, and make presentations.

■ **Plan for your financial future.** Ask yourself, "How can I spend less, earn more, and manage better?" Often, people make job decisions based on financial decisions, which makes them feel trapped instead of secure.

■ **Develop multiple options.** The career survivalist looks at multiple options constantly. Moving up is only one option. Being aware of emerging trends in nursing, adjacent fields, lateral moves, and special projects presents other options.

■ **Build a safety net.** Networking is extremely important to the career survivalist. Joining professional organizations, taking time to build long-term nursing relationships, and getting to know other career survivalists will make your career path more enjoyable and successful.

What do employers think you need to be ready to work for them? In addition to passing the National Council Licensure Examination (NCLEX), employers cite the following skills as desirable in job candidates (Cazacu, 2010):

■ Oral and written communication skills
■ Responsibility and accountability
■ Integrity
■ Interpersonal skills
■ Proficiency in field of study/technical competence
■ Teamwork ability
■ Willingness to work hard
■ Leadership abilities
■ Motivation, initiative, and flexibility
■ Critical thinking and analytical skills
■ Self-discipline
■ Organizational skills

In today's world there are multiple approaches to looking for a nursing position. The traditional approaches include looking through newspapers, professional magazines, and school career placement offices. Newer electronic methods include career search engines (Kluemper, 2009). Contacting specific health-care institutions and organizations and filling out a job application lets employers know that you are interested in working with them.

Some Internet sites that post nursing opportunities are:

■ www.careerbuilders.com
■ www.nurse.com
■ www.healthcareersinteraction.com

In recent years, three trends have emerged related to recruiting. First, employers are being more creative by using alternative sources to increase the diversity of employees. They commonly place advertisements in minority newspapers and magazines and recruit nurses at minority organizations. Second, employers are using more temporary help as a way to evaluate potential employees. Nursing staffing agencies are common in most areas of the county. Third, the Internet is being used more frequently for advertising and recruitment.

Regardless of where you begin your search, explore the market vigorously and thoroughly. Looking only in the classified ads on Sunday morning is a limited search. Instead, speak to everyone you know about your job search. Encourage classmates and colleagues to share contacts with you, and do the same for them. Also, when possible, try to speak directly with the person who is looking for a nurse when you hear of a possible opening. The people in human resources offices may reject a candidate on a technicality that a nurse manager would realize does not affect that person's ability to handle the job if he or she is otherwise a good match for the position. For example, experience in day surgery prepares a person to work in other surgery-related settings, but a human resources interviewer may not know this.

Try to obtain as much information as you can about the available position. Is there a match between your skills and interests and the position? Ask yourself whether you are applying for this position because you really want it or just to gain interview experience. Be careful about going through the interview process and receiving job offers only to turn them down. Employers may share information with one another, and you could end up being denied the position you really want. Regardless of where you explore potential opportunities, use these "pearls of wisdom" from career nurses:

■ Know yourself.
■ Seek out mentors and wise people.
■ Be a risk taker.

- Never, ever stop learning.
- Understand the business of health care.
- Involve yourself in community and professional organizations.
- Network.
- Understand diversity.
- Be an effective communicator.
- Set short- and long-term goals, and strive continually to achieve them.

Researching Your Potential Employer

You have spent time taking a look at yourself and the climate of the health-care job market. You have narrowed your choices to the organizations that really interest you. Now is the time to find out as much as possible about these organizations.

It is important to evaluate your values and goals when researching an organization. Ownership of the company may be public or private, foreign or American. The company may be local or regional, a small corporation or a division of a much larger corporation. Depending on the size and ownership of the company, information may be obtained from the public library, chamber of commerce, government offices, or company Web site.

Has the organization recently gone through a merger, a reorganization, or downsizing? Information from current and past employees is valuable and may provide you with more details about whether the organization might be suitable for you. Be wary of gossip and half-truths that may emerge, however, because they may discourage you from applying to an excellent health-care facility. In other words, if you hear something negative about an organization, investigate it for yourself. Often, individuals jump at work opportunities before doing a complete assessment of the culture and politics of the institution.

The first step in assessing the culture is to review a copy of the company's mission statement. The mission statement reflects what the institution considers important to its public image. What are the core values of the institution?

The department of nursing's philosophy and objectives indicate how the department defines nursing; they identify what the department's important goals are for nursing. The nursing philosophy and goals should reflect the mission of the organization. Where is nursing administration on the organizational chart of the institution? To whom does the chief nursing officer report?

Although much of this information may not be obtained until an interview, a preview of how the institution views itself and the value it places on nursing will help you decide if your philosophy of health care and nursing is compatible with that of a particular organization. To find out more about a specific health-care facility, you can (Zedlitz, 2003):

- Talk to nurses currently employed at the facility.
- Access the facility's Web site for information on its mission, philosophy, and services.
- Check the library for newspaper and magazine articles related to the facility.

Writing a Résumé

Your résumé is your personal data sheet and a way of marketing yourself. It is the first impression the recruiter or your potential employer has about you. Consider your résumé your time to shine. The résumé highlights your skills, talents, and abilities. You may decide to prepare your own résumé or have it prepared by a professional service. Regardless of who prepares it, the purpose of a résumé is to get a job interview.

Many people dislike the idea of writing a résumé. After all, how can you sum up your entire career in a single page? You want to scream at the printed page, "Hey, I'm bigger than that! Look at all I have to offer!" However, this one-page summary has to work well enough to get you the position you want. Chestnut (1999) summarized résumé writing by stating, "Lighten up. Although a very important piece to the puzzle in your job search, a résumé is not the only ammunition. What's between your ears is what will ultimately lead you to your next career" (p. 28). Box 12-1 summarizes reasons for preparing a well-considered, up-to-date résumé.

Although you might labor intensively over preparing your résumé, most job applications live or die within 10–30 seconds as the receptionist or applications examiner decides whether your résumé should be forwarded to the next step or rejected. In many places, nonnursing personnel first screen your résumé. Some beginning helpful tips include the following (Ervin, Bickes, & Schim, 2006).

- Keep the résumé to one or two pages. Do not use smaller fonts to cram more information on the page. Proofread, proofread, proofread. Typing errors, misspelled words, and poor

box 12-1

Reasons for Preparing a Résumé

Assists in completing an employment application quickly and accurately

Demonstrates your potential

Focuses on your strongest points

Gives you credit for all your achievements

Identifies you as organized, prepared, and serious about the job search

Serves as a reminder and adds to your self-confidence during the interview

Provides initial introduction to potential employers in seeking the interview

Serves as a guide for the interviewer

Functions as a tool to distribute to others who are willing to assist you in a job search

Adapted from Marino, K. (2000). Resumes for the health care professional. New York: John Wiley & Sons; and Zedlitz, R. (2003). How to get a job in health care. New York: Delmar Learning.

grammar act as red flags. Use action verbs when possible. Do not substitute quantity of words for quality.

■ Itemize your educational experiences on your résumé. Also include any certifications you may have. As a new graduate, it may be helpful to highlight specific clinical experiences as they relate to the position you wish to obtain.

■ State your objective. Although you know very well what position you are seeking, the individual conducting the initial screening does not want to take the time to determine this. Tailor your résumé to the institution and position to which you are applying.

■ Employers care about what you can do for them and your potential for future success with their company. Your résumé must answer those questions.

Essentials of a Résumé

Most résumés follow one of four formats: standard, chronological, functional, or a combination. There are several Web sites on resume writing. Many of these offer free templates to assist you with this skill. Regardless of the type of résumé, basic elements of personal information, education, work experience, qualifications for the position, and references should be included (Marino, 2000; Zedlitz, 2003):

■ **Standard.** The standard résumé is organized by categories. By clearly stating your personal information, job objective, work experience, education and work skills, memberships, honors, and special skills, you give the

employer a "snapshot" of the person requesting entrance into the workforce. This is a useful résumé for first-time employees or recent graduates.

■ **Chronological.** The chronological résumé lists work experiences in order of time, with the most recent experience listed first. This style is useful in showing stable employment without gaps or many job changes. The objective and qualifications are listed at the top.

■ **Functional.** The functional résumé also lists work experience but in order of importance to your job objective. List the most important work-related experience first. This is a useful format when you have gaps in employment or lack direct experience related to your objective.

■ **Combination.** The combination résumé is a popular format, listing work experience directly related to the position but in a chronological order.

Most professional recruiters and placement services agree on the following tips in preparing a résumé (Korkki, 2010):

■ *Make sure your résumé is readable.* Is the type large enough for easy reading? Are paragraphs indented or bullets used to set off information, or does the entire page look like a gray blur? Using bold headings and appropriate spacing can offer relief from lines of gray type, but be careful not to get so carried away with graphics that your résumé becomes a new art form. The latest trends in résumé writing are using fonts such as Arial or Century New Gothic over the standard Times New Roman (James, 2003). The paper should be an appropriate color such as cream, white, or off-white. Use easily readable fonts and a laser printer. If a good computer and printer are not available, most printing services prepare résumés at a reasonable cost. Résumés may also be sent electronically. Some organizations require applicants to upload their resumes into their application system. Another way is to attach a resume to an introductory e-mail. It is often recommended that you convert your resume to a portable document format (PDF). This format is readable by most systems and also allows for greater protection, as word processing documents (Microsoft Word, WordPerfect) are easily altered.

- *Make sure the important facts are easy to spot.* Education, current employment, responsibilities, and facts to support the experience you have gained from previous positions are important. Put the strongest statements at the beginning. Avoid excessive use of the word "I." If you are a new nursing graduate and have little or no job experience, list your educational background first. Remember that positions you held before you entered nursing might support experience that will be relevant in your nursing career. Be sure to let your prospective employer know how to contact you.
- *Do a spelling and grammar check.* Use simple terms, action verbs, and descriptive words. Check your finished résumé for spelling, style, and grammar errors. If you are not sure if the grammar or style is correct, get another opinion.
- *Follow the do nots.* Do not include pictures, fancy binders, salary information, or hobbies (unless they have contributed to your work experience). Do not include personal information such as weight, marital status, and number of children. Do not repeat information just to make the résumé longer. A good résumé is concise and focuses on your strengths and accomplishments.

No matter which format you use, it is essential to include the following:

- A clearly stated job objective
- Highlighted qualifications
- Directly relevant skills and experience
- Chronological work history
- Relevant education and training

How to Begin

Start by writing down every applicable point you can think of in the preceding five categories. Work history is usually the easiest place to begin. Arrange your work history in reverse chronological order, listing your current job first. Account for all your employable years. Short lapses in employment are acceptable, but give a brief explanation for longer periods (e.g., "maternity leave"). Include employer, dates worked (years only, e.g., 2001–2002), city, and state for each employer you list. Briefly describe the duties and responsibilities of each position. Emphasize your accomplishments, any special techniques you learned, or changes you implemented. Use action verbs, such as those listed in Table 12-1, to describe your accomplishments. Also cite any special awards or committee chairs. If a previous position was not in the health field, try to relate your duties and accomplishments to the position you are seeking.

Education

Next, focus on your education. Include the name and location of every educational institution you attended; the dates you attended; and the degree, diploma, or certification attained. Start with your most recent degree. It is not necessary to include your license number because you will give a copy of the license when you begin employment. If you are

table 12-1			
Action Verbs			
Management Skills	**Communication Skills**	**Accomplishments**	**Helping Skills**
Attained	Collaborated	Achieved	Assessed
Developed	Convinced	Adapted	Assisted
Improved	Developed	Coordinated	Clarified
Increased	Enlisted	Developed	Demonstrated
Organized	Formulated	Expanded	Diagnosed
Planned	Negotiated	Facilitated	Expedited
Recommended	Promoted	Implemented	Facilitated
Strengthened	Reconciled	Improved	Motivated
Supervised	Recruited	Instructed	Represented
		Reduced (losses)	
		Resolved (problems)	
		Restored	

Source: Adapted from Parker, Y. (1989). The Damn Good Résumé Guide. Berkeley, CA: Ten Speed Press.

still waiting to take the National Council Licensure Examination (NCLEX), you need to indicate when you are scheduled for the examination. If you are seeking additional training, such as for intravenous certification, include only what is relevant to your job objective.

Your Objective

It is now time to write your job objective. Write a clear, brief job objective. To accomplish this, ask yourself: What do I want to do? For or with whom? When? At what level of responsibility? For example (Parker, 1989; Hart, 2006):

- **What:** RN
- **For whom:** Pediatric patients
- **Where:** Large metropolitan hospital
- **At what level:** Staff

A new graduate's objective might read: "Position as staff nurse on a pediatric unit" or "Graduate nurse position on a pediatric unit." Do not include phrases such as "advancing to neonatal intensive care unit." Employers are trying to fill current openings and do not want to be considered a stepping stone in your career.

Skills and Experience

Relevant skills and experience are included in your résumé not to describe your past but to present a "word picture of you in your proposed new job, created out of the best of your past experience" (Parker, 1989, p. 13; Impollonia, 2004). Begin by jotting down the major skills required for the position you are seeking. Include five or six major skills such as:

- Administration/management
- Teamwork/problem solving
- Patient relations
- Specialty proficiency
- Technical skills

Other

Academic honors, publications, research, and membership in professional organizations may be included. Were you active in your school's student nurses association, or in a church or community organization? Were you on the dean's list? What if you were "just a housewife" for many years? First, do an attitude adjustment: you were not "just a

housewife" but a family manager. Explore your role in work-related terms such as *community volunteer, personal relations, fund-raising, counseling,* or *teaching.* A college career office, women's center, or professional résumé service can offer you assistance with analyzing the skills and talents you shared with your family and community. A student who lacks work experience has options as well. Examples of nonwork experiences that show marketable skills include (Eubanks, 1991; Parker, 1989):

- Working on the school paper or yearbook
- Serving in the student government
- Leadership positions in clubs, bands, or church activities
- Community volunteer
- Coaching sports or tutoring children in academic areas

After you have jotted down everything relevant about yourself, develop the highlights of your qualifications. This area could also be called the *Summary of Qualifications,* or just *Summary.* The highlights should be immodest one-liners designed to let your prospective employer know that you are qualified and talented and the best choice for the position. A typical group of highlights might include (Parker, 1989):

- Relevant experience
- Formal training and credentials, if relevant
- Significant accomplishments, very briefly stated
- One or two outstanding skills or abilities
- A reference to your values, commitment, or philosophy, if appropriate

A new graduate's highlights could read:

- Five years of experience as a licensed practical nurse in a large nursing home
- Excellent patient/family relationship skills
- Experience with chronic psychiatric patients
- Strong teamwork and communication skills
- Special certification in rehabilitation and reambulation strategies

Tailor the résumé to the job you are seeking. Include only relevant information, such as internships, summer jobs, inter-semester experiences, and volunteer work. Even if your previous work experience is not directly related to nursing, it can show transferable skills, motivation, and your potential to be a great employee.

Regardless of how wonderful you sound on paper, if the résumé itself is not high quality, it may end up in a trash can. Also let your prospective employer know whether you wish to have a response on an answering machine or fax.

Job Search Letters

The most common job search letters are the cover letter, thank-you letter, and acceptance letter. Job search letters should be linked to your SWOT analysis. Regardless of their specific purpose, letters should follow basic writing principles (Banis, 1994):

- State the purpose of your letter.
- State the most important items first, and support them with facts.
- Keep the letter organized.
- Group similar items together in a paragraph, and then organize the paragraphs to flow logically.

Business letters are formal, but they can also be personal and warm but professional.

- Avoid sending an identical form letter to everyone. Instead, personalize each letter to fit each individual situation.
- As you write the letter, keep it work-centered and employment-centered, not self-centered.
- Be direct and brief. Keep your letter to one page.
- Use the active voice and action verbs and have a positive, optimistic tone.
- If possible, address your letters to a specific individual, using the correct title and business address. Letters addressed to "To Whom It May Concern" do not indicate much research or interest in your prospective employer.
- A timely (rapid) response demonstrates your knowledge of how to do business.
- Be honest. Use specific examples and evidence from your experience to support your claims.

Cover Letter

You have spent time carefully preparing the résumé that best sells you to your prospective employer. The cover letter will be your introduction. If it is true that first impressions are lasting ones, the cover letter will have a significant impact on your prospective employer. The purposes of the cover letter include (Beatty, 1989):

- Acting as a transmittal letter for your résumé
- Presenting you and your credentials to the prospective employer
- Generating interest in interviewing you

Regardless of whether your cover letter will be read first by human resources personnel or by the individual nurse manager, its effectiveness cannot be overemphasized. A poor cover letter can eliminate you from the selection process before you even have an opportunity to compete. A sloppy, disorganized cover letter and résumé may suggest you are sloppy and disorganized at work. A lengthy, wordy cover letter may suggest a verbose, unfocused individual (Beatty, 1991). Your cover letter should do the following (Anderson, 1992):

- **State your purpose in applying and your interest in a specific position.** Also identify how you learned about the position.
- **Emphasize your strongest qualifications that match the requirements for the position.** Provide evidence of experience and accomplishments that relate to the available position, and refer to your enclosed résumé.
- **Sell yourself.** Convince this employer that you have the qualifications and motivation to perform in this position.
- **Express appreciation to the reader for consideration.**

If possible, address your cover letter to a specific person. If you do not have a name, call the healthcare facility and obtain the name of the human resources supervisor. If you still can't get a name, create a greeting that includes the word *manager:* for example, Dear Human Resources Manager or Dear Personnel Manager (Zedlitz, 2003, p. 19).

Thank-You Letter

Thank-you letters are important but seldom used tools in a job search. You should send a thank-you letter to everyone who has helped in any way in your job search. As stated earlier, promptness is important. Thank-you letters should be sent within

24 hours to anyone who has interviewed you. The letter (Banis, 1994, p. 4) should:

- Express appreciation
- Reemphasize your qualifications and the match between your qualifications and the available position
- Restate your interest in the position
- Provide any supplemental information not previously stated

Acceptance Letter

Write an acceptance letter to accept an offered position; confirm the terms of employment, such as salary and starting date; and reiterate the employer's decision to hire you. The acceptance letter often follows a telephone conversation in which the terms of employment are discussed.

Rejection Letter

Although not as common as the first three job search letters, you should send a rejection letter if you are declining an employment offer. When rejecting an employment offer, indicate that you have given the offer careful consideration but have decided that the position does not fit your career objectives and interests at this time. As with your other letters, thank the employer for his or her consideration and offer.

Using the Internet

Performing Internet searches for positions offers greater opportunities and the ability to see what types of jobs are available. Numerous sites either post positions or assist potential employees in matching their skills with available employment. More and more corporations are using the Internet to reach wider audiences. If you use the Internet in your search, it is always wise to follow up with a hard copy of your résumé if an address is listed. Mention in your cover letter that you sent your résumé via the Internet and the date you did so. If you are using an Internet-based service, follow up with an e-mail to ensure that your résumé was received. Table 12-2 summarizes the major "do's and don'ts" when using the Internet to job search.

The Interview Process

Initial Interview

Your first interview may be with the nurse manager, someone in the human resources office, or an interviewer at a job fair or even over the telephone. Regardless of with whom or where you interview, preparation is the key to success.

You began the first step in the preparation process with your SWOT analysis. If you did not obtain any of the following information regard-

table 12-2	
Do's and Don'ts of Internet Job Searching	
Do	**Don't**
Focus on selling yourself: "My clinical practicum in the ICU at a major health center and my strong organizational skills fit with the entry-level ICU position posted in Nursing Spectrum."	Use many "I"s in the message: "I saw your job posting in Nursing Spectrum, and I have attached my résumé."
Use short paragraphs; keep the message short.	Long messages probably will not even be read.
Use highlighting and bullets.	Forget to format for e-mail.
Use an appropriate e-mail address: DKWhitehead431@. . ..	Use a silly or inappropriate e-mail: smartypants@. . . or partyanimal@. . .
Use an effective subject: ICU RN position.	Use subjects used by computer viruses or junk e-mailers: Hi, Important, Information.
Send your message to the correct e-mail address.	Assume; if the address is not indicated, call to see what person/address is appropriate.
Send messages individually.	Send a blast message to many recipients; it may be discarded as junk mail.
Treat e-mail with the same care you treat a traditional business application.	Slip into informality—remember spelling and grammar checks.
Keep your résumé "cyber-safe."	Remove your standard contact information and replace it with your e-mail address.
Change the format of your resume: save your Word document as an HTML file or an ASCII text file.	Assume that everyone is using the same word processing program.

Source: Adapted from Job Hunt: The Online Job Search Guide. Retrieved October 1, 2013, from www.job-hunt.org/

ing your prospective employer at that time, it is imperative that you do it now (Impollonia, 2004):

■ Key people in the organization
■ Number of patients and employees
■ Types of services provided
■ Reputation in the community
■ Recent mergers and acquisitions
■ Other recent news

Much of this information will be available on the prospective employer's Web site. Other potential sources of information are local newspapers and magazines, either in print or on the publications; websites.

You also need to review your qualifications for the position. What does your interviewer want to know about you? Consider the following:

■ Why should I hire you?
■ What kind of employee will you be?
■ Will you get things done?
■ How much will you cost the company?
■ How long will you stay?
■ What have you not told us about your weaknesses?

Answering Questions

The interviewer may ask background questions, professional questions, and personal questions. If you are especially nervous about interviewing, role-play your interview with a friend or family member acting as the interviewer. Have this person help you evaluate not just what you say but how you say it. Voice inflection, eye contact, and friendliness are demonstrations of your enthusiasm for the position (Costlow, 1999).

Whatever the questions, know your key points and be able to explain in the interview why the company will be glad it hired you, say, 4 years from now. Never criticize your current employer before you leave. Personal and professional integrity will follow you from position to position. Many companies count on personal references when hiring, including those of faculty and administrators from your nursing program. When leaving positions you held during school or on graduating from your program, it is wise not to take parting shots at someone. Doing a professional program evaluation is fine, but "taking cheap shots" at faculty or other employees is unacceptable (Costlow, 1999).

Background Questions

Background questions usually relate to information on your résumé. If you have no nursing experience, relate your prior school and work experience and other accomplishments in relevant ways to the position you are seeking without going through your entire autobiography with the interviewer. You may be asked to expand on the information in your résumé about your formal nursing education. Here is your opportunity to relate specific courses or clinical experiences you enjoyed, academic honors you received, and extracurricular activities or research projects you pursued. The background questions are an invitation for employers to get to know you. Be careful not to appear inconsistent with this information and what you say later.

Professional Questions

Many recruiters are looking for specifics, especially those related to skills and knowledge needed in the position available. They may start with questions related to your education, career goals, strengths, weaknesses, nursing philosophy, style, and abilities. Interviewers often open their questioning with phrases such as "review," "tell me," "explain," and "describe," followed by "How did you do it?" or "Why did you do it that way?" (Mascolini & Supnick, 1993). How successful will you be with these types of questions?

When answering "how would you describe" questions, it is especially important that you remain specific. Cite your own experiences, and relate these behaviors to a demonstrated skill or strength. Examples of questions in this area include the following (Bischof, 1993):

■ **What is your philosophy of nursing?** This question is asked frequently. Your response should relate to the position you are seeking.
■ **What is your greatest weakness? Your greatest strength?** Do not be afraid to present a weakness, but present it to your best advantage, making it sound like a desirable characteristic. Even better, discuss a weakness that is already apparent, such as lack of nursing experience, stating that you recognize your lack of nursing experience but that your own work or management experience has taught you skills that will assist you in this position. These skills might include organization, time management, team spirit, and communication.

If you are asked for both strengths and weaknesses, start with your weaknesses and end on a positive note with your strengths. Do not be too modest, but do not exaggerate. Relate your strengths to the prospective position. Skills such as interpersonal relationships, organization, and leadership are usually broad enough to fit most positions.

■ **Where do you see yourself in 5 years?** Most interviewers want to gain insight into your long-term goals as well as some idea whether you are likely to use this position as a brief stop on the path to another job. It is helpful for you to know some of the history regarding the position. For example, how long have others usually remained in that job? Your career planning should be consistent with the organization's needs.

■ **What are your educational goals?** Be honest and specific. Include both professional education, such as RN or bachelor of science in nursing, and continuing education courses. If you want to pursue further education in related areas, such as a foreign language or computers, include this as a goal. Indicate schools to which you have applied or in which you are already enrolled.

■ **Describe your leadership style.** Be prepared to discuss your style in terms of how effectively you work with others, and give examples of how you have implemented your leadership in the past.

■ **What can you contribute to this position? What unique skill set do you offer?** Review your SWOT analysis as well as the job description for the position before the interview. Be specific in relating your contributions to the position. Emphasize your accomplishments. Be specific and convey that, even as a new graduate, you are unique.

■ **What are your salary requirements?** You may be asked about a minimum salary range. Try to find out the prospective employer's salary range before this question comes up. Be honest about your expectations but make it clear that you are willing to negotiate.

■ **What-if questions.** Prospective employers are increasingly using competency-based interview questions to determine people's preparation for a job. There is often no single correct answer

to these questions. The interviewer may be assessing your clinical decision-making and leadership skills. Again, be concise and specific, aligning your answer with the organizational philosophy and goals. If you do not know the answer, tell the interviewer how you would go about finding the answer. You cannot be expected to have all the answers before you begin a job, but you can be expected to know how to obtain answers once you are in the position.

Personal Questions

Personal questions deal with your personality and motivation. Common questions include the following:

■ **How would you describe yourself?** This is a standard question. Most people find it helpful to think about an answer in advance. You can repeat some of what you said in your résumé and cover letter, but do not provide an in-depth analysis of your personality.

■ **How would your peers describe you?** Ask them. Again, be brief, describing several strengths. Do not discuss your weaknesses unless you are asked about them.

■ **What would make you happy with this position?** Be prepared to discuss your needs related to your work environment. Do you enjoy self-direction, flexible hours, and strong leadership support? Now is the time to cite specifics related to your ideal work environment.

■ **Describe your ideal work environment.** Give this question some thought before the interview. Be specific but realistic. If the norm in your community is two RNs to a floor with licensed practical nurses and other ancillary support, do not say that you believe a staff consisting only of RNs is needed for good patient care.

■ **Describe hobbies, community activities, and recreation.** Again, brevity is important. Many times this question is used to further observe the interviewee's communication and interpersonal skills.

Never pretend to be someone other than who you are. If pretending is necessary to obtain the position, then the position is not right for you.

Additional Points About the Interview

Federal, state, and local laws govern employment-related questions. Questions asked on the job application and in the interview must be related to the position advertised. Questions or statements that may lead to discrimination on the basis of age, gender, race, color, religion, or ethnicity are illegal. If you are asked a question that appears to be illegal, you may wish to take one of several approaches:

■ You may answer the question, realizing that it is not a job-related question. Make it clear to the interviewer that you will answer the question even though you know it is not job-related.
■ You may refuse to answer. You are within your rights but may be seen as uncooperative or confrontational.
■ Examine the intent of the question and relate it to the job.

Just as important as the verbal exchanges of the interview are the nonverbal aspects. These include appearance, handshake, eye contact, posture, and listening skills.

Appearance

Dress in business attire. For women, a skirted suit, pants suit, or tailored jacket dress is appropriate. Men should wear a classic suit, light-colored shirt, and conservative tie. For both men and women, gray or navy blue clothing is rarely wrong. Shoes should be polished, with appropriate heels. Nails and hair for both men and women should reflect cleanliness, good grooming, and willingness to work. The 2-inch red dagger nails worn on prom night will not support an image of the professional nurse. In many institutions, even clear, acrylic nails are not allowed. Paint stains on the hands from a weekend of house maintenance are equally unsuitable for presenting a professional image.

Handshake

Arrive at the interview 10 minutes before your scheduled time. (Allow yourself extra time to find the place if you have not previously been there.) Introduce yourself courteously to the receptionist. Stand when your name is called, smile, and shake hands firmly. If you perspire easily, wipe your palms just before handshake time.

Eye Contact

During the interview, use the interviewer's title and last name as you speak. Never use the interviewer's first name unless specifically requested to do so. Use good listening skills (all those leadership skills you have learned). Smile and nod occasionally, making frequent eye contact. Do not fold your arms across your chest, but keep your hands at your sides or in your lap. Pay attention, and sound sure of yourself.

Posture and Listening Skills

Phrase your questions appropriately and relate them to yourself as a candidate: "What would be my responsibility?" instead of "What are the responsibilities of the job?" Use appropriate grammar and diction. Words or phrases such as "yeah," "uh-huh," "uh," "you know," or "like" are too casual for an interview.

Do not say "I guess" or "I feel" about anything. These words make you sound indecisive. Remember your action verbs—I analyzed, organized, developed. Do not evaluate your achievements as mediocre or unimpressive.

Asking Questions

At some point in the interview, you will be asked if you have any questions. Knowing what questions you want to ask is just as important as having prepared answers for the interviewer's questions. The interview is as much a time for you to learn the details of the job as it is for your potential employer to find out about you. You will need to obtain specific information about the job, including the type of patients for whom you would care, the people with whom you would work, the salary and benefits, and your potential employer's expectations of you. Be prepared for the interviewer to say, "Is there anything else I can tell you about the job?" Jot down a few questions on an index card before going for the interview. You may want to ask a few questions based on your research, demonstrating knowledge about and interest in the company. In addition, you may want to ask questions similar to the ones listed next. Above all, be honest and sincere (Bhasin, 1998; Bischof, 1993; Johnson, 1999).

■ What is this position's key responsibility?
■ What kind of person are you looking for?
■ What are the challenges of the position?

- Why is this position open?
- To whom would I report directly?
- Why did the previous person leave this position?
- What is the salary for this position?
- What are the opportunities for advancement?
- What kind of opportunities are there for continuing education?
- What are your expectations of me as an employee?
- How, when, and by whom are evaluations done?
- What other opportunities for professional growth are available here?
- How are promotion and advancement handled within the organization?

The following are a few additional tips about asking questions during a job interview:

- *Do not* begin with questions about vacations, benefits, or sick time. This gives the impression that these are the most important part of the job to you, rather than the work itself.
- *Do* begin with questions about the employer's expectations of you. This gives the impression that you want to know how you can contribute to the organization.
- *Do* be sure you know enough about the position to make a reasonable decision about accepting an offer if one is made.

- *Do* ask questions about the organization as a whole. The information is useful to you and demonstrates that you are able to see the big picture.
- *Do* bring a list of important points to discuss as an aid to you if you are nervous.

During the interview process, there are a few red flags to be alert for (Tyler, 1990):

- Much turnover in the position
- A newly created position without a clear purpose
- An organization in transition
- A position that is not feasible for a new graduate
- A "gut feeling" that things are not what they seem

The exchange of information between you and the interviewer will go more smoothly if you review Box 12-2 before the interview.

After the Interview

If the interviewer does not offer the information, ask about the next step in the process. Thank the interviewer, shake hands, and exit. If the receptionist is still there, you may quickly smile and say thank you and good-bye. Do not linger and chat, and do not forget to send your thank-you letter.

---

box 12-2

Do's and Don'ts for Interviewing

Do:
Shake the interviewer's hand firmly, and introduce yourself.
Know the interviewer's name in advance, and use it in conversation.
Remain standing until invited to sit.
Use eye contact.
Let the interviewer take the lead in the conversation.
Talk in specific terms, relating everything to the position.
Support responses in terms of personal experience and specific examples.
Make connections for the interviewer. Relate your responses to the needs of the individual organization.
Show interest in the facility.
Ask questions about the position and the facility.

Come across as sincere in your goals and committed to the profession.
Indicate a willingness to start at the bottom.
Take any examinations requested.
Express your appreciation for the time.

Do Not:
Place your purse, briefcase, papers, etc., on the interviewer's desk. Keep them in your lap or on the floor.
Slouch in the chair.
Play with your clothing, jewelry, or hair.
Chew gum or smoke, even if the interviewer does.
Be evasive, interrupt, brag, or mumble.
Gossip about or criticize former agencies, schools, or employees.

Adapted from Bischof, J. (1993). Preparing for job interview questions. Critical Care Nurse, 13(4), 97–100; Krannich, C., & Krannich, R. (1993). Interview for success. New York: Impact Publications; Mascolini, M., & Supnick, R. (1993). Preparing students for the behavioral job interview. Journal of Business and Technical Communication, 7(4), 482–488; and Zedlitz, R. (2003). How to get a job in health care. New York: Delmar Learning.

The Second Interview

Being invited for a second interview means that the first interview went well and that you made a favorable impression. Second visits may include a tour of the facility and meetings with a higher-level executive or a supervisor in the department in which the job opening exists and perhaps several colleagues. In preparation for the second interview, review the information about the organization and your own strengths. It does not hurt to have a few résumés and potential references available. Pointers to make your second visit successful include the following (Knight, 2005; Muha & Orgiefsky, 1994):

- Dress professionally. Do not wear "trendy" outfits, sandals, or open-toed shoes. Minimize jewelry and makeup.
- Be professional and pleasant with everyone, including administrative assistants and housekeeping and maintenance personnel.
- Do not smoke.
- Remember your manners.
- Avoid controversial topics for small talk.
- Obtain answers to questions you might have considered since your first visit.

In most instances, the personnel director or nurse manager will let you know how long it will be before you are contacted again. It is appropriate to ask for this information before you leave the second interview. If you do receive an offer during this visit, graciously say "thank you" and ask for a little time to consider the offer (even if this is the offer you have anxiously been awaiting).

If the organization does not contact you by the expected date, do not panic. It is appropriate to call your contact person, state your continued interest, and tactfully express the need to know the status of your application so that you can respond to other deadlines.

Making the Right Choice

You have interviewed well, and now you have to decide among several job offers. Your choice will not only affect your immediate work but also influence your future career opportunities. The nursing shortage has led to greatly enhanced workplace enrichment programs and nurse residencies as a recruitment and retention strategy. Career ladders, shared governance, participatory management, staff nurse presence on major hospital committees, decentralization of operations, and a focus on quality interpersonal relationships are among some of these features. Be sure to inquire about the components of the professional practice environment (Joel, 2003). There are several additional factors to consider.

Job Content

The immediate work you will be doing should be a good match with your skills and interests. Although your work may be personally challenging and satisfying this year, what are the opportunities for growth? How will your desire for continued growth and challenge be satisfied?

Development

You should have learned from your interviews whether your initial training and orientation seem sufficient. Inquire about continuing education to keep you current in your field. Is tuition reimbursement available for further education? Is management training provided, or are supervisory skills learned on the job?

Direction

Good supervision and mentors are especially important in your first position. You may be able to judge prospective supervisors throughout the interview process, but you should also try to get a broader view of the overall philosophy of supervision. You may not be working for the same supervisor in a year, but the overall management philosophy is likely to remain consistent.

Work Climate

The daily work climate must make you feel comfortable. Your preference may be formal or casual, structured or unstructured, complex or simple. It is easy to observe the way people dress, the layout of the unit, and lines of communication. It is more difficult to observe company values, factors that will affect your work comfort and satisfaction over the long term. Try to look beyond the work environment to get an idea of values. What is the unwritten message? Is there an open-door policy sending a message that "everyone is equal and important," or does the nurse manager appear too busy to be concerned with the needs of the employees? Is your supervisor the kind of person for whom you could work easily?

Compensation

In evaluating the compensation package, starting salary should be less important than the organization's philosophy on future compensation. What is the potential for salary growth? How are individual increases determined? Can you live on the wages being offered? Also review the organization's package regarding retirement and health insurance.

I Cannot Find a Job (or I Moved)

It is often said that finding the first job is the hardest. Many employers prefer to hire seasoned nurses who do not require a long orientation and mentoring, particularly in specialty areas. Some require new graduates to do postgraduate internships. Changes in skill mix with the implementation of various types of care delivery influence the market for the professional nurse. The new graduate may need to be armed with a variety of skills, such as intravenous certification, home assessment, advanced rehabilitation skills, and various respiratory modalities, to even warrant an initial interview. Keep informed about the demands of the market in your area, and be prepared to be flexible in seeking your first position. Even with the continuing nursing shortage, hiring you as a new graduate will depend on you selling yourself.

After all this searching and hard work, you still may not have found the position you want. You may be focusing on work arrangements or benefits rather than on the job description. Your lack of direction may come through in your résumé, cover letter, and personal presentation. As a new graduate, you may also have unrealistic expectations or be trying to cut corners, ignoring the basic rules of marketing yourself discussed in this chapter. Go back to your SWOT analysis. Take another look at your résumé and cover letter. Become more assertive as you start again.

The Critical First Year

Why a section on the "first year"? Working hard is important; however, some of the behaviors that were rewarded in school are not rewarded on the job. There are no syllabi, study questions, or extra-credit points. Only As are acceptable, and there do not appear to be many completely correct answers. Quality is the expectation with little room for error. Discovering this has been called "reality shock" (Kramer, 1974). Voluminous concept maps and meticulous medication cards are out; multiple responsibilities and thinking on your feet are in. What is the new graduate to do?

Your first year will be a transition year. You are no longer a college student. You are a novice nurse. You are "the new kid on the block," and people will respond to you differently and judge you differently than when you were a student. To be successful, you have to respond differently. You may be thinking, "Oh, they always need nurses—it doesn't matter." Yes, it does matter. Many of your career opportunities will be influenced by the early impressions you make. The following section addresses what you can do to help ensure first-year success.

Attitude and Expectations

Adopt the right attitudes, and adjust your expectations. Now is the time to learn the art of being new. You felt like the most important, special person during the recruitment process. Now, in the real world, neither you nor the position may be as glamorous as you once thought. In addition, although you thought you learned much in school, your decisions and daily performance do not always warrant an A. Above all, people shed the company manners they displayed when you were interviewing, and organizational politics eventually surface. Your leadership skills and commitment to teamwork will get you through this transition period.

Impressions and Relationships

Manage a good impression, and build effective relationships. Remember, you are being watched: by peers, subordinates, and superiors. Because you as yet have no track record, first impressions are magnified. Although every organization is different, most are looking for someone with good judgment, a willingness to learn, a readiness to adapt, and a respect for the expertise of more experienced employees. Most people expect you to "pay your dues" to earn respect from them.

Organizational Savvy

Develop organizational savvy. An important person in this first year is your immediate supervisor. Support this person. Find out what is important to your supervisor and what he or she needs and expects from the team. Become a team player.

When confronted with an issue, present solutions, not problems, as often as you can. You want to be a good leader someday; learn first to be a good follower. Finding a mentor is another important goal of your first year. Mentors are role models and guides who encourage, counsel, teach, and advocate for their mentee. In these relationships, both the mentor and mentee receive support and encouragement (Klein & Dickenson-Hazard, 2000).

The spark that ignites a mentoring relationship may come from either the protégé or the mentor. Protégés often view mentors as founts of success, a bastion of life skills they wish to learn and emulate. Mentors often see the future that is hidden in another's personality and abilities (Klein & Dickenson-Hazard, 2000, pp. 20–21).

Skills and Knowledge

Master the skills and knowledge of the position. Technology is constantly changing, and contrary to popular belief, you did not learn everything in school. Be prepared to seek out new knowledge and skills on your own. This may entail extra hours of preparation and study, but no one ever said learning stops after graduation. Lifelong learning is key to being a successful nurse.

Advancing Your Career

Many of the ideas presented in this chapter will continue to be helpful as you advance in your nursing career. Continuing to develop your leadership and patient care skills through practice, and further education will be the keys to your professional growth. The RN is expected to develop and provide leadership to other members of the healthcare team while providing safe, effective, and quality care to patients. According to the Health Resources and Services Administration (HRSA) (2010), the number of licensed RNs in the United States increased to a record high level. This increase reflects a larger number of younger nurses entering the workforce along with older experienced nurses. Getting your first job within this environment due to the increased demand for nurses may not be so difficult, but you hold the responsibility for advancing your career.

Conclusion

Finding your first position is more than being in the right place at the right time. It is a complex combination of learning about yourself and the organizations you are interested in and presenting your strengths and weaknesses in the most positive manner possible. Keeping the first position and using the position to grow and learn are also part of a planning process. Recognize that the independence you enjoyed through college may not be the skill you need to keep your first position. There is an important lesson to be learned: becoming a team player and being savvy about organizational politics are as important as becoming proficient in nursing skills. Take the first step toward finding a mentor—before you know it, you will become one yourself.

Study Questions

1. Using the SWOT analysis worksheet developed for this chapter, how will you articulate your strengths and weaknesses during an interview?

2. Design a one- to two-page résumé to use in seeking your first position. Are you able to "sell yourself" in one or two pages? If not, what adjustments are you going to make? Develop a cover letter, thank-you letter, acceptance letter, and rejection letter that you can use during the interview process.

3. Using the interview preparation worksheet developed for this chapter, formulate responses to the questions. How comfortable do you feel answering these questions? Share your responses with other classmates to get additional ideas.

4. Evaluate the job prospects in the community where you now live. What areas could you explore in seeking your first position?

5. What plans do you have for advancing your career? What plans do you have for finding a mentor?

Case Study to Promote Critical Reasoning

Paul Delane is interviewing for his first nursing position after obtaining his RN license. He has been interviewed by the nurse recruiter and is now being interviewed by the nurse manager on the pediatric floor. After a few minutes of social conversation, the nurse manager begins to ask some specific nursing-oriented questions: How would you respond if a mother of a seriously ill child asks you if her child will die? What attempts do you make to understand different cultural beliefs and their importance in health care when planning nursing care? How does your philosophy of nursing affect your ability to deliver care to children whose mothers are HIV-positive?

Paul is very flustered by these questions and responds with "it depends on the situation," "it depends on the culture," and "I don't ever discriminate."

1. What responses would have been more appropriate in this interview?

2. How could Paul have used these questions to demonstrate his strengths, experiences, and skills?

References

Anderson, J. (1992). Tips on résumé writing. *Imprint, 39*(1), 30–31.

Arvidsson, B., Skarsater, I., Oijervall, J., & Friglund, B. (2008). Process-oriented group supervision during nursing education: Nurses' conception one year after their nursing degree. *Journal of Nursing Management, 16*(7), 868–875.

Banis, W. (1994). The art of writing job-search letters. In College Placement Council, Inc. (ed.), *Planning Job Choices*. Philadelphia: College Placement Council, 44–51.

Beatty, R. (1991). *Get the right job in 60 days or less*. New York: John Wiley & Sons.

Beatty, R. (1989). *The Perfect cover letter*. New York: John Wiley & Sons.

Bhasin, R. (1998). Do's and don'ts of job interviews. *Pulp & Paper, 72*(2), 37.

Bischof, J. (1993). Preparing for job interview questions. *Critical Care Nurse, 13*(4), 97–100.

Cazacu, A. (2010). What are employers looking for in a candidate? Retrieved on October 1, 2013, from http://ezinearticles.com/?What-Are-Employers-Looking-For-in-a-Candidate?&id=4738932

Chestnut, T. (1999). Some tips on taking the fear out of résumé writing. *Phoenix Business Journal, 19*(47), 28.

Christie, I. (2012). Analyze your career with a personal SWOT. Retrieved on October 1, 2013, from http://career-advice.monster.com

Costlow, T. (1999). How not to create a good first impression. *Fairfield County Business Journal, 38*(32), 17.

Ervin, E.E., Bickes, J.T., & Schim, S.M. (2006). Environments of care: A curriculum model for preparing a new generation of nurses. *Journal of Nursing Education, 45*(2). 75–80.

Eubanks, P. (1991). Experts: Making your résumé an asset. *Hospitals, 5*(20), 74.

Goal setting using the SMART acronym (n.d.). Retrieved October 1, 2013, from health.mo.gov/living/families/wic/wicupdates/. . ./GoalSetting-SMART.doc

Hart, K. (2006). Student extra: The employment interview: Tips for success selecting an employer for the perfect fit. *American Journal of Nursing, 106*(4), 72AAA–72CCC.

Health Resources and Services Administration. (HRSA). (2010). HRSA study finds nursing workforce is growing. Retrieved on October 1, 2013, from www.hrsa.gov/about/news/pressreleases/2010/100922/nursingworkforce

Impollonia, M. (2004), How to impress nursing recruiters to get the job you want. *Imprint*, March.

Institute of Medicine. (2001). Crossing the quality chasm: A new health system for the 21st century. National Academies Press.

Jackson, D., Firtko, A., & Edinborough, M. (2007). Personal resilience as a strategy for surviving and thriving in the face of workplace diversity: A literature review. *Journal of Advanced Nursing, 60*(1), 1–9.

James, L. (2003). Vitae statistics. *Travel Weekly, 1695*, 70.

Job Hunt: The online job search guide. Retrieved October 1, 2013, from www.job-hunt.org/

Joel, L. (2003). The role of the workplace in your transition from student to nurse. *Imprint*, April.

Johnson, K. (1999). Interview success demands research, practice, preparation. *Houston Business Journal, 30*(23), 38.

Klein, E., & Dickenson-Hazard, N. (2000). The spirit of mentoring. *Reflections on Nursing Leadership, 26*(3), 18–22.

Kluemper, D.H. (2009) Future employment selection methods: Evaluating social networking web sites. *Journal of Managerial Psycholog,*. 24(6), 567–580.

Knight, K. (2005). New grad? Be prepared to look great. *Imprint*, January.

Kramer, M. (1974). *Reality shock: Why nurses leave nursing*. St. Louis: C.V. Mosby.

Krannich, C., & Krannich, R. (1993). *Interview for success*. New York: Impact Publications.

Korkki, P. (2010). Writing a résumé that shouts 'Hire Me.' *New York Times*. February 27, 2010.

Marino, K. (2000). *Resumes for the health care professional*. New York: John Wiley & Sons.

Mascolini, M., & Supnick, R. (1993). Preparing students for the behavioral job interview. *Journal of Business and Technical Communication, 7*(4), 482–488.

Morgan, H. (2013). The 8 new rules of a career survivalist. *U.S. News and World Report*, June 26, 2013. Retrieved October 1, 2013, from http://money.usnews.com/money/blogs/outside-voices-careers/2013/06/26/the-8-new-rules-of-a-career-survivalist

Muha, D., & Orgiefsky, R. (1994). The 2nd interview: The plant or office visit. In College placement council, inc. (ed.), *Planning Job Choices*. Philadelphia: College Placement Council, 58–60.

Parker, Y. (1989). *The damn good résumé guide*. Berkeley, CA: Ten Speed Press.

Schoessler, M., & Waldo, M. (2006). The first 18 months in practice: A development transition model for the newly graduated nurse. *Journal of Nurses in Staff Development, 22*(2), 47–52.

Tyler, L. (1990). Watch out for "red flags" on a job interview. *Hospitals, 64*(14), 46–47.

Zedlitz, R. (2003). *How to get a job in health care*. New York: Delmar Learning.

chapter 13

Evolution of Nursing as a Profession

Introduction

It is often said that you do not know where you are going until you know where you have been. Over 40 years ago, Beletz (1974) wrote that most people thought of nurses in gender-linked, task-oriented terms: "a female who performs unpleasant technical jobs and functions as an assistant to the physician" (p. 432). Interestingly, physicians in the 1800s viewed nursing as a complement to medicine. According to Warrington (1839), ". . . the prescriptions of the best physician are useless unless they be timely and properly administered and attended to by the nurse" (p. iv).

In its earliest years, most nursing care occurred at home. Even in 1791 when the first hospital opened in Philadelphia, nurses continued to care for patients in their own home settings. It took almost another century before nursing moved into hospitals. These institutions, mostly dominated by male physicians, promoted the idea that nurses acted as the "handmaidens" to the better educated, more capable men in the medical field.

The level of care differed greatly in these early health-care institutions. Those operated by the religious nursing orders gave high-quality care to patients. In others, care varied greatly from good to almost none at all. Although the image of nurses and nursing has advanced considerably since then, some still think of nurses as helpers who carry out the physician's orders.

Throughout its history, the nursing profession provided many great leaders who participated in social change and health-care reform. These nurse leaders initiated change within the social environment of the time, using the strategies of change and conflict resolution discussed earlier in the text.

It comes as no surprise that nursing and health care have converged and reached a crossing point. Nurses face a new age for human experience; the very foundations of health practices and therapeutic interventions continue to be dramatically altered by significantly transformed scientific, technological, cultural, political, and social realities (Porter-O'Grady, 2003). The global environment needs nurses more than ever to meet the health-care needs of all. This chapter discusses nurse leaders of the past and present and how nursing itself has changed. Chapter 14 discusses changes to the overall health-care system and their implications for nurses.

Nursing Defined

The changes that have occurred in nursing are reflected in the definitions of nursing that have developed over time. In 1859, Florence Nightingale defined the goal of nursing as putting the client "in the best possible condition for nature to act upon him" (Nightingale, 1859, p. 79). In 1966, Virginia Henderson focused her definition on the uniqueness of nursing:

> *The unique function of the nurse is to assist the individual, sick or well, in the performance of those activities contributing to health or its recovery (or to peaceful death) that he would perform unaided if he had the necessary strength, will or knowledge. And to do this in such a way as to help him gain independence as rapidly as possible (Henderson, 1966, p. 21).*

Martha Rogers defined nursing practice as "the process by which this body of knowledge, nursing science, is used for the purpose of assisting human beings to achieve maximum health within the potential of each person" (Rogers, 1988, p. 100). Rogers emphasized that nursing is concerned with *all* people, only some of whom are ill.

In the modern nursing era, nurses are viewed as collaborative members of the health-care team. Nursing has emerged as a strong field of its own in which nurses have a wide range of obligations, responsibilities, and accountability. Recent polls show that nurses are considered the most trusted group of professionals because of their knowledge, expertise, and ability to care for diverse populations.

Early and Modern Nurse Leaders

The 19th and 20th Centuries

Florence Nightingale, immortalized by Henry Wadsworth Longfellow in his poem *The Lady with the Lamp* (Longfellow, 1868), remains the best known of the historic nursing leaders and is considered the founder of modern nursing. Nightingale brought about changes in the care of soldiers, the keeping of hospital records, the status of nurses, and even the profession itself. On her return home after the Crimean War she had two goals: to reform military health care and to establish an official training school for nurses. The British public contributed more than $220,000 (a great sum of money at that time) to the Nightingale Fund for the purpose of establishing the school.

Nightingale's concepts of nursing care became the basis of modern theory development and, in today's language, used evidence-based practice to promote nursing. Her book *Notes on Nursing: What It Is and What It Is Not* laid the foundation for modern nursing education and practice. Many nursing theorists have used Nightingale's thoughts as a basis for constructing their view of nursing.

Nightingale believed that schools of nursing must be independent institutions and that women who were selected to attend the schools should be from the higher levels of society. Many of Nightingale's beliefs about nursing education are still applicable, particularly those involved with the progress of students, the use of diaries kept by students, and the need for integrating theory into clinical practice (Roberts, 1937).

The Nightingale school served as a model for nursing education. Its graduates were sought worldwide. Many of them established schools and became matrons (superintendents) in hospitals in other parts of England, the British Commonwealth, and the United States. However, very few schools were able to remain financially independent of the hospitals and thus lost much of their autonomy. This was in contradiction to Nightingale's philosophy that the training schools were educational institutions, not part of any service agency.

Other well-known nurse leaders include the following people:

Lillian Wald, who founded the Henry Street Settlement, provided a role model for contemporary community health nursing. She developed a system for bringing health care back to people within their homes, schools, and neighborhoods. She focused on health teaching and health promotion for families, particularly women and children.

Wald and her colleagues brought basic nursing care to the people in their home environment. These nurses were independent practitioners who made their own decisions and followed up on their own assessments of families' needs. Like Nightingale, they were very aware of the effect of the environment on the health of their clients and worked hard to improve their clients' surroundings.

Wald was convinced that many illnesses resulted from causes outside individual control and that treatment needed to be holistic. She said she chose the title *public health nurse* to emphasize the value of the nurse whose work was built on an understanding of the social and economic problems that inevitably accompanied the clients' ills (Bueheler-Wilkerson, 1993). The success of the nurses of the

Henry Street Settlement laid the groundwork for school nurses placed in the New York City school system (www.henrystreet.org/about/history/).

Margaret Sanger, a political activist like many of the others, is best known for her courageous fight to make birth control information available to everyone who needed or wanted it. She had a tremendous impact on contemporary society. Through enabling women to control their fertility and giving them access to contraception, as advocated by Sanger, it is possible for women to have a broader set of life options, particularly in the areas of education and employment (Malveaux, 2013).

Sanger was very concerned about the working conditions faced by people living in poverty. Her fight to make Congress aware of the plight of children in the labor force is less well known but led to important changes in the child labor laws. A major strike of industrial workers in Lawrence, Massachusetts, marked the beginning of Sanger's career as an advocate and social reformer. The workers had previously attempted a strike for better conditions, but they conceded because of threatening starvation. If the workers went on strike, then there was no money for food. Strike sympathizers in New York offered to help the workers and to take the children from Lawrence into their homes. Because of her interest in the situation of the underpaid workers and her involvement with New York laborers, Sanger was asked to assist in the evacuation of children from the unsettled and sometimes violent conditions in Lawrence. Following an outbreak of serious rioting, she was called to Washington to testify before the House Committee on Rules about the children's condition. She testified that the children were poorly nourished, ill, ragged, and living in conditions worse than those in impoverished city slums.

Two months later, the owners of the mills sat down to talk with the workers and gave in to their demands. Sanger's interventions on behalf of children had brought the workers' plight to the attention of the general public and to people in Washington. Sanger may have been the first nurse lobbyist.

Mary Eliza Mahoney was the first African-American registered nurse (RN) in the United States. Her professional attitude helped to change the status of black nurses in this country. In 1878, at the age of 33, she applied to the hospital's nursing program and was accepted as a student. She spent her training days washing, ironing, and cleaning, expected competencies of that time. Sixteen months later, of the 43 students who began the rigorous course, Mahoney and four white students were the only ones who completed it.

Mahoney recognized the need for nurses to work together to advance the status of black nurses within the profession. In 1896 Mahoney became one of the original members of the predominately white Nurses Associated Alumnae of the United States and Canada (later known as the American Nurses Association [ANA]). She cofounded the National Association of Colored Graduate Nurses (NACGN). Mahoney delivered the welcoming speech at the first convention of the NACGN and served as its national chaplain.

Mildred Montag is attributed with developing the associate degree in nursing. In her dissertation, "The Education of Nursing Technicians," Montage suggested two levels of nursing. The technical nurse could be educated in 2 years. World War II created a nursing shortage which was then compounded by the Korean War. At the time it took a minimum of 3 to 4 years to educate a nurse. Her dissertation described a shorter nursing education program that would provide a sound base for students and help alleviate the nursing shortage plaguing the nation (Boyd, 2011).

The associate degree program proved successful because it attracted a wide range of nontraditional students, including men, married people, and minorities, who could financially afford this academic option. Associate degree nursing education has had a profound effect on nursing education. Montag's achievement also advanced the shift of nursing education from the hospital to institutions of higher learning. It should be noted that Montag did not see the associated degree as a replacement for baccalaureate nursing degrees.

Virginia Henderson has often been considered a 20th-century Florence Nightingale. Ms. Henderson was an early advocate of autonomy for nurses and the importance of nursing scholarship. She wrote the nursing fundamentals textbook most commonly used by nurse educators throughout the country for most of the last century. Virginia Henderson's most important publication, *Principles and Practice of Nursing,* is considered the 20th century's equivalent to Nightingale's *Notes on Nursing.* Nightingale had emphasized nature as the primary healer but, with the advent of antibiotic therapy and other technological advances, this approach needed expansion (Henderson, 1955).

Henderson's beginnings were in public health, and this influenced her definition of nursing. Because of this background, Henderson was a proponent of publicly financed, universally accessible health-care services. She understood that nurses maintained roots in the communities where they lived, and she believed that nursing belonged in the forefront of health-care reform. She also believed that nurses should take every opportunity to advance the profession by becoming leaders in developing plans for implementing accessible health care.

Nurse Leaders in the 21st Century

Linda Aiken

The 21st century also boasts several nurse leaders who have brought the need for change to the attention of the public. Dr. Linda Aiken is one of the nation's most influential nurse leaders in health care. She holds the title of Director of the Center for Health Outcomes and Policy Research, and is the Claire M. Fagin Leadership Professor of Nursing and Professor of Sociology at the University of Pennsylvania.

Dr. Aiken has made major contributions to studies of health-care workers and outcomes research (Aiken et al., 2002; Kelly, McHugh, & Aiken 2011). She is recognized for pioneering research using statistical data to link nurse-to-patient ratios and patient safety. Her influential work also includes the development of magnet hospitals across the nation. She directed a multistate study of nursing care and patient safety in the field. The study offered important information linking nursing practice and patient outcomes in hospitals, nursing homes, and home care, in addition to providing information on why some nurses choose to leave nursing.

Dr. Aiken's research on quality and safety in health care extends beyond the borders of this country and into the global health-care system. She co-directs RN4CAST, a study of the nursing workforce and quality of hospital care in 14 countries in Europe, China, South Africa, and Botswana. She serves as an advisory for the China Medical Board (www.researchamerica.org/bio_aiken).

Dr. Beverly Malone

Another prominent nurse leader is Dr. Beverly Malone. In the year 2000, Dr. Malone became deputy assistant secretary for health within the U.S. Department of Health and Human Services, the highest position so far held by any nurse in the U.S. government. In 2007, she assumed the role of chief executive officer of the National League for Nursing.

Dr. Malone is "among America's most vocal leaders in the national conversations concerning nursing, the nurse educator shortage, and the role of nursing in ensuring access to safe, quality, culturally competent care to diverse patient populations, domestically and globally" (NLN, 2012). She saw a need for change in nursing education and continues to work toward restructuring nursing curricula and entry into practice, and advancing nursing's role within this health-care environment.

Dr. Tim Porter-O'Grady

Dr. Tim Porter-O'Grady has also contributed greatly to nursing and health care. Currently the senior partner of Tim Porter-O'Grady Associates, an international health consulting practice, he has served in many positions from clinical provider to both hospital and health service executive in a variety of health services and is a principal in an international health consulting practice.

Dr. Porter-O'Grady's work in health systems' futures, governance, leadership, and conflict issues has contributed to changes in practice and nursing education. Most of his effort continues to focus on health systems innovation and creativity as applied to the design and delivery of health services. He is considered an expert on health futures and innovative health service models. Dr. Porter-O'Grady has a strong commitment to building healthy communities and facilitating the partnerships necessary to sustain them. His most prominent contributions have been in the area of shared governance, which helps nurses oversee and regulate the practice of nursing, and challenges traditional behaviors and roles (Dashnaw, 2010).

The previous paragraphs named a few prominent nurse leaders in the early part of the 21st century. Nurse leaders come in the form of teachers, chief nursing officers, and nurses who deliver direct patient care. They are members of the profession who think outside the box, embrace change, and contribute to the health and well-being of the community.

Political Influences and the Advance of Nursing as a Profession

Nursing made many advances during the time of social upheaval and change. The passing of the Social Security Act in 1935 strengthened public health services. Public health nursing found itself in an ideal position to step up and assume responsibility for providing care to dependent mothers and children, the blind, and disabled children (Black, 2014). In 1965, under President Lyndon B. Johnson, amendments to the Social Security Act designed to ensure access to health care for the elder adult, the poor, and the disabled resulted in the creation of Medicare and Medicaid (CMS, 2013). Health insurance companies emerged and increased in number during this time as well. Hospitals started to rely on Medicare, Medicaid, and insurance reimbursement for services. Care for the sick and new opportunities and roles emerged for nurses within this environment.

Historically, nursing has made most of its advances during times of social change. The 1960s through the 1980s brought many changes for both women and nursing. In 1964, President Johnson signed the Civil Rights Act, which guaranteed equal treatment for all individuals and prohibited gender discrimination in the workplace. However, the law lacked enforcement. During this time the feminist movement gained momentum and the National Organization for Women was founded to help women achieve equality and give women a voice. Nursing moved forward as well. Specialty care disciplines developed. Advances in technology gave way to the more complex medical–surgical treatments such as cardiothoracic surgery, complex neurosurgical techniques, and the emergence of intensive care environments to care for these patients. These changes fostered the development of specialization for nurses and physicians, creating a shortage of primary care physicians. The public demanded increased access to health care, and nursing again stepped forward by developing an advanced practice role for nurses to meet the primary health-care needs of the public.

Throughout the years, wars created situations that facilitated changes in nursing and its role within society. Wars increase the nation's need for nurses and the public's awareness of nursing's role in society (Kalisch & Kalisch, 2004). Nurses served in the military during both world wars and the Korean War. The Korean War changed nursing practice during the time of war. For the first time, nurses were close to the front and worked in mobile hospital units. Often they lacked necessary supplies and equipment (Kalisch & Kalisch, 2004). They found themselves in situations where they needed to function independently and make immediate decisions, often assuming roles normally associated with the physicians and surgeons.

The Vietnam War afforded nurses opportunities to push beyond the boundaries as they functioned in mobile hospital units in the war theater, often without direct supervision of physicians. These nurses performed emergency procedures such as tracheostomies and chest tube insertions in order to preserve the lives of the wounded soldiers (www.vietnam.ttu.edu/exhibits/nurses/). After functioning independently in the field, many nurses felt restricted by the practice limits placed on them when they returned home.

Challenges for society and nurses continued from the 1980s through 2000. The 1980s were marked by the emergence of the human immunodeficiency virus (HIV) and acquired immunodeficiency syndrome (AIDS). Although we know more about HIV/AIDs today than we knew more than 30 years ago, society's fear of the disease stigmatized groups of individuals and created fear among global populations and health-care providers. Nurses became instrumental in educating the public and working directly with infected individuals.

The increase in available technology allowed for the widespread use of life support systems. Nurses working in critical care areas often faced ethical dilemmas involving the use of these technologies. During this time period, nurses voiced their opinions and concerns and helped in formulating policies addressing these issues within their communities and institutions. The field of hospice nursing received a renewed interest and support (www.nhpco.org/history-hospice-care). The number of hospice care providers grew and opened new opportunities for nurses.

The first part of the 21st century introduced nurses to situations beyond anyone's imagination. Nursing's response to the attack on the World Trade Center and during the onset and aftermath of Hurricane Katrina raised multiple questions regarding nurses' abilities to react to major disasters. Nurses, physicians, and other health-care providers attempted to care for and protect patients under horrific conditions. Nurses found themselves trying to function "during unfamiliar and unusual conditions with the health care environment that may necessitate adaptations to recognized standards of nursing practice" (ANA, 2006).

Nursing has recognized the need for the profession to understand and function during human-caused and natural disasters such as 9/11 and hurricanes. The profession has answered the call by increasing disaster preparedness training for nurses.

Nursing and Health Care Reform

For more than 40 years, Florence Nightingale played an influential part in most of the important health-care reforms of her time. Her accomplishments went beyond the scope of nursing and nursing education, affecting all aspects of health-care and social reform.

Nightingale contributed to health-care reform through her work during the Crimean War, where she greatly improved the health and well-being of the British soldiers. She kept accurate records and accountings of her interventions and outcomes, and on her return to England she continued this work and reformed the conditions in hospitals and health care.

Lillian Wald and the Henry Street Settlement demonstrated nursing's commitment to social justice and that health care is a right for all, not just a privilege for some. These nurses provided health teaching and services to the poor and immigrants who came to America in search of better lives. Their commitment to this endeavor provided the impetus for school nursing and health promotion and disease prevention.

The 21st century brings both challenges and opportunities for nursing. It is estimated that more than 434,000 nurses will be needed by the year 2020 (Stokowski, 2004). The severe nursing shortage has increased the demand for more nurses, while the passing of the Affordable Care Act offers opportunities for nurses to take the lead in providing primary health care to those who need it. More advanced practice nurses will be needed to address the needs of the diverse population in this country. Health-care reform is discussed in more detail in Chapter 14.

Nursing Today

Issues specific to nursing reflect the problems and concerns of the health-care system as a whole. The average age of nurses in the United States is 46.8 years, and approximately 40% of the nursing workforce is over 50 (Lillis & O'Brien, 2007; Spiva, Hart, & McVay, 2011). Due to changes in the economy, many nurses who planned to retire have instead found it necessary to remain in the workforce.

Researchers project that more than 80% of nurses aged 40 and older will retire within the next 20 years. Ninety percent of nurses are female, although the number of men is gradually increasing (Dougherty, 2008). Concerns about the supply of RNs and staffing shortages persist in both the United States and abroad. For the first time, multiple generations of nurses find themselves working together within the health-care environment. The oldest of the generations, the early baby boomers, planned to retire over the last several years; however, economics have forced many to remain in the workplace. They presently work alongside Generation X (born between 1965 and 1979) and the generation known as the millennials (born in 1980 and later). Nurses from the baby boomer generation and Generation X provide the majority of bedside care. Where the millennials find themselves comfortable with technology, the baby boomers feel the "old ways" worked well.

Generational issues in the nursing workforce present potential conflicts in the work environment as these generations come with differing viewpoints as they attempt to work together within the health-care environment (Wieck, 2008). Each generation brings its own set of core values to the workplace. In order to be successful and work together as cohesive teams, each generation needs to value the others' skills and perspectives. This requires active and assertive communication, recognizing the individual skill sets of the generations, and placing individuals in positions that fit their specific characteristics.

The related issues of excessive workload, mandatory overtime, scheduling, abuse, workplace violence, and lack of professional autonomy contribute to the concerns regarding the nursing shortage (Villeneuve & MacDonald, 2006). On the bright side, there are also some indications of increasing interest in a nursing career as salaries improve and job opportunities expand.

Health Care in the Future

The changes in health care and the increased need for primary care providers has opened the door for nursing. The Institute of Medicine (IOM) (2010) report specifically stated that nurses should be permitted to practice to the full extent of their education. Nurses are educated to care for individuals who have chronic illnesses and need health teaching and monitoring.

Advance practice nurses (APRNs) are qualified to diagnose and treat certain conditions. These highly educated nurses are more than physician extenders as they sit for board certification examinations and are licensed by the states in which they practice. Educational requirements for APRNs include a minimum of a master's degree in nursing with a clinical focus, and a designated number of clinical hours. Many nurse practitioners are obtaining the Doctor of Nursing Practice (DNP) degree. The American Association of Critical-Care Nurses (AACN) and the National League for Nursing (NLN) both promote this as the terminal degree for nurse practitioners. Areas of advanced practice include family nurse practitioner, acute care nurse practitioner, pediatric nurse practitioner, and certified nurse midwife.

Conclusion

As nursing moves forward in the 21st century, the need for courageous and innovative nurse leaders is greater than ever. Society's demand for high-quality health care at an affordable cost is now law and an impetus for change in how nurses function in the new environment.

Nurses began in hospitals, moved to the community, moved back into the hospitals, and are now seeing a move back to the community. The Affordable Care Act has opened doors for more opportunities for nurses, and the IOM report on the *Future of Nursing* states that nurses need to be permitted to use their educational skills in the health-care environment.

Often students ask the question: "So what can I do? I am a new graduate." Get involved in your profession by joining organizations and becoming politically active. Ask the questions and seek the answers. You will be the Nightingales, Walds, Sangers, Mahoneys, Montags, and Hendersons of the future; the creativity and dedication of these nurses are part of everyone.

Study Questions

1. Read *Notes on Nursing: What It Is and What It Is Not* by Florence Nightingale. How much of its content is still true today?

2. If Margaret Sanger were alive, how do you think she would view the issue of teaching schoolchildren about HIV/AIDS?

3. What do you think Lillian Wald would say about the status of hospitals and health care today?

4. If you were Margaret Sanger, would you have decided to stop teaching women about birth control? Explain your answer.

5. What is your definition of nursing? How does it compare or contrast with Virginia Henderson's definition?

6. Review the mission and purpose of the ANA or another national nursing organization online. Do you believe that nurses should belong to these organizations? Explain your answer.

Case Study #1 to Promote Critical Reasoning

Thomas went to nursing school on a U.S. Public Health Service scholarship. He has been directed to go to a rural village in a small Central American country to work in a local health center. Several other nurses have been sent to this village, and the residents forced them to leave.

The village lacks electricity and plumbing; water comes from in-ground wells. The villagers and children suffer from frequent episodes of gastrointestinal disorders.

1. How do you think Florence Nightingale would have approached these issues?

2. What do you think Thomas should do first to gain the trust of the residents of the village?

3. Explain how advance practice nurses would contribute to the health and welfare of the residents of the village.

Case Study #2 to Promote Critical Reasoning

The younger nurses in your health-care institution have created a petition to change the dress code policy. They feel it is antiquated and rigid. Rather than wearing uniforms or scrubs on the nursing units, they would like to wear more contemporary clothing such as khakis and nice shirts with lab coats. The older generation nurses feel that this will detract from the nursing image, as patients expect nurses to dress in uniforms or scrubs and this is what defines them as a "profession."

1. What are your thoughts regarding the image of nursing and uniforms?

2. Do you feel that uniforms define nurses? Explain your reason.

3. Explain the reasons certain generations may see this as a threat to their professionalism.

4. Which side would you support? Explain your answer with current research.

References

Aiken, L., Clarke, S.P., Sloane, D., Sochalski, J., et al. (2002). Hospital nurse staffing and patient mortality, nurse burnout and job dissatisfaction. *Journal of the American Medical Association, 288*(16), 1987–1993.

American Nurses Association. (2006). Retrieved on October 16, 2007, from www.nursingworld.org/FunctionalMenuCategories/About ANA.aspx

American Nurses Association. (2008a). Health reform: The 2008 elections and beyond. *The American Nurse,* September/October.

American Nurses Association. (2008b). Safe staffing save lives. *The American Nurse,* March/April.

American Nurses Association. (2012). Healthcare transformation the Affordable Care Act and more. Retrieved on October 3, 2013. from www.nursingworld.org/MainMenuCategories/Policy-Advocacy/HealthSystemReform/AffordableCareAct.pdf

Beletz, E. (1974). Is nursing's public image up-to-date? *Nursing Outlook, 22,* 432–435.

Black, B.P. (2014). Professional nursing: Concepts and challenges (7th ed.). Philadelphia: Saunders-Elsevier, Inc.

Boyd, T. (2011). Profile: Mildred Montag. April 29, 2011. Retrieved October 2, 2013. from http://news.nurse.com/article/20110429/NATIONAL02/305020027/-1/frontpage#.UliMRCSr_UQ

Bucheler Williamson. (1993). Bring care to the people: Lillian Wald's legacy to public health nursing. *American Journal of Public Health, 83,* 1778–1785.

Centers for Medicare and Medicaid Services (CMS). (2013). History of medicare and medicaid. Retrieved October 2, 2013, from www.cms.gov/About-CMS/Agency-Information/History/index.html?redirect=/history/

Dashnaw, C.C. (2010). A legacy lives on: Tim Porter-O'Grady. *Nurse.com.* Retrieved October 2, 2013, from http://news.nurse.com/article/20100628/NATIONAL02/100628005/-1/frontpage#.UlmbWySr9ok

Dougherty, C. (2008, May 7). Slowdown's side effect: More nurses. *Wall Street Journal,* pp. D1, D8.

Henderson, V. (1966). *The nature of nursing.* New York: Macmillan.

Henderson, V. (1955). *The principles and practice of nursing.* ualberta.ca/~jmorris/nt/henderson.htm. Retrieved on May 9, 2000, from www.unc.edu/ehallora/henderson.htm

History of Hospice Care (2012). Hospice: A historical perspective. Retrieved October 2, 2013, from www.nhpco.org/history-hospice-care

Institute of Medicine. (2010). *The future of nursing: Leading change, advancing health.* Retrieved from http://books.nap.edu/openbook.php?record_id=12956&page=R1

Kalisch, B.J., Ischannen, D., & Lee K.H. (2011). Do staffing levels predict missed nursing care? *International Journal for Quality in Health Care, 23*(3), 302–308.

Kalisch, P.A., & Kalisch, B.J. (2004). *American nursing: A history.* Philadelphia: Lippincott, Williams & Wilkins.

Kelly, L.A., McHugh, M.D., & Aiken, L.H. (2011).Nurse outcomes in magnet and non-magnet hospitals. *Journal of Nursing Administration, 4*(10). 428–433.

Lillis, K., & O'Brien, A. (2007, February 12). Salary survey 2007. *Advance for Nurses,* pp. 11–18.

Longfellow, H.W. (1868). The lady with the lamp. In Williams, M. (1975). *How does a poem mean?* Boston: Houghton Mifflin.

Malveaux, J. (2013). Sanger's legacy is reproductive freedom and racism. *We-news.* October, 11, 2013. Retrieved October 11, 2013, from www.womensenews.org/article.cfm/dyn/aid/618

National League for Nursing. Retrieved on May 4, 2006, from www.nln.org/aboutnln/info-history.htm

National League for Nursing (NLN). (2012). Retrieved October 1, 2013, from www.nln.org/aboutnln/bio_bev.htm.

Nightingale, F. (1859). *Notes on nursing: What it is and what it is not.* Reprinted 1992. Philadelphia: J.B. Lippincott.

Porter-O'Grady, T. (2003). A different age for leadership, Part 1: New context, new content. *Journal of Nursing Administration, 33*(2), 105–110.

Roberts, M. (1937). Florence Nightingale as a nurse educator. *American Journal of Nursing, 37,* 775.

Rogers, M.E. (1988). Nursing science and art: A perspective. *Nursing Science Quarterly, 1,* 99–102.

Schuyler, C.B. (1992). Florence Nightingale. In *Notes on nursing: What it is and what it is not.* Philadelphia: J.B. Lippincott.

Spiva, L., Hart, P., & McVay, F. (2011). Discovering ways that influence the older nurse to continue bedside practice. *Nursing Research and Practice,* Article ID 840120, doi:10.1155/2011/840120. Retrieved on October 3, 2013, from www.hindawi.com/journals/nrp/2011/840120/cta/

Stowkowski, L., (2004). Trends in nursing: 2004 and beyond. *Topics in Advanced Practice Nursing eJournal.* 4(1).

Villeneuve, M., & MacDonald, J. (2006). *Toward 2020: Visions of nursing.* Ottawa: Canadian Nurses Association.

Warrington, J. (1839). The nurse's guide: A series of instructions to females who wish to engage in the important business of nursing mother and child in the lying-in chamber. Philadelphia: Thomas Cowperthwait and Co. Retrieved on October 1, 2013, from www.nursing.upenn.edu.

Wieck, K.L. (2008). Managing the millennials. *Nurse Leader, 6*(6). 26–29.

OBJECTIVES

After reading this chapter, the student should be able to:

- Differentiate the roles of the American Nurses Association, National League for Nursing, National Organization for Associate Degree Nursing, American Academy of Nursing, and National Institute for Nursing Research.
- Discuss current efforts to achieve health-care reform.
- Describe an ideal health-care system.
- Discuss some of the issues faced by the nursing profession today.
- List changes that may affect nursing's future.
- Describe actions every nurse can take to promote the profession and high quality of care.

OUTLINE

Professional Organizations
American Nurses Association (ANA)
National League for Nursing

National Organization for Associate Degree Nursing
National Student Nurses Association
American Academy of Nursing
National Institute for Nursing Research
Specialty Organizations
Health Care Today
Health-Care Reform
Nursing Today
Trends in Nursing and Health Care
Health Care in the Future
Nursing in the Future
Conclusion

As a new graduate nurse, you are about to enter a proud profession, one that ranks high in the public's trust and fills a great societal need. Although most of your attention will be focused on learning your new role and caring for your patients, we encourage you to join your professional organization and at least be aware of the many political and economic issues that affect nurses and the nursing profession. You will be introduced to them in this chapter.

Professional Organizations

American Nurses Association (ANA)

In 1896, delegates from 10 nursing schools' alumnae associations met to organize a national professional association for nurses. The constitution and bylaws were completed in 1907, and the Nurses Associated Alumnae of the United States and Canada was created. The name was changed in 1911 to the American Nurses Association, which in 1982 became a federation of constituent state nurses associations. In 1908, the Canadian Association of Nursing Education created the Canadian National Association of Trained Nurses, which became the

Canadian Nurses Association in 1924 (Mansell & Dodd, 2005).

The purposes of the ANA are to:

1. Foster high standards of nursing practice
2. Promote the rights of nurses in the workplace
3. Project a positive and realistic view of nursing
4. Lobby the Congress and regulatory agencies on health-care issues affecting nurses and the public

These purposes, reviewed during each biennial meeting by the House of Delegates, are unrestricted by consideration of age, color, creed, disability, gender, health status, lifestyle, nationality, religion, race, or sexual orientation (ANA, 2013).

The core policy issues identified by the ANA in 2011 were:

- Nursing Ethics
- Leadership
- Fixing the Health-Care System
- Nursing and Environmental Health
- Public Health
- Emergency Preparedness
- Improve Your Workplace

- Patient Safety
- Nursing Informatics
- Global Health Issues

The goals of the Canadian Nurses Association are to:

1. Advance the discipline of nursing in the interest of the public
2. Advocate for policy that incorporates the principles of primary health care (access, interprofessional approach, patient and community involvement, health promotion) and respects the Canada Health Act
3. Advance the regulation of RNs in the interest of the public
4. Collaborate with nurses, other providers, stakeholders, and the public to achieve and sustain quality practice environments and positive client outcomes
5. Advance international health
6. Promote awareness of the profession so that the roles and expertise of RNs are understood, respected, and optimized (abbreviated statements CAN-AIIC at www.cna-aiic.ca/en/on-the-issues/cna-position-statements/)

Although there are approximately 2.9 million nurses in the United States, only about 10% are members of their professional organization. The many different subgroups and numerous specialty nursing organizations contribute to this fragmentation, which causes difficulty in presenting a united front from which to advocate for nursing. As the ANA works on the goal of preparing nurses for the demands of the 21st century, nurses need to work together in their efforts to identify and promote their unique, autonomous role within the health-care system.

Membership in the ANA offers benefits such as informative publications, group life and health insurance, access to malpractice insurance, and continuing education courses. As the primary voice of nursing in the United States, ANA lobbies legislators to influence the passage of laws that affect the practice of nursing and the safety of consumers. The power of the ANA was apparent when nurses lobbied against the American Medical Association's (AMA) proposal to create a new category of health-care worker, the registered care technician, as an answer to the nursing shortage of the 1980s.

The registered care technician category was never established despite the AMA's vigorous support.

The ANA frequently publishes position statements outlining the organization's position on particular topics important to the health and welfare of the public and/or the nurse. Box 14-1 summarizes some of the current position statements available from the ANA, which can be accessed on the ANA Web site (www.nursingworld.org/position statements). Likewise, the Canadian Nurses Association publishes position statements on such issues as education, ethics, healthy public policy, leadership, practice, primary health care, protection of the public, and research (Box 14-2) (Nursing Now, 2005; CNA, 2011).

The ANA also offers certification in various specialty areas through its subsidiary, the American Nurses Credentialing Center (ANCC) (www.nursecredentialing.org). Certification is a formal but voluntary process by which the professional nurse demonstrates knowledge of and expertise in a specific area of practice. It is a way to establish the nurse's expertise beyond the basic requirements for licensure and is an important part of peer recognition for nurses. In many facilities, certification entitles the nurse to salary increases and position advancement. Some specialty nursing organizations also have certification programs.

National League for Nursing

Another large nursing organization in the United States is the National League for Nursing (NLN). Unlike ANA membership, NLN membership is open to other health professionals and interested consumers. Over 1,500 nursing schools and health-care agencies and more than 5,000 nurses, educators, administrators, consumers, and students are members of the NLN (www.nln.org/aboutnln/info-history.htm).

NLN participates in test services, research, and publication. It also lobbies actively for nursing issues and is currently working cooperatively with the ANA and other nursing organizations on health-care reform issues. To do such things more effectively, the ANA, NLN, American Association of Colleges of Nursing, and American Organization of Nurse Executives have formed a coalition called the TriCouncil for the purpose of dealing with issues that are important to all nurses.

The NLN formed a separate accrediting agency, the National League for Nursing Accred-

American Nurses Association (ANA) Position Statements

Bloodborne and Airborne Diseases
Needle Exchange and HIV
HIV Exposure from Rape/Sexual Assault
HIV Disease and Correctional Inmates
HIV Infection and Nursing Students
Education and Barrier Use for Sexually Transmitted Diseases and HIV Infection
Equipment/Safety Procedures to Prevent Transmission of Bloodborne Diseases
Personnel Policies and HIV in the Workplace
Post-Exposure Programs in the Event of Occupational Exposure to HIV/HBV
HIV Testing

Consumer Advocacy
Mercury in Vaccines

Drug and Alcohol Abuse
Drug Testing for Health Care Workers
Abuse of Prescription Drugs

Environmental Health
Pharmaceutical Waste

Ethics and Human Rights
Constituent/State Nurses Associations (C/SNAs) as Ethics Resources, Educators, and Advocates
Non-punitive Alcohol and Drug Treatment for Pregnant and Breast-feeding Women and their Exposed Children
Nursing Care and Do Not Resuscitate (DNR) and Allow Natural Death (AND) Decisions
Reduction of Patient Restraint and Seclusion in Health Care Settings
Foregoing Nutrition and Hydration
Protecting and Promoting Individual Worth, Dignity, and Human Rights in Practice Settings
In Support of Patients' Safe Access to Therapeutic Marijuana
Stem Cell Research
Privacy and Confidentiality
Assuring Patient Safety: The Employers' Role in Promoting Healthy Nursing Work Hours
Assuring Patient Safety: Registered Nurses' Responsibility to Guard Against Working When Fatigued
Risk and Responsibility in Providing Nursing Care
Discrimination and Racism in Health Care
Assisted Suicide
Cultural Diversity in Nursing Practice
Nursing and the Patient Self-Determination Acts
Active Euthanasia
The Nonnegotiable Nature of the ANA Code of Ethics for Nurses
Nurses' Role in Capital Punishment

Nursing Practice
The Role of the Registered Nurse in Ambulatory Care
One Perioperative Registered Nurse Circulator Dedicated to Every Patient Undergoing an Invasive Procedure
Care Coordination and Registered Nurses' Essential Role

Competencies for Nurse Practitioners in Emergency Care
The Doctor of Nursing Practice: Advancing the Nursing Profession
Emergency Care Psychiatric Clinical Framework
Association of Operating Room Nurses Official Statement on RN First Assistants
Electronic Health Record
Additional Access to Care: Supporting Nurse Practitioners in Retail-Based Health Clinics
Determining a Standard Order of Credentials for the Professional Nurse
Establishing a Culturally Competent Master's and Doctorally Prepared Nursing Workforce
The Mayday Fund Report: A Call to Revolutionize Chronic Pain Care in America
Promoting Safe Medication Use in the Older Adult
Safe Practices for Needle and Syringe Use
Professional Role Competence
Procedural Sedation Consensus Statement
Elimination of Manual Patient Handling to Prevent Work-Related Musculoskeletal Disorders
Safety Issues Related to Tubing and Catheter Misconnections
Principles of Fatigue that Impact Safe Nursing Practice
Assuring Safe, High Quality Health Care in Pre-K Through 12 Educational Setting
Credentialing of Advanced Practice Registered Nurses

Social Causes and Health Care
Reproductive Health
NAPNAP Position Statement on Immunizations
Nursing Leadership in Global and Domestic Tobacco Control
Elimination of Violence in Advertising Directed Toward Children, Adolescents and Families
Violence Against Women
Adolescent Health
Uses of Placebos for Pain Management in Patients with Cancer
Promotion and Disease Prevention
Lead Poisoning and Screening

Unlicensed Personnel
Registered Nurses Utilization of Nursing Assistive Personnel in All Settings
Registered Nurse Education Relating to the Utilization of Unlicensed Assistive Personnel
Joint Statement on Delegation

Workplace Advocacy
Just Culture
Patient Safety: Rights of Registered Nurses When Considering a Patient Assignment
Employers' Guidelines for Work Release During a Disaster
Registered Nurses' Rights and Responsibilities Related to Work Release During a Disaster
Sexual Harassment

American Nurses Association. (2013). Official ANA Position Statements. *Retrieved from www.nursingworld.org/positionstatements*

---

iting Agency (NLNAC) which is now called The Accreditation Commission for Education in Nursing (ACEN) (http://acenursing.org; NLN, 2013a, 2013b). The ACEN provides for the specialized accreditation of nursing education schools and programs, both post-secondary and higher degree (master's degree, baccalaureate degree, associate degree, diploma, and practical nursing programs).

box 14-2

Canadian Nurses Association (CNA) Position Statements

Nurse Practitioners and Clinical Nurse Specialists
Clinical Nurse Specialist
Advanced Nursing Practice
The Nurse Practitioner

RN Licensing
Canadian Regulatory Framework for Registered Nurses
Accountability: Regulatory Framework
Regulation and Integration of International Nurse Applicants into the Canadian Health System

Nursing Ethics
Spirituality, Health and Nursing Practice
Ethical Nurse Recruitment
Ethical Practice: *Code of Ethics for Registered Nurses*
Global Health Partnerships
Nurses' Involvement in Screening for Alcohol or Drugs in the Workplace
Privacy of Personal Health Information
Providing Nursing Care at the End of Life

Leadership
Nurses and Midwives Collaborate on Client-Centered Care
Nursing Leadership
Interprofessional Collaboration
The Nurse Practitioner
Global Health and Equity
Clinical Nurse Specialist
Advanced Nursing Practice
The Value Of Nursing History Today
Nursing Information and Knowledge Management

Fixing the Health Care System
Nurses and Midwives Collaborate on Client-Centered Care
Financing Canada's Health System
Overcapacity Protocols and Capacity in Canada's Health System

Primary Health Care
Telehealth: The Role of the Nurse
The Role of Health Professionals in Tobacco Cessation
Interprofessional Collaboration
Mental Health Services
Determinants of Health

Nursing and Environmental Health
Nurses and Environmental Health
Toward an Environmentally Responsible Canadian Health Sector
Environmentally Responsible Activity in the Health-Care Sector
Climate Change and Health

Public Health
Joint Statement on Breastfeeding
Physical Activity
Determinants of Health
The Role of Health Professionals in Tobacco Cessation
Problematic Substance Use by Nurses
Direct-to-Consumer Advertising
Joint Position Statement on Harm Reduction
Influenza Immunization of Registered Nurses

Mental Health
Mental Health Services

Emergency Preparedness
Emergency Preparedness and Response

Improve Your Workplace
Workplace Violence
Practice Environments: Maximizing Client, Nurse and System Outcomes
Evidence-informed Decision-making and Nursing Practice
Taking Action on Nurse Fatigue
Interprofessional Collaboration
Promoting Cultural Competence in Nursing
Problematic Substance Use by Nurses
Patient Safety
Staffing Decisions for the Delivery of Safe Nursing Care
Scopes of Practice
Nursing Information and Knowledge Management

Staffing
Pan-Canadian Health Human Resources Planning
Staffing Decisions for the Delivery of Safe Nursing Care
Scopes of Practice

Patient Safety
Interprofessional Collaboration
Patient Safety
Nurse Fatigue & Patient Safety
Workplace Violence
Staffing Decisions for the Delivery of Safe Nursing Care
Influenza Immunization of Registered Nurses

Nursing Informatics
Nursing Information and Knowledge Management
Telehealth: The Role of the Nurse

Global Health Issues
Global Health Partnerships
Global Health and Equity
International Trade and Labor Mobility
Peace and Health
Registered Nurses, Health and Human Rights

Canadian Nurses Association. (2013). CNA Position Statements. Retrieved from www.cna-aiic.ca/en/on-the-issues/cna-position-statements/

National Organization for Associate Degree Nursing

Associate-degree nursing programs prepare the largest number of new graduates for RN licensure. Many of these individuals would never have had the opportunity to become RNs without the access afforded by the community college system. The move to begin a national organization to address associate degree nursing began in 1986. The organization identified two major goals: to maintain eligibility for licensure for associate degree graduates and to interact with other nursing organizations. Today, the mission of the National Organization for Associate Degree Nursing (N-OADN) is to promote associate degree nursing "through collaboration, advocacy and education to ensure excellence in the future of healthcare and professional nursing practice." The N-OADN joined the ANA as an organizational affiliate in 2013.

National Student Nurses Association

The National Student Nurses Association (NSNA) has 60,000 members across the United States. Students enrolled in associate degree, baccalaureate, and diploma programs are eligible for membership. NSNA conferences offer opportunities to hear renowned leaders in nursing, panels on career development, and state board exam mini-reviews (www.nsna.org).

American Academy of Nursing

The American Academy of Nursing consists of more than 2,100 nursing leaders in practice, education, management, and research. Its mission is to advance health policy and practice through the generation, synthesis, and dissemination of nursing knowledge. The mission is accomplished through *Nursing Outlook*, a professional journal; expert panels composed of members of the academy, a Scholar in Residence program, and supporting appointments of nurses to key policy positions. Membership is through nomination and election by current Fellows of the Academy (www.aannet .org).

National Institute for Nursing Research

The National Institute for Nursing Research (NINR), unlike the other associations described here, is an arm of the federal government, one of the 27 institutes and centers of the National Institutes of Health (NIH). The NINR supports and conducts basic and clinical research and provides research training in health promotion, disease and disability prevention, quality of life, health disparities, management of symptoms, and end-of-life care encompassing the entire life span (www.ninr .nih.gov).

Specialty Organizations

In addition to the national nursing organizations, nurses may join specialty practice organizations focused on practice areas (e.g., critical care, nephrology, obstetrics) or special interest groups (e.g., male nurses, Hispanic nurses, Philippine nurses, Aboriginal nurses). These organizations provide nurses with information regarding evidence-based practice, trends in the field, and approved standards of specialty practice. Links to nursing organizations may be found at www.nursingsociety.org/career/ nursing_orgs.html or www.cna-nurses.ca.

Health Care Today

The United States has technologically advanced, highly sophisticated health care and spends more per capita (per person) on health care than most countries. Yet, among the industrialized countries of the world, the United States is the only one that does not provide basic health-care coverage to every citizen (Lieberman, 2003). Eighty-one million Americans age 19–64 are underinsured or uninsured (Schoen et al., 2011). Many report going without care, skipping doses of medication, or not filling a prescription because they could not afford it. One third of them report using credit card debt or a loan to pay health-care bills. Sixty-two percent of personal bankruptcies in the United States (2007 figures) were due to individuals' health problems, even though 78% of these individuals had health insurance (ANA, 2009).

If the United States has the most advanced knowledge and equipment and spends a great deal of money on health care, then why the cause for alarm? What is wrong? Why doesn't everyone have health insurance? Why are people so worried about the quality of care? The answer is complex.

For most people, health insurance comes through their place of employment. One problem with this is that many employers are motivated to keep the cost as low as possible or transfer much of the cost to the employee. Another problem is that if one loses one's job, health insurance is also lost.

Managed care was originally designed to reduce the amount spent on health care by emphasizing prevention. Some believe that it has become a way to limit choices and ration care (Mechanic, 2002) rather than prevent illness. As managed care plans have grown and spread across the country, these companies have become powerful enough to negotiate reduced rates (discounts) from local hospitals (Trinh & O'Connor, 2002). They can, in effect, say, "We can get an appendectomy for $2,300 at hospital A; why should we pay you $2,700?" If hospital B does not agree, the hospital may lose all the patients enrolled in that managed care plan. This pressures hospital B to reduce costs and spread staff even thinner than before.

Similar price pressures come from the government-supported programs of Medicare, Medicaid, and other health insurance companies. To keep costs under control, some states have cut benefits for people receiving Medicaid (which is state-supported health benefits for low-income people) (Pear, 2002).

With the upsurge in for-profit health plans and the purchase of not-for-profit hospitals by for-profit companies, U.S. health care has become increasingly "corporatized." It was thought that this would yield a highly efficient, responsive system ("the customer is always right"). That has not happened, because the "customer" who pays for insurance coverage is usually the employer or the government, not the individual patient. The care provided by the for-profits, in general, appears to be of lesser quality than the old not-for-profit or fee-for-service plans (Mechanic, 2002).

There is a limit to the extent to which cost cutting can increase efficiency without endangering patient safety. For many years, the United States has been trying to fix its health-care system by applying patches over its worst cracks, but this apparently has not worked very well. Does the system need a major overhaul? Yes. But first, there needs to be a clear vision of what it should be and what it should do (O'Connor, 2002). However these changes develop, it is certain that nurses will have an important role in a future health-care system. Research studies consistently find that nursing input contributes to better patient outcomes (Ryerson, 2013). As Aiken and colleagues (2002) wrote, "nurses contribute importantly to surveillance, early detection and timely interventions that save lives" (p. 18).

The ANA, among others, has described the current health-care system in the United States as "sick" and "broken" (ANA, 2008). Nearly 52 million Americans, including 9 million children, have no health-care insurance (AFL-CIO, 2009; Schoen et al., 2011). Even worse, two-thirds of the working-age population have a health-care–related financial problem such as unpaid medical bills, being under-insured, or being uninsured. A survey of more than 26,000 Americans, half of whom belonged to a union, found that one in three had decided to do without care because of the cost. Half had stayed in a job just to keep their health-care benefits. More than half reported that their health-care insurance did not cover the care they needed at a price they could afford (Currie, 2008b). More detail about the survey can be found at www.healthcaresurvey.aflcio.org.

The quality of the care provided is a second major concern. A 1999 report issued by the Institute of Medicine (IOM) estimated that 100,000 deaths in hospitals every year were due to errors that could have been prevented (ANA, 2008). Hospital-acquired, drug-resistant infections have become a major problem, having increased a hundredfold over the last 10 years or so. In 1993 there were 3,000 hospital discharges that included a diagnosis of drug-resistant microorganism. In 2005 there were 394,000 of these discharges (Currie, 2008a).

Additional concerns include fragmented, impersonal care; failure to consider the whole person when treating a problem; and continuations of an illness focus rather than prevention focus. Furthermore, the United States faces what Buchan called a "demographic double whammy" of an aging population that will need more health care and, at the same time, an aging workforce (Hewison & Wildman, 2008).

In Canada, a debate over privatization versus public funding of health care continues (Villeneuve & MacDonald, 2006). Health care is still illness- and disease-focused as in the United States. Although there is interest in complementary and alternative treatments, they have not been integrated into general care. Disparities in care of members of minority groups threaten to increase if not addressed more effectively.

Global interconnectedness has brought new concerns about how quickly and easily infectious diseases can cross national borders. Human immunodeficiency virus (HIV), severe acute respiratory syndrome, Ebola, Chikungunya, and the annual waves of influenza that cross the globe are just a few reminders of how vulnerable populations remain. These risks create an increased need for health-care provider surveillance across continents.

Health-Care Reform

There have been many attempts to address the problems described in the previous section. After lengthy arguments and despite some strenuous opposition, the Patient Protection and Affordable Care Act, known familiarly as Obamacare after the president who promoted it, was enacted in 2012 (Rosenbaum, 2011). This complex legislation contains provisions for sweeping changes in health care (see Table 14-1). The following are some of the changes of most interest to nurses:

■ Insurance reforms that prohibit cancellation if the person is ill, eliminate preexisting

table 14-1	

Provisions of the Affordable Care Act 2010–2015

2010	Young adults can be covered by parents' health insurance to age 26 instead of 19. Insurers will eventually be prohibited from denying coverage for preexisting conditions. In the meantime, the government will provide coverage.
2011	Insurers are required to spend 80% of their premiums on patient care or reimburse policyholders for the excess. Reimbursement for Medicare Advantage plans (HMOs) is frozen at 2010 rates.
2012	Hospitals with high readmission rates will be penalized by Medicare. States are expected to submit plans for insurance exchanges.
2013	Tax increases on medical devices and for Medicare on high-income wage earners. Sales to begin enrolling people through their insurance exchanges.
2014	State health exchanges up and running. Preexisting condition rule effective. Medicaid expanded to those earning 133% of poverty level wage. Businesses with more than 50 employees must provide health insurance. Uninsured individuals will pay increased taxes.
2015	Added tax on so-called "Cadillac" insurance plans.

Source: Adapted from Leonard, D. (2012/October 11). Obamacare is not an epithet. Bloomberg/BusinessWeek. Additional references from American Nurses Association (2010, April).

condition clauses, and prohibit lifetime limits

■ Creation of state health insurance exchanges to offer affordable insurance coverage
■ Support for nursing education and nursing students
■ Nurse-managed clinics that will be eligible for federal funding
■ Expansion of school-based health centers
■ Support for transitional care and chronic disease management
■ Creation of accountable care organizations and medical homes that bridge the gap between hospital, nursing home, and home and medical office care (Webb & Marshall, 2010)
■ Free preventive services for women, including HIV screening, contraception, breastfeeding, and domestic violence services
■ A standardized report of their health insurance coverage so that consumers can compare different plans (ANA, 2013).

There has been much controversy surrounding the Affordable Care Act. The right of the government to require people to have health insurance—that is, to tax people to pay for health care—was even challenged in the Supreme Court. The Affordable Care Act was found to be constitutional on a close vote of 5–4 (von Drehle, 2012). There was also a strong protest over coverage for contraception (birth control) when it was categorized as preventive care in the Affordable Care Act. So far, fewer people

than expected have applied for coverage of preexisting conditions, and some insurers have threatened to drop individual policies for children if they had to cover preexisting conditions (Adamy & Radnofsky, 2012). A number of states have also resisted setting up the proposed health exchanges (Anonymous, 2013).

Some call the Affordable Care Act socialized medicine and are strongly opposed to it; others think it is a much needed step in the direction of ensuring that everyone can afford the health care they need. Some might even say it does not go far enough. The second opinion seems to be in line with the World Health Assembly resolution supporting universal coverage:

> [E]nsuring that all people have access to needed health services—prevention, promotion, treatment and rehabilitation—without facing financial ruin because of the need to pay for them (World Health Organization, 2012, p. 38).

Nursing Today

As discussed in Chapter 13, issues specific to nursing reflect the problems and concerns about the system as a whole. The related issues of excessive workload, mandatory overtime, incivility, workplace violence, and lack of professional autonomy contribute to these concerns (Villeneuve & MacDonald, 2006), along with an aging workforce. On the bright side, there are also some indications of increasing interest in a nursing career as salaries improve and job opportunities expand.

Safe staffing, defined as the appropriate number and mix of nursing staff, is a critical issue for nurses and the people who need their care. A series of research studies has demonstrated the importance of adequate nurse staffing. There is powerful evidence that nurses save lives: for each additional patient assigned to a nurse, there is a 7% increase in the likelihood of a patient dying within 30 days of admission (Aiken, Clarke, Sloane, Sochalski et al., 2002; Potter & Mueller, 2007). Nurses cannot gain in-depth understanding of their patients, protect their patients, or catch early warning signs if they are overwhelmed by the number of patients for whom they are responsible. Adequate numbers of nurses affect patient mortality, length of stay, prevalence of urinary tract infections, fall rates, incidence of hospital-acquired pneumonia, and more. For further information, see www.safestaffingsaveslives .org.

In a related finding, recent reports demonstrate that increased surveillance and improved infection control techniques decreased the number of methicillin-resistant *staphylococcus aureus* (MRSA) from 2005 through 2011 (Dantes et al., 2013). This decrease is partly attributed to an increase in nursing interventions, such as patient teaching both within acute care settings and in the community.

Trends in Nursing and Health Care

Changes and innovation are constants in health care. The following are trends that are expected to affect the nursing profession and the care nurses provide to their patients in the near future:

- The continued aging of the nursing workforce will increase the need for new nurses across the globe (Lu, Barriball, Zhang, & While, 2012).
- The aging of the large baby boomer generation will cause a demand for more health-care services.
- Evidence-based practice will become integrated into nursing education programs and eventually become standard nursing practice (Melnyk et al., 2012).
- Efforts to ensure patient safety, especially in acute care, will continue to be emphasized, including reduction of nosocomial infections, medication errors, failure to rescue, and other serious adverse events.
- Quality improvement efforts will also continue to increase, along with the drive for patient safety.

- The use of electronic health records will become standard practice in hospitals, nursing homes, and community settings along with other technological innovations (computerized provider order entry, telehealth, mobile devices, sensors, webcams, etc.) designed to improve care (Cornell, Riorden, & Herrin-Griffith, 2010; Matthews, 2012).
- Alternative and complementary approaches (such as meditation, use of nutraceuticals, etc.), already widely accepted by many members of the public, will be integrated into standard medical and nursing practice.
- Increased focus on care transitions (from hospital to home, from the nursing home back to the hospital, etc.) will involve nurses in better preparing patients for these transitions.
- Whenever and wherever possible, care will move out of the hospital into the community (Firger, 2012).
- Hospitals and nursing homes are anticipating further cuts in reimbursement from Medicare and Medicaid. In response, they are looking for additional ways to reduce costs and diversify into community-based services, such as hospice and rehab (Flavelle, 2012).
- Continued cost cutting will increase use of "physician extenders" (nurse practitioners and physician assistants, etc.) but may also put additional strain on current nursing staff.
- Improved communication and increased travel bring increased exposure to disease from other parts of the world (Johnson, 2011).

What does all of this mean for the new nurse? Many opportunities for nurses will open up in community-based care, transitional care, quality improvement efforts, telehealth, and nontraditional roles. But there will also be challenges ahead as cost cutting increases the demand on individual staff members and tolerance of errors that threaten patient safety and well-being becomes very limited.

Health Care in the Future

Ideally, a new model of health care is needed that offers the following:

- Holistic, person-centered care
- Seamless connections across community, acute-care, and long-term care settings (Pogue, 2007)

- Elimination of health disparities
- Guaranteed accessible, affordable care for everyone
- Safe care that heals and does not harm the patient
- Equal support for prevention, health promotion, and mental health care
- Creation of a healthy environment from green buildings to the elimination of air, water, soil, and other forms of pollution
- Attention to global health concerns: global warming, hunger, poverty, and disease at home and in developing countries

While provisions in the Affordable Care Act address some of these concerns, there is still much work to do on health-care reform.

Nursing in the Future

Within the nursing profession, there is also much work to do. Too often members of the public and colleagues in other professions think of nurses in only an assistive role (Bleich, 2012). This limited view ignores our unique perspective that encompasses the whole person within his or her family and community. Nurses think differently from other health-care providers. Michael Bleich (2012, p. 184) says we need to "publicly give voice to the value of this perspective," particularly during this time of health-care reform. If we do not, we "will be left to react to models that may stymie our capacity to influence health," until the next wave of health reform occurs.

Cohen (2007) addressed the issue of the image that many nurses present to their public. One is professional appearance and behavior. She quotes Dumont on the question of dress, particularly wearing uniforms covered with cartoon characters: "You're the only thing between the patient and death, and you're covered in cartoons. No wonder you have no authority." The following are some additional suggestions to improve nursing's image:

- Always introduce yourself as a registered nurse.
- Define professional appearance appropriate to your workplace and enforce it.
- Define professional behavior and enforce it.
- Take every opportunity to speak to the public about nursing.
- Document what nurses do and how important they are (Cohen, 2007).

What else can nurses do? It is important that more members of minority groups be brought into nursing so that nursing better reflects the increasing diversity of the population. Collaboration with colleagues in other health professions is also vital to improving health care. Physicians, therapists, social workers, psychologists, aides, assistants, and technicians are concerned about the quality of care provided. Patients and their families are also concerned and personally affected by the quality of care provided. All these groups together would have a stronger voice in health-care reform.

Nurses are the largest professional group within health care in terms of numbers. They spend the most time with patients and receive top ranking for having the public's trust according to Gallup polls. These are significant accomplishments. But a national Gallup poll of 1,500 opinion leaders revealed a serious lack of nursing representation and influence at the highest policy levels. These opinion leaders thought that government and health insurance executives have the most influence on health-care reform. Only 14% of them thought that nurses would be influential. It was also noted that nurses did not have a single, unified voice and seemed disinterested and uninvolved for the most part (Khoury, Blizzard, Moore, & Hassmiller, 2011). There was a more positive side to these disturbing survey results. Many of the opinion leaders interviewed thought more nurses should get involved. Issues on which nurses should have a say include patient safety, quality of care, reducing medical errors, health promotion, and prevention (Hassmiller, 2011). The urgency of making our voices heard is undisputable. Hassmiller (2011) writes that "right now is the right time to tackle the difficult and essential work of bringing nursing perspectives, knowledge, and voices into health policy decision making" (p. 308).

The following are some specific actions you can take to exert leadership in supporting your profession and improving health care:

- Learn more about the health-care system and your role in it.
- Join your professional association and specialty association and support their efforts to improve care.
- Talk about these issues with everyone and anyone who will listen.

- Write letters to the editor, speak on local radio and television programs, and participate in online discussions.
- Speak to your local, state, and national representatives about these concerns.

In summary, be "visible and vocal" in your support of nursing and improved health care (ANA, 2008).

Conclusion

As nursing moves forward in the 21st century, the need for courageous and innovative nurse leaders is greater than ever. Society's demand for high-quality health care at an affordable cost is a contemporary force for change.

Nurses began in hospitals, moved to the community, moved back into the hospitals, and are now seeing a move back to the community. Men were the earliest nurses, then left the profession and have now returned, bringing with them new ideas and leadership abilities. Nursing is becoming as diversified as the populations it serves.

Study Questions

1. Review the mission and purpose of the ANA or another national nursing organization online. Do you believe that nurses should belong to these organizations? Why or why not? Explain your answer.

2. Describe your ideal health-care system of the future. Compare it with the description in this chapter. What is different? What is similar?

3. Write an "elevator speech" (30 seconds to 2 minutes in length) that describes the value of the care nurses provide. (An elevator speech or elevator pitch is speech that describes the value of something so quickly that it can be delivered during an elevator ride.)

Case Study to Promote Critical Reasoning

Alina went to nursing school on a U.S. Air Force scholarship. She has been directed to lead the planning for establishing a comprehensive primary care and health promotion program clinic on board the National Aeronautics and Space Administration's (NASA) newest international space station. The crew is to remain on board the station for 6 months at a time. The crew will consist of military men and women from three countries.

1. What type of care will be needed by the crew of the space station? How much of this will be provided by nurses?

2. What medical and nursing technology and equipment should Alina plan to have in this center?

3. Develop a nursing research topic for this situation that Alina could study when the space station becomes a reality.

References

Accreditation Commission for Education in Nursing. (2013, December). Important update from the ACEN. Retrieved from http://acenursing.org/update-092613

Adamy, J., & Radnofsky, L. (2012). Health law slow to win favor. *Wall Street Journal,* A1, A12.

AFL-CIO. (2009). Resolution 34, the social insurance model for health care reform. Alameda Labor Council (CA), *California Nurses Association/National Nurses Organizing Committee and International Longshore and Warehouse Union,* 35.

Aiken, L., Clarke, S.P., Sloane, D., Sochalski, J., et al. (2002). Hospital nurse staffing and patient mortality, nurse burnout and job dissatisfaction. *Journal of the American Medical Association, 288*(16), 1987–1993.

American Academy of Nursing. (2013, December). About the academy. Retrieved from www.aannet.org/about-the -academy

American Nurses Association. (2013). ANA position statements. Retrieved from www.nursingworld.org/ positionstatements

American Nurses Association. (2013, December). Associate degree nursing organization joins ANA as affiliate. Retrieved from https://www.noadn.org/dmdocuments/ Release_ANAGainsNewAffiliate_AssocDegreeNsg.pdf

American Nurses Association. (2013, July). Health care reform. Retrieved from www.nursingworld.org/ MainMenuCategories/Policy-Advocacy/ HealthSystemReform/Health-Care-Law.pdf

American Nurses Association. (2008). Health reform: The 2008 elections and beyond. *The American Nurse,* September/October.

American Nurses Association. (2010, April). Selected patient protection and affordable care act (PPACA) implementation dates of interest to RNs as caregivers, RNS as patients, and RNs as employees. Retrieved from www.nursingworld.org/MainMenuCategories/Policy -Advocacy/HealthSystemReform/Health-Care-Reform -Legislation-Timeline.pdf

American Nurses Association. (2009/September 15). Testimony before the democratic steering and policy committee, U.S. House of Representatives forum on the urgent need for health care reform. Retrieved from www .nursingworld.org/DemocraticSteeringPolicy.aspx

American Nurses Credentialing Center. (ANCC). (December 2013). About ANCC. Retrieved from http:// nursecredentialing.org/FunctionalCategory/AboutANCC

Anonymous. (2013). Utah faces off with Obama over health care exchanges. *Huffington Post.* Retrieved January 4, 2013, from www.huffingtonpost .com/2013/01/03 ut-health-care-reform_n_2403294 .html

Bleich, M.R. (2012). Leadership responses to the future of nursing: Leading change, advancing health 10M report. *Journal of Nursing Administration, 42*(4), 108–184.

Canadian Nurses Association. (2011). CNA Position statements. Retrieved January 4, 2012, from www.cna- aiic.ca/en/on-the-issues/cna-position-statements/

Cohen, S. (2007). The image of nursing: How do others see us? How do we see ourselves? *American Nurse Today, 2*(5), 24–26.

Cornell, P., Riorden, M., & Herrin-Griffith, D. (2010). Transforming nursing workflow, part 2: The impact of technology on nurse activities. *Journal of Nursing Administration, 40*(10), 432–439.

Currie, D. (2008a). Drug-resistant tests could lower costs. *The Nation's Health, 38*(4), 8.

Currie, D. (2008b). One in three forgo care because of cost. *The Nation's Health, 38*(4), 8.

Dantes, R., Mu, Y., Belflower, R., Aragon, D., Dumyati, G., Harrison, L.H., Lessa, F.C., & Nadle, J. (2013). National burden of invasive Methicillin-resistant *Staphylococcus aureas* infections, United States, 2011. *Journal of the American Medical Association,* September 16, 2013. doi: 10.1001. Retrieved October 4, 2013, from http://archinte.jamanetwork.com/article. aspx?articleid=1738718

Firger, J. (2012/June 12). Bringing the hospital home for the tiniest of patients. *Wall Street Journal,* D1–D2.

Flavelle, C. (2012/October 8–14). A nip and a tuck? Or open heart surgery? *Bloomberg/BusinessWeek,* 59–60.

Hassmiller, S.B. (2011). Nursing leadership from bedside to boardroom. *Journal of Nursing Administration, 41*(7/8), 306–308.

Hewison, A., & Wildman, S. (2008). Looking back, looking forward: Enduring issues in nursing management. *Journal of Nursing Management, 16*(1), 1–3.

Johnson, T.D. (2011). Measles cases in the U.S. rise as travelers bring the disease with them. *The Nation's Health, 41*(7), 1, 16–17.

Khoury, C.M., Blizzard, R., Moore, L.W., & Hassmiller, S. (2011). Nursing leadership from beside to boardroom. *Journal of Nursing Administration, 41*(7/8), 299–305.

Leonard, D. (2012/October 11). Obamacare is not an epithet. *Bloomberg/BusinessWeek.*

Lieberman, T. (2003). Bruised and broken: The US health system. *AARP Bulletin, 44*(3), 3–5.

Lu, H., Barriball, K.L., Zhang, I., & While, A.E. (2012). Job satisfaction among hospital nurses revisited. *International Journal of Nursing Studies, 49,* 1017–1038.

Mansell, D., & Dodd, D. (2005). Professionalism and Canadian nursing. In Bates, C., Bates, D., & Rousseau, N. (eds.), *On all frontiers: Four centuries of Canadian nursing* (pp. 197–211). Ottawa: University of Ottawa Press.

Matthews, A.W. (2012/December 21). Doctors move to webcams. *Wall Street Journal,* B1, B5.

Mechanic, D. (2002). Sociocultural implications of changing organizational technologies in the provision of care. *Social Science and Medicine, 54,* 459–467.

Melnyk, B.M., Fineout-Overholt, E., Gallagher-Ford, L., & Kaplan, L. (2012). The state of evidence-based practice in U.S. nurses. *Journal of Nursing Administration, 42*(9), 410–417.

National League for Nursing a. (2013a, August). New York Supreme Court Upholds NLN Position in Ongoing Litigation with ACEN (formerly NLNAC). NLN News Releases. Retrieved from www.nln.org

National League of Nursing b. (2013b, December). NLN accreditation services: FAQs. Retrieved from www.nln .org/aboutnln/PDF/accreditationfaq8_1.pdf

National Student Nurses' Association. (December, 2013) About Us. Retrieved from www.nsna.org/AboutUs.aspx

Nursing leadership in a changing world. (2005, January). *Nursing Now: Issues and Trends in Canadian Nursing,* Number 18.

O'Connor, K. (2002, April 8). Healthcare in need of a fix. *Modern Healthcare,* 27.

Pear, R. (2002, November 20). Report: Health system in crisis. *Sun Sentinel,* 3A.

Pogue, P. (2007). The nurse practitioner role. *Into the Future Nursing Leadership, 20*(2), 34–38.

Potter, P., & Mueller, J.R. (2007). How well do you know your patients? *Nursing Management, 38*(2), 40–41.

Ryerson, N. (2013, July). Spotlight: ANA President on Health Care Reform. http://dotmed.com/legal/print/story.html?nid=21516

Rosenbaum, S. (2011). The Patient protection and affordable care act: Implications for public health policy and practice. *Public Health Reports, 126,* 130–135.

Schoen, C., Doty, M., Robertson, R.H., & Collins, S.R. Affordable care act reforms could reduce the number of underinsured US adults by 70 percent. *Health Affairs, 3*(9), 1762–1771.

Trinh, H.Q., & O'Connor, S.J. (2002). Helpful or harmful? The impact of strategic change on the performance of U.S. urban hospitals. *Health Services Research, 37*(1), 145–171.

Villeneuve, M., & MacDonald, J. (2006). *Toward 2020: Visions of nursing.* Ottawa: Canadian Nurses Association.

von Drehle, D. (2012). Roberts's rules: The upholder. *Time, 18*(3), 30–33.

Webb, J.A.K., & Marshall, D.R. (2010). Healthcare reform and nursing: What does it mean? *Journal of Nursing Administration, 40*(9), 345–347.

World Health Organization. (2012). *World health statistics 2012.* Geneva, Switzerland: WHO

Codes of Ethics for Nurses

American Nurses Association Code of Ethics for Nurses

1. The nurse, in all professional relationships, practices with compassion and respect for the inherent dignity, worth, and uniqueness of every individual, unrestricted by considerations of social or economic status, personal attributes, or the nature of health problems.
2. The nurse's primary commitment is to the patient, whether an individual, family, group, or community.
3. The nurse promotes, advocates for, and strives to protect the health, safety, and rights of the patient.
4. The nurse is responsible and accountable for individual nursing practice and determines the appropriate delegation of tasks consistent with the nurse's obligation to provide optimum patient care.
5. The nurse owes the same duties to self as to others, including the responsibility to preserve integrity and safety, to maintain competence, and to continue personal and professional growth.
6. The nurse participates in establishing, maintaining, and improving health care environments and conditions of employment conducive to the provision of quality health care and consistent with the values of the profession through individual and collective action.
7. The nurse participates in the advancement of the profession through contributions to practice, education, administration, and knowledge development.
8. The nurse collaborates with other health professionals and the public in promoting community, national, and international efforts to meet health needs.
9. The profession of nursing, as represented by associations and their members, is responsible for articulating nursing values, for maintaining the integrity of the profession and its practice, and for shaping social policy.

Approved July 2001. Web site: www.nursing world.org/ethics/chcode.htm

Reprinted with permission from American Nurses Association, Code of Ethics for Nurses with Interpretive Statements, ©2001 American Nurses Publishing, American Nurses Foundation/ American Nurses Association, Washington, DC.

Canadian Nurse Association Code of Ethics for Registered Nurses

The Code of Ethics for Registered Nurses (CNA, 2008) serves as a foundation for nurses' ethical practice. CNA believes that the follow ing seven values, which are described in the code, are central to ethical nursing practice. In the code, each of these values is accompanied by a number of responsibility statements, and together they outline the ethical practice that is expected of registered nurses. CNA believes that the quality of the work environment in which nurses practice is also fundamental to their ability to practice ethically.

1. Providing safe, compassionate, competent and ethical care

Nurses provide safe, compassionate, competent and ethical care.

2. Promoting health and well-being

Nurses work with people to enable them to attain their highest possible level of health and well-being.

3. Promoting and respecting informed decision-making

Nurses recognize, respect and promote a person's right to be informed and make decisions.

4. Preserving dignity

Nurses recognize and respect the intrinsic worth of each person.

5. Maintaining privacy and confidentiality

Nurses recognize the importance of privacy and confidentiality and safeguard personal, family and community information obtained in the context of a professional relationship.

6. Promoting justice

Nurses uphold principles of justice by safeguarding human rights, equity and fairness and by promoting the public good.

7. Being accountable

Nurses are accountable for their actions and answerable for their practice. Ethical nursing practice also involves endeavoring to address broad aspects of social justice that are associated with health and well-being. These aspects relate to the need for change in systems and societal structures in order to create greater equity for all. Nurses should endeavor as much as possible, individually and collectively, to advocate for and work toward eliminating social inequities. The code contains thirteen statements entitled "ethical endeavors," which are intended to guide nurses in this area. These statements address the need for awareness and action around such areas as social inequalities, accessibility and comprehensiveness of health care, and major health concerns (e.g., poverty, violence, inadequate shelter) as well as broader global concerns (e.g., war, violations of human rights, world hunger).

Canadian Nursing Association. Web site: www.cna-nurses.ca

Reprinted with permission from the Canadian Nurses Association, 2008.

The International Council of Nurses Code of Ethics for Nurses

Nurses and People

The nurse's primary professional responsibility is to people requiring nursing care.

In providing nursing care, the nurse promotes an environment in which the human rights, values, customs, and spiritual beliefs of the individual, family, and community are respected.

The nurse ensures that the individual receives sufficient information on which to base consent for care and related treatment.

The nurse holds in confidence personal information and uses judgment in sharing this information.

The nurse shares with society the responsibility for initiating and supporting action to meet the health and social needs of the public, in particular those of vulnerable populations.

The nurse also shares responsibility to sustain and protect the natural environment from depletion, pollution, degradation, and destruction.

Nurses and Practice

The nurse carries personal responsibility and accountability for nursing practice, and for maintaining competence by continual learning.

The nurse maintains a standard of personal health such that the ability to provide care is not compromised.

The nurse uses judgment regarding individual competence when accepting and delegating responsibility.

The nurse at all times maintains standards of personal conduct which reflect well on the profession and enhance public confidence.

The nurse, in providing care, ensures that use of technology and scientific advances are compatible with safety, dignity, and rights of people.

Nurses and the Profession

The nurse assumes the major role in determining and implementing acceptable standards of clinical nursing practice, management, research, and education.

The nurse is active in developing a core research-based professional knowledge.

The nurse, acting through professional organizations, participates in creating and maintaining equitable social and economic working conditions in nursing.

Nurses and Co-Workers

The nurse sustains a co-operative relationship with co-workers in nursing and other fields.

The nurse takes appropriate action to safeguard individuals when their care is endangered by a co-worker or any other person.

Approved 2000. Web site: www.icn.ch/ethics.htm

Used with permission from the International Council of Nurses, Geneva, Switzerland, copyright 2000.

Standards Published by the American Nurses Association*

- Faith Community Nursing: Scope and Standards of Practice
- Intellectual and Developmental Disabilities Nursing: Scope and Standards of Practice
- Neonatal Nursing: Scope and Standards of Practice
- Pain Management Nursing: Scope and Standards of Practice
- Plastic Surgery Nursing: Scope and Standards of Practice
- School Nursing: Scope and Standards of Practice
- Scope and Standards for Nurse Administrators
- Scope and Standards of Addictions Nursing Practice
- Scope and Standards of College Health Nursing Practice
- Scope and Standards of Diabetes Nursing Practice
- Scope and Standards of Gerontological Nursing Practice
- Scope and Standards of Home Health Nursing Practice

- Scope and Standards of Hospice and Palliative Nursing Practice
- Scope and Standards of Neuroscience Nursing Practice
- Scope and Standards of Nursing Informatics Practice
- Scope and Standards of Pediatric Nursing Practice
- Scope and Standards of Pediatric Oncology Nursing
- Scope and Standards of Practice for Nursing Professional Development
- Scope and Standards of Psychiatric-Mental Health Nursing Practice
- Scope and Standards of Public Health Nursing Practice
- Scope and Standards of Vascular Nursing Practice
- Standards of Addictions Nursing Practice with Selected Diagnoses and Criteria

*www.nursingworld.org/books/

Guidelines for the Registered Nurse in Giving, Accepting, or Rejecting a Work Assignment*

Registered Nurses, as licensed professionals, share the responsibility and accountability along with their employer to ensure that safe, quality nursing care is provided. The scope of professional nurses' accountability involves legal, ethical, and professional guidelines for assuring safe, quality patient care. Legal responsibility for the provisions, delegation and supervision of patient care is specified in the Nurse Practice Acts and the Administrative Rules. The American Nurses Association (ANA) Code for Nurses with Interpretive Statements (2010) guides ethical conduct and decision making of professional nurses. The ANA Standards and Scope of Practice (2010) provides a systematic application of nursing process for patient care management across patient care settings. Lastly, the employer requirements for safe, competent staffing are outlined in facility policies and guidelines.

Within ethical and legal parameters the nurse exercises informed judgment and uses individual competence and qualifications as criteria in seeking consultation, accepting responsibilities and delegating nursing activities to others. The nurse's decision regarding accepting or making work assignments is based on the legal, ethical and professional obligation to assume responsibility for nursing judgment and action.

The document offers strategies for problem solving as the staff nurse, nurse manager, chief nurse executive and administrator practice within the complex environment of the health care system.

Nursing Care Delivery

Only a Registered Nurse (RN) will assess, plan and evaluate a patient's or client's nursing care needs. No nurse shall be required or directed to delegate nursing activities to other personnel in a manner inconsistent with the Nurse Practice Act, the standards of the Joint Commission on Accreditation of Health Organizations, the ANA Standards of Practice or Hospital Policy. Consistent with the preceding sentence, the individual RN has the autonomy to delegate (or not delegate) those aspects of nursing care the nurse determines appropriate based on the patient assessment.

When a nurse is floated to a unit or area where the nurse receives an assignment that is considered unsafe to perform independently, the RN has the right and obligation to request and receive a modified assignment, which reflects the RN's level of competence.

The Florida Nurses Association (FNA), the Florida Organization of Nurse Executives (FONE), and the FNA Labor Employee Relations Commission (LERC) recognize that changes in the health care delivery system have occurred and will continue to occur, while emphasizing the common goal to provide safe quality patient care. The parties also recognize that RNs have a right and responsibility to participate in decisions affecting delivery of nursing care and related terms and conditions of employment. All parties have a mutual interest in developing systems, which will provide quality care on a cost efficient basis without jeopardizing patient outcomes. Thus, commitment to measuring the impact of staffing and assignments to patient outcomes is a shared commitment of all professional nurses irrespective of organizational structure.

*Reproduced with permission of Florida Nurses Association, 1999, Orlando, Florida.
Revised 03/2014

Assignment Despite Objection (ADO)/Documentation of Practice Situation (DOPS)

Staff nurses today often face untenable assignments that need to be documented as such. Critical, clinical judgment should be utilized when evaluating the appropriateness of an assignment. Refusal to accept an assignment without appropriate discussion within the chain of command can be defined as insubordinate behavior. Each Registered Nurse should become familiar with organizational policies, procedures and documentation regarding refusal to accept an unsafe assignment. ANA has recently adopted a position statement and model ADO form available for use by SNA members. (Please contact Florida Nurses Association for further information.)

Staffing

In the event a Registered Nurse determines in his/her professional opinion that he/she has been given an assignment that does not allow for appropriate patient care, he/she shall notify the Supervisor or designee who shall review the concerns of the nurse. If the nurse's concerns cannot be resolved by telephone, the Supervisor or designee, except in instances of compelling business reasons that preclude him/her from doing so, will then come to the unit within four (4) hours of being contacted by the nurse to assess the staffing. Such assessment shall be documented with a copy given to the nurse. Nothing herein shall prohibit a Registered Nurse from completing and submitting a protest of assignment form.

Nurse Practice Act, 1994, Administrative Rules Chapt. 59s, 14.001 Definitions (4/29/96)

"Assignments" are the normal daily functions of the UAPs based on institutional or agency job duties which do not involve delegation of nursing functions or nursing judgment.

"Competency" is the demonstrated ability to carry out specified tasks or activities with reasonable skill and safety that adheres to the prevailing standard of practice in the nursing community.

"Delegation" is the transference to a competent individual the authority to perform a selected nursing task or activity in a selected situation by a nurse qualified by licensure and experience to perform the task or activity.

"Supervision" is the provision of guidance by a qualified nurse and periodic inspection by the nurse for the accomplishment of a nursing task or activity, provided the nurse is qualified and legally entitled to perform such task or activity. The supervisor may be the delegator or a person of equal or greater licensure to the delegator.

Scenario

- Suppose you are asked to care for an unfamiliar patient population or to go to a unit for which you feel unqualified—what do you do?
- Suppose you are approached by your supervisor and asked to work an additional shift. Your immediate response is that you don't want to work another shift—what do you do?

Such situations are familiar and emphasize the rights and responsibilities of the RN to make informed decisions. Yet all members of the health care team, from staff nurses to administrator, share a joint responsibility to ensure that quality patient care is provided. At times, though, difference in interpretation of legal or ethical principles may lead to conflict.

Guidelines for decision-making are offered to assist RNs problem-solve work assignment issues. Applications of these guidelines are presented in the form of scenarios, examples of unsafe assignments experienced by RNs.

Guidelines for Decision Making

The complexity of the delivery of nursing care is such that only professional nurses with appropriate education and experience can provide nursing care. Upon employment with a health care facility, the nurse contracts or enters into an agreement with that facility to provide nursing services in a collaborative practice environment.

It is the Registered Nurse's Responsibility to:

- provide competent nursing care to the patient
- exercise informed judgment and use individual competence and qualifications as criteria in seeking consultation, accepting responsibilities and delegating nursing activities to others
- clarify assignments, assess personal capabilities, jointly identify options for patient care

assignments when he/she does not feel personally competent or adequately prepared to carry out a specific function
- refuse an assignment that he/she does not feel prepared to assume after appropriate consultation with supervisor

It Is Nursing Management's Responsibility to:

- ensure competent nursing care is provided to the patient
- evaluate the nurse's ability to provide specialized patient care
- organize resources to ensure that patients receive appropriate nursing care
- collaborate with the staff nurse to clarify assignments, assess personal capabilities, jointly identify options for patient care assignments when the nurse does not feel personally competent or adequately prepared to carry out a specific function
- take appropriate disciplinary action according to facility policies
- communicate in written policies to the staff the process to make assignment and reassignment decisions
- provide education to staff and supervisory personnel in the decision making process regarding patient care assignments and reassignments, including patient placement and allocation of resources
- plan and budget for staffing patterns based upon patient's requirements and priorities for care
- provide a clearly defined written mechanism for immediate internal review of proposed assignments, which includes the participation of the staff involved, to help avoid conflict

Issues Central to Potential Dilemmas Are:

- the right of the patient to receive safe professional nursing care at an acceptable level of quality
- the responsibility for an appropriate utilization and distribution of nursing care services when nursing becomes a scare resource
- the responsibility for providing a practice environment that assures adequate nursing resources for the facility, while meeting the current socioeconomic and political realities of shrinking health care dollars

Legal Issues

Behaviors and activities relevant to giving, accepting, or rejecting a work assignment that could lead to disciplinary action include:

- practicing or offering to practice beyond the scope permitted by law, or accepting and performing professional responsibilities which the licensee knows or has reason to know that he or she is not competent to perform
- performing, without adequate supervision, professional services which the licensee is authorized to perform only under the supervision of a licensed professional, except in an emergency situation where a person's life or health is in danger
- abandoning or neglecting a patient or client who is in need of nursing care without making reasonable arrangements for the continuation of such care
- failure to exercise supervision over persons who are authorized to practice only under the supervision of the licensed professional

Of the above, the issue of abandonment or neglect has thus far proven the most legally devastating. Abandonment or neglect has been legally defined to include such actions as insufficient observation (frequency of contact), failure to assure competent intervention when the patient's condition changes (qualified physician not in attendance), and withdrawal of services without provision for qualified coverage. Since nurses at all levels most frequently act as agents of the employing facility, the facility shares the risk of liability with the nurse.

Application of Guidelines for Decision Making

Two clinical scenarios are presented for the RN to demonstrate appropriate decision making when faced with an unsafe assignment. Sometimes an example or two can help the RN objectively examine legal, ethical and professional issues prior to making a final decision. Additional resources are listed following the scenarios.

Scenario—A Question of Competence

An example of a potential dilemma is when an evening supervisor pulls a psychiatric nurse to the coronary care unit because of a lack of nursing staff.

The CCU census has risen and there is not additional qualified staff available.

Suppose you are asked to care for an unfamiliar patient population or to go to a unit for which you feel unqualified—what do you do?

1. CLARIFY what it is you are being asked to do.
   ■ How many patients will you be expected to care for?
   ■ Does the care of these patients require you to have specialty knowledge and skills in order to deliver safe nursing care?
   ■ Will there be qualified and experienced RNs on the unit?
   ■ What procedures and/or medications will you be expected to administer?
   ■ What kind of orientation do you need to function safely in the unfamiliar setting?
2. ASSESS yourself. Do you have the knowledge and skill to meet the expectations that have been outlined for you? Have you had experience with similar patient populations? Have you been oriented to this unit or a similar unit? Would the perceived discrepancies between your abilities and the expectations lead to an unsafe patient care situation?
3. IDENTIFY OPTIONS and implications of your decision.
   a) If you perceive that you can provide safe patient care, you should accept the assignment. You would now be ethically and legally responsible for the nursing care of these patients.
   b) If you perceive there is a discrepancy between abilities and the expectations of the assignment, further dialogue with the nurse supervisor is needed before you reach a decision. At this point it may be appropriate to consult the next level of management, such as the house supervisor or the chief nurse executive.

In further dialogue, continue to assess whether you are qualified to accept either a portion or the whole of the requested assignment. Also point out options which might be mutually beneficial. For example, obviously it would be unsafe for you to administer chemotherapy without prior training. However, if someone else administered the chemotherapy, perhaps you could provide the remainder of the required nursing care for that patient. If you feel unqualified for the assignment in its entirety, the dilemma becomes more complex.

At this point the RN must be aware of the legal rights of the facility. Even though the RN may have legitimate concern for patient safety and one's own legal accountability in providing safe care, the facility has legal precedent to initiate disciplinary action, including termination, if you refuse to accept an assignment. Therefore, it is important to continue to explore options in a positive manner, recognizing that both the RN and the facility have a responsibility for safe patient care.

4. POINT OF DECISION/IMPLICATIONS:
   If none of the options are acceptable, you are at your final decision point.
   a) Accept the assignment, documenting carefully your concern for patient safety and the process you used to inform the facility (manager) of your concerns. Keep a personal copy of this documentation and send a copy to the manager(s) involved. Once you have reached this decision it is unwise to discuss the situation or your feelings with other staff or patients. Now you are legally accountable for these patients. From this point, withdrawal from the agreed upon assignment may constitute abandonment.
   b) Refuse the assignment, being prepared for disciplinary action. Document your concern for patient safety and the process you used to inform the facility (manager) of your concerns. Keep a personal copy of this documentation and send a copy to the nurse executive. Courtesy suggests that you also send a copy to the manager(s) involved.
   c) Document the steps taken in making your decision. It may be necessary for you to use the facility's grievance procedure.

Scenario—A Question of an Additional Shift

An example of another potential dilemma is when a nurse who recognizes his/her fatigue and its potential for patient harm is required to work an additional shift.

Suppose you are approached by your supervisor and asked to work an additional shift. Your immediate response is that you don't want to work another shift—what do you do?

1. CLARIFY what it is you are expected to do.
   - For example, would the additional shift be with the same patients you are currently caring for, or would it involve a new patient assignment?
   - Is your reluctance to work another shift because of a new patient assignment you do not feel competent to accept? (If the answer is yes, then refer to the previous example, "A Question of Competence.")
   - Is your reluctance due to work fatigue, or do you have other plans?
   - Is this a chronic request due to poor scheduling, inadequate staffing, or chronic absenteeism?
   - Are you being asked to work because there is no relief nurse coming for your present patient assignment? Because your unit will be short of professional staff on the next shift? Because another unit will be short of professional staff on the next shift?
   - How long are you being asked to work— the entire shift or a portion of the shift?

2. ASSESS yourself.
   - Are you really tired, or do you just not feel like working? Is your fatigue level such that your care may be unsafe? Remember, you are legally responsible for the care of your current patient assignment if relief is not available.

3. IDENTIFY OPTIONS and implications of your decision.
   a) If you perceive that you can provide safe patient care and are willing to work the additional shift, accept the assignment.
   b) If you perceive that you can provide safe patient care but are unwilling to stay due to other plans or the chronic nature of the request, inform the manager of your reasons for not wishing to accept the assignment.
   c) If you perceive that your fatigue will interfere with your ability to safely care for patients, indicate this fact to the manager.

If you do not accept the assignment and the manager continues to attempt to persuade you it

may be appropriate to consult the next level of management, such as the house supervisor or the nurse executive.

In further dialogue, continue to weigh your reasons for refusal versus the facility's need for an RN. If you have a strong alternate commitment, such as no child care, or if you seriously feel your fatigue will interfere with safe patient care, restate your reasons for refusal.

At this point, it is important for you to be aware of the legal rights of the facility. Even though you may have legitimate concern for patient safety and your own legal accountability in providing safe care, or legitimate concern for the safety of your children or other commitments, the facility has legal precedent to initiate disciplinary action, including termination, if you refuse to accept an assignment. Therefore, it is important to continue to explore options in a positive manner, recognizing both you and the facility have a responsibility for safe patient care.

4. POINT OF DECISION/IMPLICATIONS
   a) Accept the assignment, documenting your professional concern for patient safety and the process you used to inform the facility (manager) of your concerns. Keep a personal copy of this documentation and send a copy to the nurse executive. Courtesy suggests that you also send a copy to the manager(s) involved. Once you have reached this decision it is unwise to discuss the situation or your feelings with other staff and/or patients.
   b) Accept the assignment, documenting your professional concerns for the chronic nature of the request and possible long-term consequences in reducing the quality of care. Documentation should follow the procedures outlined in (a).
   c) Accept the assignment, documenting your personal concerns regarding working conditions in which management decides the legitimacy of employee personal commitments. This documentation should go to your manager. You may wish to request a meeting with your manager to discuss the incident and your concerns regarding future requests.
   d) Refuse the assignment, being prepared for disciplinary action. If your reasons for

refusal were patient safety or an imperative personal commitment, document this carefully, including the process you used to inform the facility (nurse manager) of your concerns. Keep a personal copy of this documentation and send a copy to the chief nurse executive. Courtesy suggests that you also send a copy to the manager(s) involved.

e) Document the rationale for your decision. It may be necessary to use the facility's grievance procedure.

Summary

Two scenarios of how an RN may apply the guidelines for decision making in the actual work situation have been presented. Staffing dilemmas will always be present and mandate that active communication between staff nurses and all levels of nursing management be maintained to assure patient safety. The likelihood of a satisfactory solution will increase if there is prior consideration of the choices available. This consideration of available alternatives should include recognition that professional nurses are intelligent adults who should be involved in the decision-making process. Professional nurses are accountable for nursing judgments and actions regardless of the personal consequences. Providing safe nursing care to the patient is the ultimate objective of the professional nurse and the health-care facility.

The Florida Nurses Association Labor and Employment Relations Commission acknowledges:

- the Florida Organization of Nurse Executives for input and collaboration in this document and the development of the previous 1989 edition of this document.
- the **Florida Nurses Association Labor and Employment Relations Commission** for final preparation of the revised 1999 edition of this document.

Resources

To maintain current and accurate information on accountability of registered nurses for giving, accepting, or rejecting a work assignment, the following resources are suggested:

- **Health Care Facility:** Nurses are encouraged to seek consultation with their nurse manager/executives to discuss the facility's missions and goals as well as policies and procedures.
- The **Florida Nurses Association,** the largest statewide organization for registered nurses, represents nursing in the governmental, policy making arena and maintains current information and publications relative to the nurse's practice environment. Contact FNA or check out our website http://www.floridanurse .org for the benefits and services of membership, as well as priorities and activities of the Association.
- The **American Nurses Association** serves as the national clearing-house of information and offers publications on contemporary issues, including standards of practice, nursing ethics, as well as legal and regulatory issues. Contact ANA for a complimentary copy of the Publications Catalogue.
- *ANA Basic Guide to Safe Delegation* available through the American Nurses Association.
- *ANA Code of Ethics for Nurses* (2010) available through the American Nurses Association.
- *ANA Standards and Scope of Practice* (2010) available through the American Nurses Association.
- Nurse Practice Act (Florida Statutes 464, January 1994) and Administrative Rules (59S).
- Board of Nursing. A complimentary copy of the Nurse Practice Act is available to each registered nurse upon request.

Note: Page numbers followed by "b," "f," and "t" indicate boxes, figures and tables, respectively.